Graphical Models

Computational Neuroscience

Terrence J. Sejnowski and Tomaso A. Poggio, editors

Neural Nets in Electric Fish, Walter Heiligenberg, 1991

The Computational Brain, Patricia S. Churchland and Terrence J. Sejnowski, 1992

Dynamic Biological Networks: The Stomatogastric Nervous System, edited by Ronald M. Harris-Warrick, Eve Marder, Allen I. Selverston, and Maurice Moulins, 1992

The Neurobiology of Neural Networks, edited by Daniel Gardner, 1993

Large-Scale Neuronal Theories of the Brain, edited by Christof Koch and Joel L. Davis, 1994

The Theoretical Foundation of Dendritic Function: Selected Papers of Wilfrid Rall with Commentaries, edited by Idan Segev, John Rinzel, and Gordon M. Shepherd, 1995

Models of Information Processing in the Basal Ganglia, edited by James C. Houk, Joel L. Davis, and David G. Beiser, 1995

Spikes: Exploring the Neural Code, Fred Rieke, David Warland, Rob de Ruyter van Steveninck, and William Bialek, 1997

Neurons, Networks, and Motor Behavior, edited by Paul S. G. Stein, Sten Grillner, Allen I. Selverston, and Douglas G. Stuart, 1997

Methods in Neuronal Modeling: From Ions to Networks, second edition, edited by Christof Koch and Idan Segev, 1998

Fundamentals of Neural Network Modeling: Neuropsychology and Cognitive Neuroscience, edited by Randolph W. Parks, Daniel S. Levine, and Debra L. Long, 1998

Neural Codes and Distributed Representations: Foundations of Neural Computation, edited by Laurence Abbott and Terrence J. Sejnowski, 1997

Unsupervised Learning: Foundations of Neural Computation, edited by Geoffrey Hinton and Terrence J. Sejnowski, 1997

Fast Oscillations in Cortical Circuits, Roger D. Traub, John G. R. Jefferys, and Miles A. Whittington, 1999

Computational Vision: Information Processing in Perception and Visual Behavior, Hanspeter A. Mallot, 2000

Graphical Models: Foundations of Neural Computation, edited by Michael I. Jordan and Terrence J. Sejnowski, 2001

Self-Organizing Map Formation: Foundations of Neural Computation, edited by Klaus Obermayer and Terrence J. Sejnowski, 2001

Graphical Models: Foundations of Neural Computation

Edited by Michael I. Jordan and Terrence J. Sejnowski

A Bradford Book

The MIT Press
Cambridge, Massachusetts
London, England

This book was set in Palatino and printed and bound in the United States of America.

Library of Congress Cataloging-in-Publication Data

Graphical models : foundations of neural computation / edited by Michael I. Jordan and Terrence J. Sejnowski.
   p. cm. — (A Bradford book) (Computational neuroscience)
  ISBN 0-262-60042-0 (pbk. : alk. paper)
  1. Neural networks (Computer science) 2. Computer graphics. I. Jordan, Michael Irwin, 1956– II. Sejnowski, Terrence J. (Terrence Joseph) III. Series. IV. Bradford book
QA76.87 .G72   2001
006.3'2—dc21

                                    2001030212

Contents

Series Foreword

Computational neuroscience is an approach to understanding the information content of neural signals by modeling the nervous system at many different structural scales, including the biophysical, the circuit, and the systems levels. Computer simulations of neurons and neural networks are complementary to traditional techniques in neuroscience. This book series welcomes contributions that link theoretical studies with experimental approaches to understanding information processing in the nervous system. Areas and topics of particular interest include biophysical mechanisms for computation in neurons, computer simulations of neural circuits, models of learning, representation of sensory information in neural networks, systems models of sensory-motor integration, and computational analysis of problems in biological sensing, motor control, and perception.

Terrence J. Sejnowski
Tomaso A. Poggio

Sources

Smyth, P., Heckerman, D., and Jordan, M. I. 1997. Probabilistic independence networks for hidden Markov probability models. *Neural Computation* 9(2), 227–269.

Hinton, G. E., and Sejnowski, T. J. 1986. Learning and relearning in Boltzmann machines. In *Parallel Distributed Processing: Explorations in the Microstructure of Cognition, Volume 1: Foundations*, D. E. Rumelhart and J. L. McClelland, eds., pp. 282–317. MIT Press, Cambridge.

Saul, L., and Jordan, M. I. 1994. Learning in Boltzmann trees. *Neural Computation* 6(6), 1174–1184.

Hinton, G. E. 1989. Deterministic Boltzmann learning performs steepest descent in weight-space. *Neural Computation* 1(1), 142–150.

Saul, L. K., and Jordan, M. I. 2000. Attractor dynamics in feedforward neural networks. *Neural Computation* 12(6), 1313–1335.

Kappen, H. J., and F. B. Rodríguez. 1998. Efficient learning in Boltzmann machines using linear response theory. *Neural Computation* 10(5), 1137–1156.

Neal, R. 1992. Asymmetric parallel Boltzmann machines are belief networks. *Neural Computation* 4(6), 832–834.

Frey, B. J., and Hinton, G. E. 1999. Variational learning in nonlinear Gaussian belief networks. *Neural Computation* 11(1), 193–213.

Tipping, M. E., and Bishop, C. M. 1999. Mixtures of probabilistic principal component analyzers. *Neural Computation* 11(2), 443–482.

Attias, H. 1999. Independent factor analysis. *Neural Computation* 11(4), 803–851.

Jordan, M. I., and Jacobs, R. A. 1994. Hierarchical mixtures of experts and the EM algorithm. *Neural Computation* 6(2), 181–214.

Krogh, A., and Riis, S. K. 1999. Hidden neural networks. *Neural Computation* 11(2), 541–563.

Ghahramani, Z., and Hinton, G. E. 2000. Variational learning for switching state-space models. *Neural Computation* 12(4), 831–864.

Tresp, V., and Hofmann, R. 1998. Nonlinear time-series prediction with missing and noisy data. *Neural Computation* 10(3), 731–747.

Weiss, Y. 2000. Correctness of local probability propagation in graphical models with loops. *Neural Computation* 12(1), 1–41.

Introduction

A "graphical model" is a type of probabilistic network that has roots in several different research communities, including artificial intelligence (Pearl 1988), statistics (Lauritzen 1996), and neural networks (Hertz, Krogh, and Palmer 1991). The graphical models framework provides a clean mathematical formalism that has made it possible to understand the relationships among a wide variety of network-based approaches to computation and, in particular, to understand many neural network algorithms and architectures as instances of a broader probabilistic methodology. Moreover, this formal framework has made it possible to identify those features of neural network algorithms and architectures that are novel and to extend them to other more general graphical models. This interplay between the general formal framework of graphical models and the exploration of new algorithms and architectures is exemplified in the chapters included in this volume. These chapters, chosen from *Neural Computation*, include many foundational papers of historical importance as well as papers that are at the research frontier. The volume is intended for a broad range of students, researchers, and practitioners who are interested in understanding the basic principles underlying graphical models and in applying them to practical problems.

Probabilistic and information-theoretic approaches have become dominant in the neural network literature, as researchers have attempted to formalize "adaptivity" in neural computation and understand why some adaptive methods perform better than others. The probabilistic framework has also provided a guide in the exploration of new algorithms and architectures. At the same time, the notion of "locality" has continued to exert a key constraint on neural network research, restricting the kinds of architectures and algorithms that are studied. The particular relevance of graphical models to this research effort is that the graphical models framework provides formal definitions of both adaptivity and locality. It does so by forging a mathematical link between probability theory and graph theory.

Graphical models use graphs to represent and manipulate joint probability distributions. The graph underlying a graphical model may be directed, in which case the model is often referred to as a *belief network* or a *Bayesian network*, or the graph may be undirected, in which case the model is generally referred to as a *Markov random field*. A graphical model has both a structural component—encoded by the pattern of edges in the graph—and a parametric component—encoded by numerical "potentials" associated with sets of edges in the graph. The relationship between these components underlies the computational machinery associated with graphical models. In particular, general *inference algorithms* allow statistical quantities (such as likelihoods and conditional probabilities) and information-theoretic quantities (such as mutual information and conditional entropies) to be computed efficiently. *Learning algorithms* build on these inference algorithms and allow parameters and structures to be estimated from data. All of these probabilistic computations make use of data structures associated with the graph—in particular, an important data structure known as a *junction tree* (see chapter 1). The junction tree groups nodes into clusters and defines probabilistic "messages" that pass among the clusters; this essentially amounts to a graph-theoretic characterization of computational "locality" for general probabilistic inference.

Many neural network architectures,. including essentially all of the models developed under the rubric of "unsupervised learning" (Hinton and Sejnowski 1999) as well as supervised Boltzmann machines, mixtures of experts, and normalized radial basis function networks, are special cases of the graphical model formalism, both architecturally and algorithmically. Many other neural networks, including the classical multilayer perceptron, can be profitably analyzed from the point of view of graphical models.

The graphical model literature in AI and statistics has contributed the general formalism for understanding relationships between graphs and probabilities; the neural network literature has contributed a rather far-flung exploration in the space of architectures and algorithms. This exploration is the principal subject matter of this book. Before turning to specific examples, let us give a brief overview of some of the general themes that have characterized this exploration.

Classical graphical model architectures in AI have often used localist representations, in which a single node represents a complex concept, such as "chair." Neural network researchers, on the other hand, have explored *distributed* or *factorial* representations in which single nodes represent simpler properties that are broadly tuned and overlapping. This has allowed much larger problems to be tackled. Also, the graphical model literature has generally focused on exact probabilistic inference or sampling-based inference methods, whereas neural network research has studied a wider class of approximate inference methods. For example, the *mean-field*, or *variational*, methodology developed first for the Boltzmann machine and related undirected models, has flowed into the general graphical formalism and yielded fast new algorithms for approximate probabilistic inference. Finally, the neural network literature has delved deeply into nonlinear classification and regression, contributing a variety of new methods for parameter estimation and regularization in graphical models, with a particular focus on "on-line algorithms" (which can be viewed as defining another, temporal, notion of "locality"). In general, the bi-directional flow of ideas between these two fields has led to a significantly broader understanding of network-based computation. This understanding is reflected and pursued in the following chapters.

Readers new to the topic of graphical models should start with the first three sections of the chapter by Smyth, Heckerman, and Jordan (chapter 1), which provide a short overview. A full presentation can be found in any of several recent textbooks (e.g., Cowell et al. 1999). See also Jordan (1999) for several tutorial articles that provide basic background for the chapters presented here.

The Boltzmann Machine

The *Boltzmann machine* (chapter 2) is a probabilistic network of binary nodes. Historically, the Boltzmann machine played an important role in the development of the neural network field, as the first general multi-layer architecture to employ hidden units between the input and output nodes. As we discuss in this section, the Boltzmann machine is a special case of an undirected graphical model, or *Markov random field (MRF)*. The inference and learning algorithms for Boltzmann machines, and in particular the treatment of hidden units, exemplify more general solutions to the problem of inference and learning in graphical models with latent variables.

While general MRF's represent joint probability distributions as products of arbitrary local functions ("potentials") on the cliques of the graph,[1] the Boltzmann machine adopts a restricted parameterization in which the potentials are formed from *pairwise* factors. These pairwise factors take the form $\exp\{J_{ij}S_iS_j\}$, where J_{ij} is the weight on the edge between unit i and j, and S_i and S_j are the (binary) values of units i and j, respectively. (In a general MRF, higher-order interactions such as $J_{ijk}S_iS_jS_k$ would be included—when the nodes S_i, S_j, and S_k are in a clique, namely, are mutually interconnected). Taking products of these local potentials yields the total potential $\exp\{\sum_{i<j} J_{ij}S_iS_j\}$, which, when normalized, defines a Boltzmann distribution:

$$P(S) = \frac{e^{-E(S)}}{Z} \tag{1}$$

for a quadratic *energy function* $E(S) \stackrel{def}{=} -\sum_{i<j} J_{ij}S_iS_j$. From this joint probability distribution, we can define arbitrary conditional probabilities of one set of nodes given another set of nodes. Calculating these conditionals defines the *inference problem* for Boltzmann machines.

For general Boltzmann machines, in particular for the fully connected Boltzmann machines that have generally been studied in the literature, there are no structural properties (conditional independencies) to take advantage of, and the inference problem is intractable. Approximate inference techniques have generally been employed—in particular, stochastic sampling (Gibbs sampling) enhanced with simulated annealing. Although these methods do provide a way to study the Boltzmann

---

[1]A *clique* is a fully connected subgraph. A clique consisting of n binary nodes can be in one of 2^n configurations, where a *configuration* is an assignment of a binary value to each node in the clique. A *potential* is a function that assigns a nonnegative real number to each configuration.

machine empirically, they are slow and are generally viewed as complex (particularly when used in the setting of learning algorithms, where multiple simulated annealing passes are required). Historically, when the multilayer perceptron became popular, Boltzmann machines lost their luster.

The fact that the worst-case, fully connected Boltzmann machine presents no opportunities for fast inference does not imply that Boltzmann machines in general present no such opportunities. This point of view was emphasized by Saul and Jordan (chapter 3), who studied Boltzmann machines in which the hidden units form a tree. They showed that in such architectures it is not necessary to resort to Gibbs sampling to solve the inference problem; rather, a simple deterministic recursion known as *decimation* can be employed to calculate the conditional probabilities. The time required for the computation is proportional to the width of the graph. These are Boltzmann machines that can be "solved."

The decimation rule can be generalized beyond the pairwise interactions that characterize the classical Boltzmann machine, yielding an exact calculation method for general MRFs. Interestingly, this rule is a special case of the junction tree methodology that has been developed for inference in arbitrary graphical models (Cowell et al. 1999). There appears to be no particular advantage to the decimation approach, and indeed the junction tree approach has the advantage of providing an explicit method for estimating the time complexity of inference—the time complexity is exponential in the size of the largest clique in the *triangulated graph* of the network. Thus it is possible to identify systematically the classes of Boltzmann machines for which exact inference is efficient.

Mean Field Approximation

In 1987, Peterson and Anderson (1987) presented an alternative approach to inference for the Boltzmann machine that has had substantial impact. Their approach was based on an approximation known in physics as the "mean field" approximation. Under this approximation, the (approximate) mean value of the conditional probability distribution at each node is written as a function of the (approximate) mean values of its neighbors, and a so-called self-consistent set of mean values is obtained by iteratively evaluating these functions. For the Boltzmann machine, these iterative equations turn out to take a simple classical form in which each node's value is the logistic function of a weighted sum of its neighbors' values. These are the standard nonlinear equations proposed by Hopfield (1984) for the "continuous Hopfield network," and they can be shown—via Lyapunov theory—to be locally convergent (Cohen and Grossberg 1983; Hopfield 1984).

Peterson and Anderson's idea has been taken in two somewhat different directions. One line of research has focused on optimization problems, where the mean field approach has given rise to a general methodology known as *deterministic annealing* (Yuille and Kosowsky 1994). In deterministic annealing, the focus is on the energy function rather than the distribution that it defines; in particular, the goal is to find the minima of the energy function. (The probabilistic framework serves the subsidiary role of smoothing the energy function.) The mean field equations are generally derived from the point of view of saddle point approximation, which gives rise to a free "temperature" parameter that controls the degree of smoothing. In a procedure reminiscent of interior point methods, the mean field equations are solved for a gradually decreasing set of temperatures. It is possible to relate the limiting solution of these equations (as the temperature goes to zero) to the minima of the energy function (Elfadel 1995).

In a second branch of research, the focus has been on mean field theory as a methodology for approximation probabilistic inference in general graphical models. Here the emphasis has been on extending the basic approach to a wider class of architectures and on developing more refined versions of the approximation. A different point of view has proved to be fruitful in which the mean field approximation is viewed as the expression of a *variational principle*. Given a distribution $P(S)$ that is costly to calculate, approximate $P(S)$ by choosing a distribution $Q(S|\mu)$ from a family of approximating distributions, where the *variational parameter* μ indexes the family. The variational parameter is chosen so as to minimize the Kullback-Leibler (KL) divergence between Q and P:

$$\mu^* = \underset{\mu}{\operatorname{argmin}} \left\{ \sum_{\{S\}} Q(S|\mu) \ln \frac{Q(S|\mu)}{P(S)} \right\},$$

where the sum is taken over all configurations of S (assumed discrete for simplicity).

When $Q(S|\mu)$ is taken to be the completely factorized distribution, namely, $Q(S) = \prod_i Q(S_i|\mu_i)$, and when $P(S)$ is the Boltzmann distribution in equation (1), then one obtains the mean field equations of Peterson and Anderson. That is, the Peterson and Anderson equations arise by taking the derivative of the KL divergence with respect to μ_i and setting to zero.

Saul and Jordan (1996) observed that a wider class of approximations could be obtained by choosing a wider class of approximating distributions $Q(S|\mu)$. Note that a completely factorized $Q(S|\mu)$ corresponds to a subgraph of the original graphical model in which all edges are omitted. By considering subgraphs that retain some of the edges of the original graph, while maintaining tractability by restricting the subgraph to be a sparse graph (such as a chain or a tree), more refined variational approximations can be obtained. Moreover, in minimizing the KL divergence for such approximations, it is necessary to solve the inference problem for the tractable subgraph. Thus exact inference algorithms (such as the junction tree algorithm) become subroutines within an overall variational approximation. Several of the chapters included in the collection reflect this point of view.

There are other refinements to mean field theory that have been studied in the context of graphical models. Kappen and Rodríguez (chapter 6) studied the *linear response correction* (Parisi 1988) to the naive mean field approximation, which provides an improved approximation to the second-order statistics. Applying this correction to mean field equations for the Boltzmann machine, they found significant improvements in inferential accuracy.

Thus far we have focused on inference, but an equally important problem is that of learning the parameters of the model. In the setting of graphical models, the learning problem and the inference problem are closely related and learning algorithms generally make use of inference algorithms as an "inner loop." In the context of the Boltzmann machine, the classical approach is to use Gibbs sampling as an inner loop to obtain the statistics that are needed for the gradient descent procedure (the "outer loop"). There is, however, no reason to focus exclusively on sampling methods. For tractable architectures, it is preferable to calculate the necessary statistics exactly (using the junction tree algorithm). Alternatively, as shown by Hinton (chapter 4), the approximation provided by the mean field approach provides an appropriate inner loop for a gradient descent algorithm for learning. This idea has been taken further by Neal and Hinton (1999), who develop a link between approximate inference and approximate "E steps" for the EM algorithm. In general, approximate inference algorithms can be used to increase a (tractable) lower bound on an (intractable) likelihood.

Directed Graphical Models

Another point of contact between the neural network literature and the graphical model literature was made by Neal (chapter 7; see also Neal 1992 for a fuller presentation). Neal observed that certain so-called asymmetric Boltzmann machines are actually special cases of *directed graphical models*, also known as *belief networks* or *Bayesian networks*. Directed graphical models define their joint probabilities by taking products of local *conditional* probabilities. In many ways this yields a simpler entry point into the graphical model framework than the undirected formalism of Boltzmann machines.

The general definition of a joint probability distribution for a directed graphical model is given as follows:

$$P(S) = \prod_i P(S_i|\pi_i), \tag{2}$$

where π_i represents the set of parents of node S_i. Note in particular that there is no need for a normalizing constant Z in this approach to defining the joint probability.

For the special case of binary S_i, one interesting possibility is to take $P(S_i|\pi_i)$ to be the logistic function of a linear weighted sum of the parent nodes. This yields a directed graphical model known as a *sigmoid belief network*. As observed by Neal, a sigmoid belief network is a close cousin of the multilayer perceptron. Neal proposed using Gibbs sampling as the inferential engine for sigmoid belief networks, but, as in the case of the Boltzmann machine, for certain architectures (e.g., trees) one can perform exact inference efficiently using the junction tree algorithm.

Saul, Jaakkola, and Jordan (1996) derived the analog of the Peterson and Anderson mean field theory for sigmoid belief networks. The directed nature of the graph yields additional terms in the mean field equations that are not present in the undirected Boltzmann machine. Saul and Jordan (chapter 5) took this approach further in the context of large layered networks, where a central limit theorem expansion is justified. An interesting feature of their work is that the (approximate) maximum likelihood learning algorithm that they derive includes "weight-decay" terms that are familiar from statistically motivated regularization methods. Thus approximate inference based on a simplifying variational distribution can be preferable to exact inference for the purposes of parameter estimation.

Although most of the research on variational approximation algorithms has been carried out for networks of discrete nodes, Frey and Hinton (chapter 8) have developed variational algorithms for several kinds of continuous nodes. The derivation presented in their chapter includes piecewise linear nodes and nodes with continuous sigmoidal nonlinearities.

Latent Variable Models ────────────────────────────────────

The Boltzmann machine, sigmoid belief networks, and mean field or variational algorithms have provided a set of links to the graphical models literature; another link has been provided by mixture models and more general latent variable models. In the simplest cases these models are handled via exact inference methods, but in more complex cases the models shade into the layered graphical models discussed in the previous section, where sampling or variational methods are generally required.

Mixture models provide a probabilistic setting for the development of clustering algorithms, both unsupervised (Duda and Hart 1973; Nowlan 1990) and supervised (Jacobs et al. 1991). Each data point is assumed to be drawn from one of a fixed set of classes, but the class label is assumed to be "missing" or "latent" and must be inferred from the model.

As a graphical model, a classical mixture model for unsupervised clustering has a particularly simple representation (see figure 1). The unshaded ("hidden") node represents the class label, ω, and the shaded node represents the observed data point $\mathbf{y}$. The inference problem for this graphical model is that of calculating the probability of the hidden node given the observed node, namely, $P(\omega|\mathbf{y})$. The calculation of this posterior probability is the "inner loop" in a procedure (the expectation-

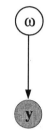

Figure 1: The graphical model representation for a mixture model, where the node labeled **y** represents an observed data point and the node labeled ω represents the (latent) class. The joint probability is given by $P(\omega)P(\mathbf{y}|\omega)$; marginalizing over ω yields a mixture.

maximization or "EM" algorithm) that estimates the parameters of the model.

An alternative latent variable model is provided by factor analysis (FA), where the underlying variable is a continuous rather than a discrete vector. This model can also be represented as the two-node graphical structure in figure 1 (although this representation hides the independencies among the components of the vectors). The model is parameterized by letting the latent variable be Gaussian with diagonal covariance matrix, and by letting the observed variable be Gaussian with a mean that is a linear function of the latent variable.

Factor analysis provides a technique for dimensionality reduction in which the data are assumed to lie near a low-dimensional hyperplane. A closely related model involving a probabilistic variant of principal component analysis (PCA) has been developed by Roweis (1998) and Tipping and Bishop (chapter 9); this model can also be represented as the two-node graphical structure in figure 1.

A number of authors, including Ghahramani and Hinton (1998), Hinton, Dayan, and Revow (1997), and Tipping and Bishop (chapter 9), have studied mixtures of FA or PCA models. We have reprinted the latter paper, which is representative of this line of research. The basic model can be rendered as a graphical model as shown in figure 2. As in a mixture model, the latent node ω is a discrete node representing the hidden class label. For each value of ω, we obtain a FA or PCA model, where the latent node y is a continuous node representing the FA or PCA subspace. Under this model, data are assumed to form clusters, where each cluster is represented as a lower-dimensional linear manifold.

Independent components analysis (ICA) is another latent variable model with links to FA and PCA (Comon 1994; Bell and Sejnowski 1995).

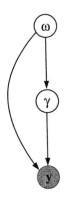

Figure 2: A graphical representation of a mixture of FA or PCA models.

As in FA, a vector of observed values is assumed to arise as a linear function of a continuous latent vector, and the components of the latent vector are assumed to be mutually independent. Whereas in FA the latent vector is assumed to be Gaussian, in ICA the latent vector is assumed to have a more general probability density—in particular, one for which the independence assumption has stronger consequences than mere decorrelation. In a nonlinear generalization of ICA (Lee, Lewicki, and Sejnowski 2000), mixtures of ICA can be used to both represent and classify data. Attias (chapter 10) proposes another generalization in which the latent density models are represented flexibly via mixture-of-Gaussian densities. Conditional on the choices of mixture components of these underlying densities, one has a FA model. The graphical model is again a three-layer directed model with a discrete node representing the mixture components in the top level and continuous nodes in the two lower levels. The exact inference algorithm for this model scales exponentially in the number of components of the latent vector. To handle large models, Attias (chapter 10) develops a variational approximation.

Finally, another line of research involving mixture models is the *mixture of experts* architecture (Jacobs et al. 1991), which is a conditional density model appropriate for supervised learning. In this model both the "mixing proportion," namely, $P(\omega)$, and the "mixing components," namely, $P(\mathbf{y}|\omega)$, are conditioned on the input vector $\mathbf{x}$. The mixture model thus takes the form $P(\mathbf{y}|\mathbf{x}) = \sum_{\omega} P(\omega|\mathbf{x})P(\mathbf{y}|\omega, \mathbf{x})$. The conditioning allows the input space to be partitioned adaptively into a set of regions (via the $P(\omega|\mathbf{x})$ term) in which different regression or classification surfaces are fit (the $P(\mathbf{y}|\omega, \mathbf{x})$ term).

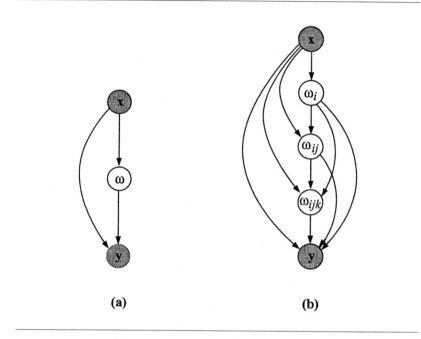

(a)   **(b)**

Figure 3: (a) The graphical representation of a mixture of experts model. This is a mixture model in which the distributions of the hidden variable ω and the output vector **y** are both conditioned on the input vector **x**. (b) The graphical model representation of a three-level hierarchical mixture of experts model. This model involves a sequence of hidden variables, ω_i, ω_{ij}, and ω_{ijk}, corresponding to a probabilistic, nested partition of the input space.

The mixture of experts is shown as a graphical model in figure 3(a). Here we see the conditional dependence of both the discrete latent variable and the observable **y** on the input vector. Note that both the input vector and the output vector are observed (shaded).

Jordan and Jacobs (chapter 11) generalized the mixture of experts to a hierarchical architecture (the *hierarchical mixture of experts*, or "HME"), in which a sequence of latent decisions are made, each of which is conditional on the input vector **x** and the previous decisions. The corresponding graphical model is shown in figure 3(b). Geometrically, the HME corresponds to· a nested partitioning of the input space (the HME is essentially a probabilistic decision tree).

Jordan and Jacobs also proposed using the EM algorithm to fit the parameters of mixture-of-experts architectures. For the HME, the inner loop of this algorithm involves a recursive pass upward in the tree to compute the posterior probabilities of the latent decision nodes (conditioned on both **x** and **y**). As should be expected from figure 3(b), this

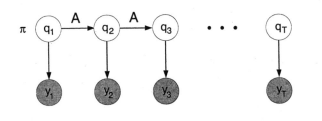

Figure 4: A hidden Markov model represented as a graphical model. Each horizontal slice corresponds to a time step and is isomorphic to the mixture model shown in figure 1. The distribution π is the *initial state distribution* and A is the *state transition matrix*. The *output sequence* $(y_0, y_1, \ldots, y_T)$ is observed and the *state sequence* $(q_0, q_1, \ldots, q_T)$ is unobserved.

recursion is a special case of the general inference algorithms for graphical models.

Dynamical Models

The hidden Markov model (HMM) is a paradigm example of a tractable graphical model. As shown in figure 4, the HMM can be viewed as a dynamical generalization of the basic mixture model in which the mixture model is copied and there are additional edges joining the hidden nodes. Each such node can be in one of M states, and there is an $M \times M$ transition matrix parameterizing these edges. The inference problem is that of calculating the probabilities of the hidden nodes given the entire sequence of observed nodes. This problem is solved via a recursive algorithm (the "alpha-beta algorithm") that proceeds forward and backward in the graph.

Smyth, Heckerman and Jordan (chapter 1) review the general graphical model formalism, describing in particular the *junction tree algorithm* for exact inference in graphical models. They then discuss HMMs, deriving the alpha-beta algorithm from the point of view of the junction tree framework. Several variants of the basic HMM architecture are also presented.

The technique of copying a basic underlying graphical model and linking nodes in the copies to obtain a Markovian dynamical model is widespread (Dean and Kanazawa 1989). Pursuing this approach in the case of factor analysis yields the classical linear-Gaussian Markov model, much studied in systems theory (cf. Roweis and Ghahramani 1999). The inference problem is solved by an analog of the forward-backward algorithm in which the "forward" algorithm is the classical Kalman filter. Both this forward recursion and any of a number of backward algorithms (e.g., the Rauch-Tung-Striebel smoother) can be derived from the perspective of the junction tree algorithm.

While the HMM and the linear-Gaussian model provide paradigm cases of graphical model technology, they also suffer from a number of limitations, and much research has been devoted to exploration of wider classes of graphical models.

One such extension involves the notion of *discriminative training*. HMMs are widely used in classification problems, such as in speech recognition, where one HMM is trained for each class. The classical approach to training such a bank of HMMs is to train each HMM separately (via the EM algorithm) with data from its class. A more successful approach in practice (Juang and Rabiner 1991) is to *decrease* the probability for the incorrect HMM models while increasing the probability for the correct HMM model. As shown by Krogh and Riis (chapter 12), this discriminative approach can be accommodated in the graphical model framework by considering a single global model in which the class labels are explicitly incorporated. The undirected graphical model (MRF) formalism provides a more satisfactory framework in which to express this model. Moreover, given that the potential function representation of MRFs does not require local normalization, it is straightforward to utilize (unnormalized) neural networks for the transition matrices and emission matrices of the HMM (see also Baldi and Chauvin 1996). The result is an interesting merger of graphical model and neural network methodology.

Ghahramani and Hinton (chapter 13) review other architectural extensions to the classical HMM and linear-Gaussian Markov models and present a new hybrid model that combines HMM and linear-Gaussian dynamics. In their model, a discrete Markovian switching variable determines which of several alternative linear-Gaussian Markov models produces the output at any given time step. While exact inference is exponentially costly under this model, a variational approach that decouples the discrete and continuous dynamics provides a computationally tractable approximation.

Some of the most challenging time series problems are those involving nonlinear models and arbitrary patterns of missing data. In these problems stochastic sampling methods are often the inference methods of choice, due to their simplicity and generality. Tresp and Hofmann (chapter 14) address missing data problems and the problem of assessing prediction accuracy for nonlinear time series, in both cases demonstrating the virtues of stochastic sampling approaches.

Probability Propagation _____

An alternative to stochastic sampling and variational approaches to approximate inference is the *probability propagation* method discussed by Weiss (chapter 15). This approach is based on the existence of a simple algorithm for exact inference in graphs without (undirected) cycles

(Pearl 1988). In the case of graphs *with* undirected cycles, rather than forming cliques and propagating in a junction tree as in the exact inference methods, the probability propagation approach simply ignores the cycles and iterates the propagation equations. Such an approach turns out to work empirically in a number of cases. In particular, for "turbo codes" and "Gallager codes," which are graphical models for error-correcting coding, probability propagation is quite successful (McEliece, MacKay, and Cheng 1998). Weiss (chapter 15) gives an analysis of probability propagation for graphs with a single loop, providing an analytical expression relating the approximate and correct conditional probabilities.

References

Baldi, P., and Chauvin, Y. 1996. Hybrid modeling, HMM/NN architectures, and protein applications. *Neural Computation* 8(7), 1541–1565.

Bell, A. J., and Sejnowski, T. J. 1995. An information-maximizaition approach to blind separation and blind deconvolution. *Neural Computation* 7(6), 1129–1159.

Cohen, M. A., and Grossberg, S. 1983. Absolute stability of global pattern formation and parallel memory storage by competitive neural networks. *IEEE Transactions on Systems, Man, and Cybernetics*, SMC-13, 815–826.

Comon, P. 1994. Independent component analysis, a new concept? *Signal Processing* 36, 287–314.

Cowell, R., Dawid, P., Lauritzen, S. L., and Spiegelhalter, D. 1999. *Probabilistic Networks and Expert Systems*. New York: Springer Verlag.

Dean, T., and Kanazawa, K. 1989. A model for reasoning about causality and persistence. *Computational Intelligence* 5, 142–150.

Duda, R. O., and Hart, P. E. 1973. *Pattern Classification and Scene Analysis*. New York: John Wiley and Sons.

Elfadel, I. M. 1995. Convex potentials and their conjugates in analog mean-field computation. *Neural Computation* 7(5), 1079–1104.

Ghahramani, Z., and Hinton, G. E. 1998. *The EM algorithm for mixtures of factor analyzers*. University of Toronto Technical Report CRG-TR-96-1, Department of Computer Science.

Hertz, J., Krogh, A., and Palmer, R. G. 1991. *Introduction to the Theory of Neural Computation*. Redwood City, CA: Addison-Wesley.

Hinton, G. E., and Sejnowski, T. 1999. *Unsupervised Learning: Foundations of Neural Computation*. Cambridge, MA: MIT Press.

Hinton G. E., Dayan, P., and Revow, M. 1997. Modelling the manifolds of images of handwritten digits. *IEEE Transactions on Neural Networks* 8(1), 65–74.

Hopfield, J. J. 1984. Neurons with graded response have collective computational properties like those of two-state neurons. *Proceedings of the National Academy of Sciences* 81, 3088–3092.

Jacobs, R. A., Jordan, M. I., Nowlan, S. J., and Hinton, G. E. 1991. Adaptive mixtures of local experts. *Neural Computation* 3(1), 79–87.

Jordan, M. I., ed. 1999. *Learning in Graphical Models*. Cambridge, MA: MIT Press.

Juang, B. H., and Rabiner, L. R. 1991. Hidden Markov models for speech recognition. *Technometrics* 33(3), 251–272.

Lauritzen, S. L. 1996. *Graphical Models*. Oxford: Oxford University Press.

Lee, T.-W., Lewicki, M. S., and Sejnowski, T. J. (2000). Unsupervised classification, segmentation and de-noising of images using ICA mixture models. *Advances in Neural Information Processing Systems* **12**.

McEliece, R. J., MacKay, D. J. C., and Cheng, J.-F. 1996. Turbo decoding as an instance of Pearl's "belief propagation algorithm." *IEEE Journal on Selected Areas in Communication* **16**, 140–152.

Neal, R. 1992. Connectionist learning of belief networks. *Artificial Intelligence* **56**, 71–113.

Neal, R., and Hinton, G. E. 1999. A view of the EM algorithm that justifies incremental, sparse, and other variants. In M. I. Jordan, ed., *Learning in Graphical Models*. Cambridge, MA: MIT Press.

Nowlan, S. J. 1990. Maximum likelihood competitive learning. In D. Touretzky, ed., *Neural Information Processing Systems 2*. San Mateo, CA: Morgan Kaufmann.

Parisi, G. 1988. *Statistical Field Theory*. Redwood City, CA: Addison-Wesley.

Pearl, J. 1988. *Probabilistic Reasoning in Intelligent Systems: Networks of Plausible Inference*. San Mateo, CA: Morgan Kaufmann.

Peterson, C., and Anderson, J. R. 1987. A mean field theory learning algorithm for neural networks. *Complex Systems* **1**, 995–1019.

Roweis, S. 1998. EM algorithms for PCA and SPCA. In M. I. Jordan, M. J. Kearns, and S. A. Solla, eds., *Advances in Neural Information Processing Systems 10*. Cambridge MA: MIT Press.

Roweis, S., and Ghahramani, Z. 1999. A unifying review of linear Gaussian models. *Neural Computation* **11**(2), 305–346.

Saul, L. K., Jaakkola, T., and Jordan, M. I. 1996. Mean field theory for sigmoid belief networks. *Journal of Artificial Intelligence Research* **4**, 61–76.

Saul, L. K., and Jordan, M. I. 1996. Exploiting tractable substructures in intractable networks. In D. S. Touretzky, M. C. Mozer, and M. E. Hasselmo, eds., *Advances in Neural Information Processing Systems 8*. Cambridge, MA: MIT Press.

Yuille, A. L., and Kosowsky, J. J. 1994. Statistical physics algorithms that converge. *Neural Computation* **6**(3), 341–356.

1

Probabilistic Independence Networks
for Hidden Markov Probability Models

Padhraic Smyth
Department of Information and Computer Science, University of California at Irvine,
Irvine, CA 92697-3425 USA
and
Jet Propulsion Laboratory 525-3660, California Institute of Technology,
Pasadena, CA 91109 USA

David Heckerman
Microsoft Research, Redmond, WA 98052-6399 USA

Michael I. Jordan
Department of Brain and Cognitive Sciences, Massachusetts Institute of Technology,
Cambridge, MA 02139 USA

Graphical techniques for modeling the dependencies of random variables have been explored in a variety of different areas, including statistics, statistical physics, artificial intelligence, speech recognition, image processing, and genetics. Formalisms for manipulating these models have been developed relatively independently in these research communities. In this paper we explore hidden Markov models (HMMs) and related structures within the general framework of probabilistic independence networks (PINs). The paper presents a self-contained review of the basic principles of PINs. It is shown that the well-known forward-backward (F-B) and Viterbi algorithms for HMMs are special cases of more general inference algorithms for arbitrary PINs. Furthermore, the existence of inference and estimation algorithms for more general graphical models provides a set of analysis tools for HMM practitioners who wish to explore a richer class of HMM structures. Examples of relatively complex models to handle sensor fusion and coarticulation in speech recognition are introduced and treated within the graphical model framework to illustrate the advantages of the general approach.

1 Introduction

For multivariate statistical modeling applications, such as hidden Markov modeling (HMM) for speech recognition, the identification and manipulation of relevant conditional independence assumptions can be useful for model building and analysis. There has recently been a considerable amount of work exploring the relationships between conditional independence in probability models and structural properties of related graphs. In particular, the separation properties of a graph can be directly related to conditional independence properties in a set of associated probability models.

The key point of this article is that the analysis and manipulation of generalized HMMs (more complex HMMs than the standard first-order model) can be facilitated by exploiting the relationship between probability models and graphs. The major advantages to be gained are in two areas:

- *Model description.* A graphical model provides a natural and intuitive medium for displaying dependencies that exist between random variables. In particular, the structure of the graphical model clarifies the conditional independencies in the associated probability models, allowing model assessment and revision.

- *Computational efficiency.* The graphical model is a powerful basis for specifying efficient algorithms for computing quantities of interest in the probability model (e.g., calculation of the probability of observed data given the model). These inference algorithms can be specified automatically once the initial structure of the graph is determined.

We will refer to both probability models and graphical models. Each consists of structure and parameters. The structure of the model consists of the specification of a set of conditional independence relations for the probability model or a set of (missing) edges in the graph for the graphical model. The parameters of both the probability and graphical models consist of the specification of the joint probability distribution: in factored form for the probability model and defined locally on the nodes of the graph for the graphical model. The inference problem is that of the calculation of posterior probabilities of variables of interest given observable data and a specification of the probabilistic model. The related task of maximum a posteriori (MAP) identification is the determination of the most likely state of a set of unobserved variables, given observed variables and the probabilistic model. The learning or estimation problem is that of determining the parameters (and possibly structure) of the probabilistic model from data.

This article reviews the applicability and utility of graphical modeling to HMMs and various extensions of HMMs. Section 2 introduces the basic notation for probability models and associated graph structures. Section 3 summarizes relevant results from the literature on probabilistic independence networks (PINs), in particular, the relationships that exist between separation in a graph and conditional independence in a probability model. Section 4 interprets the standard first-order HMM in terms of PINs. In Section 5 the standard algorithm for inference in a directed PIN is discussed and applied to the standard HMM in Section 6. A result of interest is that the forward-backward (F-B) and Viterbi algorithms are shown to be special cases of this inference algorithm. Section 7 shows that the inference algorithms for undirected PINs are essentially the same as those already discussed for directed PINs. Section 8 introduces more complex HMM structures for speech modeling and analyzes them using the graphical model framework. Section 9 reviews known estimation results for graphical models and discusses their potential implications for practical problems in the estimation of HMM structures, and Section 10 contains summary remarks.

2 Notation and Background

Let $U = \{X_1, X_2, \ldots, X_N\}$ represent a set of discrete-valued random variables. For the purposes of this article we restrict our attention to discrete-valued random variables; however, many of the results stated generalize directly to continuous and mixed sets of random variables (Lauritzen and Wermuth 1989; Whittaker 1990). Let lowercase x_i denote one of the values of variable X_i: the notation $\sum_{x_1}$ is taken to mean the sum over all possible values of X_1. Let $p(x_i)$ be shorthand for the particular probability $p(X_i = x_i)$, whereas $p(X_i)$ represents the probability function for X_i (a table of values, since X_i is assumed discrete), $1 \le i \le N$. The full joint distribution function is $p(U) = p(X_1, X_2, \ldots, X_N)$, and $p(u) = (x_1, x_2, \ldots, x_N)$ denotes a particular value assignment for U. Note that this full joint distribution $p(U) = p(X_1, X_2, \ldots, X_N)$ provides all the possible information one needs to calculate any marginal or conditional probability of interest among subsets of U.

If $A, B,$ and C are disjoint sets of random variables, the conditional independence relation $A \perp B|C$ is defined such that A is independent of B given C, that is, $p(A, B|C) = p(A|C)p(B|C)$. Conditional independence is symmetric. Note also that marginal independence (no conditioning) does not in general imply conditional independence, nor does conditional independence in general imply marginal independence (Whittaker 1990).

With any set of random variables U we can associate a graph G defined as $G = (V, E)$. V denotes the set of vertices or nodes of the graph such that there is a one-to-one mapping between the nodes in the graph and the random variables, that is, $V = \{X_1, X_2, \ldots, X_N\}$. E denotes the set of edges, $\{e(i, j)\}$, where i and j are shorthand for the nodes X_i and X_j, $1 \le i, j \le N$. Edges of the form $e(i, i)$ are not of interest and thus are not allowed in the graphs discussed in this article.

An edge may be directed or undirected. Our convention is that a directed edge $e(i, j)$ is directed from node i to node j, in which case we sometimes say that i is a parent of its child j. An ancestor of node i is a node that has as a child either i or another ancestor of i. A subset of nodes A is an ancestral set if it contains its own ancestors. A descendant of i is either a child of i or a child of a descendant of i.

Two nodes i and j are adjacent in G if E contains the undirected or directed edge $e(i, j)$. An undirected path is a sequence of distinct nodes $\{1, \ldots, m\}$ such that there exists an undirected or directed edge for each pair of nodes

$\{l, l+1\}$ on the path. A directed path is a sequence of distinct nodes $\{1, \ldots, m\}$ such that there exists a directed edge for each pair of nodes $\{l, l + 1\}$ on the path. A graph is singly connected if there exists only one undirected path between any two nodes in the graph. An (un)directed cycle is a path such that the beginning and ending nodes on the (un)directed path are the same.

If E contains only undirected edges, then the graph G is an undirected graph (UG). If E contains only directed edges then the graph G is a directed graph (DG).

Two important classes of graphs for modeling probability distributions that we consider in this paper are UGs and acyclic directed graphs (ADGs)—directed graphs having no directed cycles. We note in passing that there exists a theory for graphical independence models involving both directed and undirected edges (chain graphs, Whittaker 1990), but these are not discussed here.

For a UG G, a subset of nodes C separates two other subsets of nodes A and B if every path joining every pair of nodes $i \in A$ and $j \in B$ contains at least one node from C. For ADGs, analogous but somewhat more complicated separation properties exist.

A graph G is complete if there are edges between all pairs of nodes. A cycle in an undirected graph is chordless if none other than successive pairs of nodes in the cycle are adjacent. An undirected graph G is triangulated if and only if the only chordless cycles in the graph contain no more than three nodes. Thus, if one can find a chordless cycle of length four or more, G is not triangulated. A clique in an undirected graph G is a subgraph of G that is complete. A clique tree for G is a tree of cliques such that there is a one-to-one correspondence between the cliques of G and the nodes of the tree.

3 Probabilistic Independence Networks ⸻

We briefly review the relation between a probability model $p(\mathbf{U}) = p(X_1, \ldots, X_N)$ and a probabilistic independence network structure $G = (V, E)$ where the vertices V are in one-to-one correspondence with the random variables in $\mathbf{U}$. (The results in this section are largely summarized versions of material in Pearl 1988 and Whittaker 1990.)

A PIN structure G is a graphical statement of a set of conditional independence relations for a set of random variables $\mathbf{U}$. Absence of an edge $e(i, j)$ in G implies some independence relation between X_i and X_j. Thus, a PIN structure G is a particular way of specifying the independence relationships present in the probability model $p(\mathbf{U})$. We say that G implies a set of probability models $p(\mathbf{U})$, denoted as $\mathcal{P}_G$, that is, $p(\mathbf{U}) \in \mathcal{P}_G$. In the reverse direction, a particular model $p(\mathbf{U})$ embodies a particular set of conditional independence assumptions that may or may not be representable in a consistent graphical form. One can derive all of the conditional independence

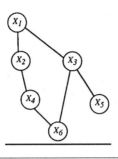

Figure 1: An example of a UPIN structure G that captures a particular set of conditional independence relationships among the set of variables $\{X_1, \ldots, X_6\}$—for example, $X_5 \perp \{X_1, X_2, X_4, X_6\} \mid \{X_3\}$.

properties and inference algorithms of interest for $\mathbf{U}$ without reference to graphical models. However, as has been emphasized in the statistical and artificial intelligence literature, and as reiterated in this article in the context of HMMs, there are distinct advantages to be gained from using the graphical formalism.

3.1 Undirected Probabilistic Independence Networks (UPINs). A UPIN is composed of both a UPIN structure and UPIN parameters. A UPIN structure specifies a set of conditional independence relations for a probability model in the form of an undirected graph. UPIN parameters consist of numerical specifications of a particular probability model consistent with the UPIN structure. Terms used in the literature to describe UPINs of one form or another include Markov random fields (Isham 1981; Geman and Geman 1984), Markov networks (Pearl 1988), Boltzmann machines (Hinton and Sejnowski 1986), and log-linear models (Bishop *et al.* 1973).

3.1.1 Conditional Independence Semantics of UPIN Structures. Let A, B, and S be any disjoint subsets of nodes in an undirected graph G. G is a UPIN structure for $p(\mathbf{U})$ if for any A, B, and S such that S separates A and B in G, the conditional independence relation $A \perp B|S$ holds in $p(\mathbf{U})$. The set of all conditional independence relations implied by separation in G constitutes the (global) Markov properties of G. Figure 1 shows a simple example of a UPIN structure for six variables.

Thus, separation in the UPIN structure implies conditional independence in the probability model; i.e., it constrains $p(\mathbf{U})$ to belong to a set of probability models $\mathcal{P}_G$ that obey the Markov properties of the graph. Note that a complete UG is trivially a UPIN structure for any $p(\mathbf{U})$ in the sense that there are no constraints on $p(\mathbf{U})$. G is a perfect undirected map for p if G is a UPIN structure for $p(\mathbf{U})$ and all the conditional independence relations present in $p(\mathbf{U})$ are represented by separation in G. For many probability models p there are no perfect undirected maps. A weaker condition is that a UPIN structure G is minimal for a probability model $p(\mathbf{U})$ if the removal of any edge from G implies an independence relation not present in the model $p(\mathbf{U})$; that is, the structure without the edge is no longer a UPIN structure for $p(\mathbf{U})$. Minimality is not equivalent to perfection (for UPIN structures) since, for example, there exist probability models with independencies that cannot be represented as UPINs except for the complete UPIN structure. For example, consider that X and Y are marginally independent but conditionally dependent given Z (e.g., X and Y are two independent causal variables with a common effect Z). In this case the complete graph is the minimal UPIN structure for $\{X, Y, Z\}$, but it is not perfect because of the presence of an edge between X and Y.

3.1.2 Probability Functions on UPIN structures.   Given a UPIN structure G, the joint probability distribution for $\mathbf{U}$ can be expressed as a simple factorization:

$$p(\mathbf{u}) = p(x_1, \ldots, x_N) = \prod_{V_C} a_C(x_C), \tag{3.1}$$

where V_C is the set of cliques of G, x_C represents an assignment of values to the variables in a particular clique C, and the $a_C(x_C)$ are non-negative clique functions. (The domain of each $a_C(x_C)$ is the set of possible assignments of values to the variables in the clique C, and the range of $a_C(x_C)$ is the semi-infinite interval $[0, \infty)$.) The set of clique functions associated with a UPIN structure provides the numerical parameterization of the UPIN.

A UPIN is equivalent to a Markov random field (Isham 1981). In the Markov random field literature the clique functions are generally referred to as potential functions. A related terminology, used in the context of the Boltzmann machine (Hinton and Sejnowski 1986), is that of energy function. The exponential of the negative energy of a configuration is a Boltzmann factor. Scaling each Boltzmann factor by the sum across Boltzmann factors (the partition function) yields a factorization of the joint density (the Boltzmann distribution), that is, a product of clique functions.[1] The advantage of defining clique functions directly rather than in terms of the exponential of an energy function is that the range of the clique functions can be allowed

---

[1] A Boltzmann machine is a special case of a UPIN in which the clique functions can be decomposed into products of factors associated with pairs of variables. If the Boltzmann machine is augmented to include "higher-order" energy terms, one for each clique in the graph, then we have a general Markov random field or UPIN, restricted to positive probability distributions due to the exponential form of the clique functions.

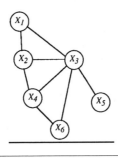

Figure 2: A triangulated version of the UPIN structure G from Figure 1.

to contain zero. Thus equation 3.1 can represent configurations of variables having zero probability.

A model p is said to be decomposable if it has a minimal UPIN structure G that is triangulated (see Fig. 2). A UPIN structure G is decomposable if G is triangulated. For the special case of decomposable models, G can be converted to a junction tree, which is a tree of cliques of G arranged such that the cliques satisfy the running intersection property, namely, that each node in G that appears in any two different cliques also appears in all cliques on the undirected path between these two cliques. Associated with each edge in the junction tree is a separator S, such that S contains the variables in the intersection of the two cliques that it links. Given a junction tree representation, one can factorize $p(\mathbf{U})$ as the product of clique marginals over separator marginals (Pearl 1988):

$$p(\mathbf{u}) = \frac{\prod_{C \in V_C} p(x_C)}{\prod_{S \in V_S} p(x_S)}, \tag{3.2}$$

where $p(x_C)$ and $p(x_S)$ are the marginal (joint) distributions for the variables in clique C and separator S, respectively, and V_C and V_S are the set of cliques and separators in the junction tree.

This product representation is central to the results in the rest of the article. It is the basis of the fact that globally consistent probability calculations on $\mathbf{U}$ can be carried out in a purely local manner. The mechanics of these local calculations will be described later. At this point it is sufficient to note that the complexity of the local inference algorithms scales as the sum of the sizes of the clique state-spaces (where a clique state-space is equal to the product over each variable in the clique of the number of states of each variable). Thus, local clique updating can make probability calculations on $\mathbf{U}$ much more tractable than using "brute force" inference if the model decomposes into relatively small cliques.

Many probability models of interest may not be decomposable. However, we can define a decomposable cover G' for p such that G' is a triangulated, but not necessarily minimal, UPIN structure for p. Since any UPIN G can be triangulated simply by the addition of the appropriate edges, one can always identify at least one decomposable cover G'. However, a decomposable cover may not be minimal in that it can contain edges that obscure certain independencies in the model p; for example, the complete graph is a decomposable cover for all possible probability models p. For efficient inference, the goal is to find a decomposable cover G' such that G' contains as few extra edges as possible over the original UPIN structure G. Later we discuss a specific algorithm for finding decomposable covers for arbitrary PIN structures. All singly connected UPIN structures imply probability models $\mathcal{P}_G$ that are decomposable.

Note that given a particular probability model p and a UPIN G for p, the process of adding extra edges to G to create a decomposable cover does not change the underlying probability model p; that is, the added edges are a convenience for manipulating the graphical representation, but the underlying numerical probability specifications remain unchanged.

An important point is that decomposable covers have the running intersection property and thus can be factored as in equation 3.2. Thus local clique updating is also possible with nondecomposable models by this conversion. Once again, the complexity of such local inference scales with the sum of the size of the clique state-spaces in the decomposable cover.

In summary, any UPIN structure can be converted to a junction tree permitting inference calculations to be carried out purely locally on cliques.

3.2 Directed Probabilistic Independence Networks (DPINs). A DPIN is composed of both a DPIN structure and DPIN parameters. A DPIN structure specifies a set of conditional independence relations for a probability model in the form of a directed graph. DPIN parameters consist of numerical specifications of a particular probability model consistent with the DPIN structure. DPINs are referred to in the literature using different names, including Bayes network, belief network, recursive graphical model, causal (belief) network, and probabilistic (causal) network.

3.2.1 Conditional Independence Semantics of DPIN Structures. A DPIN structure is an ADG $G^D = (V, E)$ where there is a one-to-one correspondence between V and the elements of the set of random variables $\mathbf{U} = \{X_1, \ldots, X_N\}$.

It is convenient to define the moral graph G^M of G^D as the undirected graph obtained from G^D by placing undirected edges between all nonadjacent parents of each node and then dropping the directions from the remaining directed edges (see Fig. 3b for an example). The term *moral* was coined to denote the "marrying" of "unmarried" (nonadjacent) parents. The motivation behind this procedure will become clear when we discuss the differ-

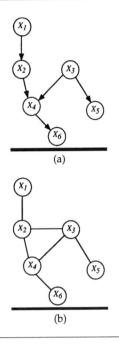

Figure 3: (a) A DPIN structure G^D that captures a set of independence relationships among the set $\{X_1, \ldots, X_5\}$—for example, $X_4 \perp X_1 | X_2$. (b) The moral graph G^M for G^D, where the parents of X_4 have been linked.

ences between DPINs and UPINs in Section 3.3. We shall also see that this conversion of a DPIN into a UPIN is a convenient way to solve DPIN inference problems by "transforming" the problem into an undirected graphical setting and taking advantage of the general theory available for undirected graphical models.

We can now define a DPIN as follows. Let A, B, and S be any disjoint subsets of nodes in G^D. G^D is a DPIN structure for $p(\mathbf{U})$ if for any $A, B,$ and S such that S separates A and B in G^D, the conditional independence relation $A \perp B | S$ holds in $p(\mathbf{U})$. This is the same definition as for a UPIN structure except that separation has a more complex interpretation in the directed context: S separates A from B in a directed graph if S separates A from B in the moral (undirected) graph of the smallest ancestral set containing $A, B,$ and S (Lauritzen et al. 1990). It can be shown that this definition of a DPIN structure is equivalent to the more intuitive statement that given the values of its parents, a variable X_i is independent of all other nodes in the directed graph except for its descendants.

Thus, as with a UPIN structure, the DPIN structure implies certain conditional independence relations, which in turn imply a set of probability models $p \in \mathcal{P}_{G^D}$. Figure 3a contains a simple example of a DPIN structure.

There are many possible DPIN structures consistent with a particular probability model $p(\mathbf{U})$, potentially containing extra edges that hide true conditional independence relations. Thus, one can define minimal DPIN structures for $p(\mathbf{U})$ in a manner exactly equivalent to that of UPIN structures: Deletion of an edge in a minimal DPIN structure G^D implies an independence relation that does not hold in $p(\mathbf{U}) \in \mathcal{P}_{G^D}$. Similarly, G^D is a perfect DPIN structure G for $p(\mathbf{U})$ if G^D is a DPIN structure for $p(\mathbf{U})$ and all the conditional independence relations present in $p(\mathbf{U})$ are represented by separation in G^D. As with UPIN structures, minimal does not imply perfect for DPIN structures. For example, consider the independence relations $X_1 \perp X_4 | \{X_2, X_3\}$ and $X_2 \perp X_3 | \{X_1, X_4\}$: the minimal DPIN structure contains an edge from X_3 to X_2 (see Fig. 4b). A complete ADG is trivially a DPIN structure for any probability model $p(\mathbf{U})$.

3.2.2 Probability Functions on DPINs. A basic property of a DPIN structure is that it implies a direct factorization of the joint probability distribution $p(\mathbf{U})$:

$$p(\mathbf{u}) = \prod_{i=1}^{N} p(x_i \mid pa(x_i)), \qquad (3.3)$$

where $pa(x_i)$ denotes a value assignment for the parents of X_i. A probability model p can be written in this factored form in a trivial manner by the conditioning rule. Note that a directed graph containing directed cycles does not necessarily yield such a factorization, hence the use of ADGs.

3.3 Differences between Directed and Undirected Graphical Representations. It is an important point that directed and undirected graphs possess different conditional independence semantics. There are common conditional independence relations that have perfect DPIN structures but no perfect UPIN structures, and vice versa (see Figure 4 for examples).

Does a DPIN structure have the same Markov properties as the UPIN structure obtained by dropping all the directions on the edges in the DPIN structure? The answer is yes if and only if the DPIN structure contains no subgraphs where a node has two or more nonadjacent parents (Whittaker 1990; Pearl et al. 1990). In general, it can be shown that if a UPIN structure G for p is decomposable (triangulated), then it has the same Markov properties as some DPIN structure for p.

On a more practical level, DPIN structures are frequently used to encode causal information, that is, to represent the belief formally that X_i precedes X_j in some causal sense (e.g., temporally). DPINs have found application in causal modeling in applied statistics and artificial intelligence. Their popularity in these fields stems from the fact that the joint probability model can

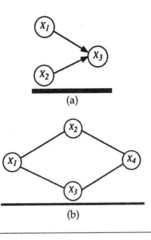

(a)

(b)

Figure 4: (a) The DPIN structure to encode the fact that X_3 depends on X_1 and X_2 but $X_1 \perp X_2$. For example, consider that X_1 and X_2 are two independent coin flips and that X_3 is a bell that rings when the flips are the same. There is no perfect UPIN structure that can encode these dependence relationships. (b) A UPIN structure that encodes $X_1 \perp X_4 | \{X_2, X_3\}$ and $X_2 \perp X_3 | \{X_1, X_4\}$. There is no perfect DPIN structure that can encode these dependencies.

be specified directly by equation 3.3, that is, by the specification of conditional probability tables or functions (Spiegelhalter *el al.* 1991). In contrast, UPINs must be specified in terms of clique functions (as in equation 3.1), which may not be as easy to work with (cf. Geman and Geman 1984, Modestino and Zhang 1992, and Vandermeulen *et al.* 1994 for examples of ad hoc design of clique functions in image analysis). UPINs are more frequently used in problems such as image analysis and statistical physics where associations are thought to be correlational rather than causal.

3.4 From DPINs to (Decomposable) UPINs. The moral UPIN structure G^M (obtained from the DPIN structure G^D) does not imply any new independence relations that are not present in G^D. As with triangulation, however, the additional edges may obscure conditional independence relations implicit in the numeric specification of the original probability model p associated with the DPIN structure G^D. Furthermore, G^M may not be triangulated (decomposable). By the addition of appropriate edges, the moral graph can be converted to a (nonunique) triangulated graph G', namely, a decomposable cover for G^M. In this manner, for any probability model p for which G^D is a DPIN structure, one can construct a decomposable cover G' for p.

This mapping from DPIN structures to UPIN structures was first discussed in the context of efficient inference algorithms by Lauritzen and

Spiegelhalter (1988). The advantage of this mapping derives from the fact that analysis and manipulation of the resulting UPIN are considerably more direct than dealing with the original DPIN. Furthermore, it has been shown that many of the inference algorithms for DPINs are in fact special cases of inference algorithms for UPINs and can be considerably less efficient (Shachter *et al.* 1994).

4 Modeling HMMs as PINs

4.1 PINs for HMMs. In hidden Markov modeling problems (Baum and Petrie 1966; Poritz 1988; Rabiner 1989; Huang *et al.* 1990; Elliott *et al.* 1995) we are interested in the set of random variables $\mathbf{U} = \{H_1, O_1, H_2, O_2, \ldots, H_{N-1}, O_{N-1}, H_N, O_N\}$, where H_i is a discrete-valued hidden variable at index i, and O_i is the corresponding discrete-valued observed variable at index i, $1 \leq i \leq N$. (The results here can be directly extended to continuous-valued observables.) The index i denotes a sequence from 1 to N, for example, discrete time steps. Note that O_i is considered univariate for convenience: the extension to the multivariate case with d observables is straightforward but is omitted here for simplicity since it does not illuminate the conditional independence relationships in the HMM.

The well-known simple first-order HMM obeys the following two conditional independence relations:

$$H_i \perp \{H_1, O_1, \ldots, H_{i-2}, O_{i-2}, O_{i-1}\} \mid H_{i-1}, \qquad 3 \leq i \leq N \tag{4.1}$$

and

$$O_i \perp \{H_1, O_1, \ldots, H_{i-1}, O_{i-1}\} \mid H_i, \qquad 2 \leq i \leq N. \tag{4.2}$$

We will refer to this "first-order" hidden Markov probability model as HMM(1,1): the notation HMM(K, J) is defined such that the hidden state of the model is represented via the conjoined configuration of J underlying random variables and such that the model has state memory of depth K. The notation will be clearer in later sections when we discuss specific examples with $K, J > 1$.

Construction of a PIN for HMM(1,1) is simple. In the undirected case, assumption 1 requires that each state H_i is connected to H_{i-1} only from the set $\{H_1, O_1, \ldots, H_{i-2}, O_{i-2}, H_{i-1}, O_{i-1}\}$. Assumption 2 requires that O_i is connected only to H_i. The resulting UPIN structure for HMM(1,1) is shown in Figure 5a. This graph is singly connected and thus implies a decomposable probability model p for HMM(1,1), where the cliques are of the form $\{H_i, O_i\}$ and $\{H_{i-1}, H_i\}$ (see Fig. 5b). In Section 5 we will see how the joint probability function can be expressed as a product function on the junction tree, thus leading to a junction tree definition of the familiar F-B and Viterbi inference algorithms.

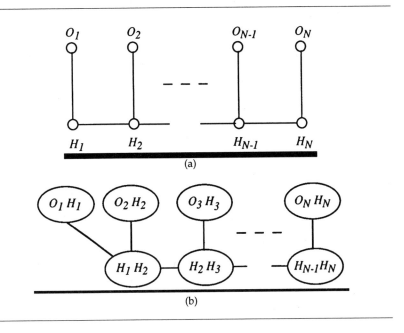

Figure 5: (a) PIN structure for HMM(1,1). (b) A corresponding junction tree.

For the directed case, the connectivity for the DPIN structure is the same. It is natural to choose the directions on the edges between H_{i-1} and H_i as going from $i - 1$ to i (although the reverse direction could also be chosen without changing the Markov properties of the graph). The directions on the edges between H_i and O_i must be chosen as going from H_i to O_i rather than in the reverse direction (see Figure 6a). In reverse (see Fig. 6b) the arrows would imply that O_i is marginally independent of H_{i-1}, which is not true in the HMM(1,1) probability model. The proper direction for the edges implies the correct relation, namely, that O_i is conditionally independent of H_{i-1} given H_i.

The DPIN structure for HMM(1,1) does not possess a subgraph with nonadjacent parents. As stated earlier, this implies that the implied independence properties of the DPIN structure are the same as those of the corresponding UPIN structure obtained by dropping the directions from the edges in the DPIN structure, and thus they both result in the same junction tree structure (see Fig. 5b). Thus, for the HMM(1,1) probability model, the minimal directed and undirected graphs possess the same Markov properties; they imply the same conditional independence relations. Furthermore, both PIN structures are perfect maps for the directed and undirected cases, respectively.

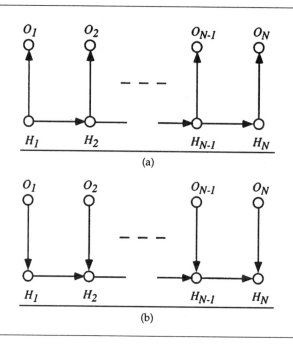

$$O_1 \quad O_2 \qquad\qquad O_{N-1} \quad O_N$$

(a)

$$O_1 \quad O_2 \qquad\qquad O_{N-1} \quad O_N$$

$$H_1 \quad H_2 \qquad\qquad H_{N-1} \quad H_N$$

(b)

Figure 6: DPIN structures for HMM(1,1). (a) The DPIN structure for the HMM(1,1) probability model. (b) A DPIN structure that is not a DPIN structure for the HMM(1,1) probability model.

4.2 Inference and MAP Problems in HMMs. In the context of HMMs, the most common inference problem is the calculation of the likelihood of the observed evidence given the model, that is, $p(o_1, \ldots, o_N|\text{model})$, where the $o_1, \ldots, o_N$ denote observed values for $O_1, \ldots, O_N$. (In this section we will assume that we are dealing with one particular model where the structure and parameters have already been determined, and thus we will not explicitly indicate conditioning on the model.) The "brute force" method for obtaining this probability would be to sum out the unobserved state variables from the full joint probability distribution:

$$p(o_1, \ldots, o_N) = \sum_{h_1, \ldots, h_N} p(H_1, o_1, \ldots, H_N, o_N), \qquad (4.3)$$

where h_i denotes the possible values of hidden variable H_i.

In general, both of these computations scale as m^N where m is the number of states for each hidden variable. In practice, the F-B algorithm (Poritz 1988; Rabiner 1989) can perform these inference calculations with much lower complexity, namely, Nm^2. The likelihood of the observed evidence can be obtained with the forward step of the F-B algorithm: calculation of the state posterior probabilities requires both forward and backward steps. The F-B algorithm relies on a factorization of the joint probability function to obtain locally recursive methods. One of the key points in this article is that the graphical modeling approach provides an *automatic* method for determining such local efficient factorizations, for an arbitrary probabilistic model, *if efficient factorizations exist* given the conditional independence (CI) relations specified in the model.

The MAP identification problem in the context of HMMs involves identifying the most likely hidden state sequence given the observed evidence. Just as with the inference problem, the Viterbi algorithm provides an efficient, locally recursive method for solving this problem with complexity Nm^2, and again, as with the inference problem, the graphical modeling approach provides an automatic technique for determining efficient solutions to the MAP problem for arbitrary models, if an efficient solution is possible given the structure of the model.

5 Inference and MAP Algorithms for DPINs

Inference and MAP algorithms for DPINs and UPINS are quite similar: the UPIN case involves some subtleties not encountered in DPINs, and so discussion of UPIN inference and MAP algorithms is deferred until Section 7. The inference algorithm for DPINs (developed by Jensen *et al.* 1990, and hereafter referred to as the JLO algorithm) is a descendant of an inference algorithm first described by Lauritzen and Spiegelhalter (1988). The JLO algorithm applies to discrete-valued variables: extensions to the JLO algorithm for gaussian and gaussian-mixture distributions are discussed in Lauritzen and Wermuth (1989). A closely related algorithm to the JLO algorithm, developed by Dawid (1992a), solves the MAP identification problem with the same time complexity as the JLO inference algorithm.

We show that the JLO and Dawid algorithms are strict generalizations of the well-known F-B and Viterbi algorithms for HMM(1,1) in that they can be applied to arbitrarily complex graph structures (and thus a large family of probabilistic models beyond HMM(1,1)) and handle missing values, partial inference, and so forth in a straightforward manner.

There are many variations on the basic JLO and Dawid algorithms. For example, Pearl (1988) describes related versions of these algorithms in his early work. However, it can be shown (Shachter *et al.* 1994) that all known exact algorithms for inference on DPINs are equivalent at some level to the JLO and Dawid algorithms. Thus, it is sufficient to consider the JLO and Dawid algorithms in our discussion as they subsume other graphical inference algorithms.[2]

---

[2] An alternative set of computational formalisms is provided by the statistical physics

The JLO and Dawid algorithms operate as a two-step process:

1. *The construction step.* This involves a series of substeps where the original directed graph is moralized and triangulated, a junction tree is formed, and the junction tree is initialized.

2. *The propagation step.* The junction tree is used in a local message-passing manner to propagate the effects of observed evidence, that is, to solve the inference and MAP problems.

The first step is carried out only once for a given graph. The second (propagation) step is carried out each time a new inference for the given graph is requested.

5.1 The Construction Step of the JLO Algorithm: From DPIN Structures to Junction Trees. We illustrate the construction step of the JLO algorithm using the simple DPIN structure, G^D, over discrete variables $\mathbf{U} = \{X_1, \ldots, X_6\}$ shown in Figure 7a. The JLO algorithm first constructs the moral graph G^M (see Fig. 7b). It then triangulates the moral graph G^M to obtain a decomposable cover G' (see Fig. 7c). The algorithm operates in a simple, greedy manner based on the fact that a graph is triangulated if and only if all of its nodes can be eliminated, where a node can be eliminated whenever all of its neighbors are pairwise-linked. Whenever a node is eliminated, it and its neighbors define a clique in the junction tree that is eventually constructed. Thus, we can triangulate a graph and generate the cliques for the junction tree by eliminating nodes in some order, adding links if necessary. If no node can be eliminated without adding links, then we choose the node that can be eliminated by adding the links that yield the clique with the smallest state-space.

After triangulation, the JLO algorithm constructs a junction tree from G' (i.e., a clique tree satisfying the running intersection property). The junction tree construction is based on the following fact: Define the weight of a link

---

literature, where undirected graphical models in the form of chains, trees, lattices, and "decorated" variations on chains and trees have been studied for many years (see, e.g., Itzykson and Drouffé 1991). The general methods developed there, notably the transfer matrix formalism (e.g., Morgenstern and Binder 1983), support exact calculations on general undirected graphs. The transfer matrix recursions and the calculations in the JLO algorithm are closely related, and a reasonable hypothesis is that they are equivalent formalisms. (The question does not appear to have been studied in the general case, although see Stolorz 1994 and Saul and Jordan 1995 for special cases.) The appeal of the JLO framework, in the context of this earlier literature on exact calculations, is the link that it provides to conditional probability models (i.e., directed graphs) and the focus on a particular data structure—the junction tree—as the generic data structure underlying exact calculations. This does not, of course, diminish the potential importance of statistical physics methodology in graphical modeling applications. One area where there is clearly much to be gained from links to statistical physics is the area of approximate calculations, where a wide variety of methods are available (see, e.g., Swendsen and Wang 1987).

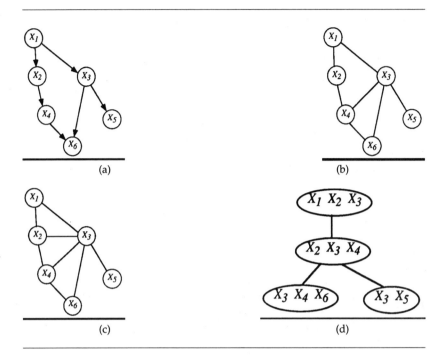

(a)

(b)

(c)

(d)

Figure 7: (a) A simple DPIN structure G^D. (b) The corresponding (undirected) moral graph G^M. (c) The corresponding triangulated graph G'. (d) The corresponding junction tree.

between two cliques as the number of variables in their intersection. Then a tree of cliques will satisfy the running intersection property if and only if it is a spanning tree of maximal weight. Thus, the JLO algorithm constructs a junction tree by choosing successively a link of maximal weight unless it creates a cycle. The junction tree constructed from the cliques defined by the DPIN structure triangulation in Figure 7c is shown in Figure 7d.

The worst-case complexity is $O(N^3)$ for the triangulation heuristic and $O(N^2 \log N)$ for the maximal spanning tree portion of the algorithm. This construction step is carried out only once as an initial step to convert the original graph to a junction tree representation.

5.2 Initializing the Potential Functions in the Junction Tree. The next step is to take the numeric probability specifications as defined on the directed graph G^D (see equation 3.3) and convert this information into the general form for a junction tree representation of p (see equation 3.2). This is achieved by noting that each variable X_i is contained in at least one clique in the junction tree. Assign each X_i to just one such clique, and for each clique define the potential function $a_C(C)$ to be either the product of $p(X_i|pa(X_i))$ over all X_i assigned to clique C, or 1 if no variables are assigned to that clique. Define the separator potentials (in equation 3.2) to be 1 initially.

In the section that follows, we describe the general JLO algorithm for propagating messages through the junction tree to achieve globally consistent probability calculations. At this point it is sufficient to know that a schedule of local message passing can be defined that converges to a globally consistent marginal representation for p; that is, the potential on any clique or separator is the marginal for that clique or separator (the joint probability function). Thus, via local message passing, one can go from the initial potential representation defined above to a marginal representation:

$$p(\mathbf{u}) = \frac{\prod_{C \in V_C} p(x_C)}{\prod_{S \in V_S} p(x_S)}.$$
(5.1)

At this point the junction tree is initialized. This operation in itself is not that useful; of more interest is the ability to propagate information through the graph given some observed data and the initialized junction tree (e.g., to calculate the posterior distributions of some variables of interest).

From this point onward we will implicitly assume that the junction tree has been initialized as described so that the potential functions are the local marginals.

5.3 Local Message Propagation in Junction Trees Using the JLO Algorithm. In general $p(\mathbf{U})$ can be expressed as

$$p(\mathbf{u}) = \frac{\prod_{C \in V_C} a_C(x_C)}{\prod_{S \in V_S} b_S(x_S)},$$
(5.2)

where the a_C and b_S are nonnegative potential functions (the potential functions could be the initial marginals described above, for example). Note that this representation is a generalization of the representations for $p(\mathbf{u})$ given by equations 3.1 and 3.2. $K = (\{a_C : C \in V_C\}, \{b_S : S \in S_C\})$ is a representation for $p(\mathbf{U})$. A factorizable function $p(\mathbf{U})$ can admit many different representations, that is, many different sets of clique and separator functions that satisfy equation 5.2 given a particular $p(\mathbf{U})$.

The JLO algorithm carries out globally consistent probability calculations via local message passing on the junction tree; probability information is passed between neighboring cliques, and clique and separator potentials are updated based on this local information. A key point is that the cliques and separators are updated in a fashion that ensures that at all times K is a representation for $p(\mathbf{U})$; in other words, equation 5.2 holds at all times. Eventually the propagation converges to the marginal representation given the initial model and the observed evidence.

The message passing proceeds as follows: We can define a flow from clique C_i to C_j in the following manner where C_i and C_j are two cliques adjacent in the junction tree. Let S_k be the separator for these two cliques. Define

$$b_{S_k}^*(x_{S_k}) = \sum_{C_i \setminus S_k} a_{C_i}(x_{C_i}) \tag{5.3}$$

where the summation is over the state-space of variables that are in C_i but not in S_k, and

$$a_{C_j}^*(x_{C_j}) = a_{C_j}(x_{C_j}) \lambda_{S_k}(x_{S_k}) \tag{5.4}$$

where

$$\lambda_{S_k}(x_{S_k}) = \frac{b_{S_k}^*(x_{S_k})}{b_{S_k}(x_{S_k})} . \tag{5.5}$$

$\lambda_{S_k}(x_{S_k})$ is the update factor. Passage of a flow corresponds to updating the neighboring clique with the probability information contained in the originating clique. This flow induces a new representation $K^* = (\{a_C^* : C \in V_C\}, \{b_S^* : S \in S_C\})$ for $p(\mathbf{U})$.

A schedule of such flows can be defined such that all cliques are eventually updated with all relevant information and the junction tree reaches an equilibrium state. The most direct scheduling scheme is a two-phase operation where one node is denoted the root of the junction tree. The collection phase involves passing flows along all edges toward the root clique (if a node is scheduled to have more than one incoming flow, the flows are absorbed sequentially). Once collection is complete, the distribution phase involves passing flows out from this root in the reverse direction along the same edges. There are at most two flows along any edge in the tree in a nonredundant schedule. Note that the directionality of the flows in the junction tree need have nothing to do with any directed edges in the original DPIN structure.

5.4 The JLO Algorithm for Inference Given Observed Evidence.

The particular case of calculating the effect of observed evidence (inference) is handled in the following manner: Consider that we observe evidence of the form $e = \{X_i = x_i^*, X_j = x_j^*, \ldots\}$, and $\mathbf{U}^e = \{X_i, X_j, \ldots\}$ denotes the set of variables observed. Let $\mathbf{U}^h = \mathbf{U} \setminus \mathbf{U}^e$ denote the set of hidden or unobserved variables and $\mathbf{u}^h$ a value assignment for $\mathbf{U}^h$.

Consider the calculation of $p(\mathbf{U}^h | e)$. Define an evidence function $g^e(x_i)$ such that

$$g^e(x_i) = \begin{cases} 1 & \text{if } x_i = x_i^* \\ 0 & \text{otherwise.} \end{cases} \tag{5.6}$$

Let

$$f^*(\mathbf{u}) = p(\mathbf{u}) \prod_{\mathbf{U}^e} g^e(x_i). \tag{5.7}$$

Thus, we have that $f^*(\mathbf{u}) \propto p(\mathbf{u}^h|e)$. To obtain $f^*(\mathbf{u})$ by operations on the junction tree, one proceeds as follows: First assign each observed variable $X_i \in \mathbf{U}^e$ to one particular clique that contains it (this is termed "entering the evidence into the clique"). Let C^E denote the set of all cliques into which evidence is entered in this manner. For each $C \in C^E$ let

$$g_C(x_C) = \prod_{\{i:\, X_i \text{ is entered into } C\}} g^e(x_i). \tag{5.8}$$

Thus,

$$f^*(\mathbf{u}) = p(\mathbf{u}) \times \prod_{C \in C^E} g_C(x_C). \tag{5.9}$$

One can now propagate the effects of these modifications throughout the tree using the collect-and-distribute schedule described in Section 5.3. Let x_C^h denote a value assignment of the hidden (unobserved) variables in clique C. When the schedule of flows is complete, one gets a new representation K_f^* such that the local potential on each clique is $f^*(x_C) = p(x_C^h, e)$, that is, the joint probability of the local unobserved clique variables and the observed evidence (Jensen et al. 1990) (similarly for the separator potential functions). If one marginalizes at the clique over the unobserved local clique variables,

$$\sum_{x_C^h} p(x_C^h, e) = p(e), \tag{5.10}$$

one gets the probability of the observed evidence directly. Similarly, if one normalizes the potential function at a clique to sum to one, one obtains the conditional probability of the local unobserved clique variables given the evidence, $p(x_C^h|e)$.

5.5 Complexity of the Propagation Step of the JLO Algorithm. In general, the time complexity T of propagation within a junction tree is $O(\sum_{i=1}^{N_C} s(C_i))$ where N_C is the number of cliques in the junction tree and $s(C_i)$ is the number of states in the clique state-space of C_i. Thus, for inference to be efficient, we need to construct junction trees with small clique sizes. Problems of finding optimally small junction trees (e.g., finding the junction tree with the smallest maximal clique) are NP-hard. Nonetheless, the heuristic algorithm for triangulation described earlier has been found to work well in practice (Jensen et al. 1990).

6 Inference and MAP Calculations in HMM(1,1) _____

6.1 The F-B Algorithm for HMM(1,1) Is a Special Case of the JLO Algorithm. Figure 5b shows the junction tree for HMM(1,1). One can apply the JLO algorithm to the HMM(1,1) junction tree structure to obtain a particular inference algorithm for HMM(1,1). The HMM(1,1) inference problem consists of being given a set of values for the observable variables,

$$e = \{O_1 = o_1, O_2 = o_2, \ldots, O_N = o_N\} \tag{6.1}$$

and inferring the likelihood of e given the model. As described in the previous section, this problem can be solved exactly by local propagation in any junction tree using the JLO inference algorithm. In Appendix A it is shown that both the forward and backward steps of the F-B procedure for HMM(1,1) are exactly recreated by the more general JLO algorithm when the HMM(1,1) is viewed as a PIN.

This equivalence is not surprising since both algorithms are solving exactly the same problem by local recursive updating. The equivalence is useful because it provides a link between well-known HMM inference algorithms and more general PIN inference algorithms. Furthermore, it clearly demonstrates how the PIN framework can provide a direct avenue for analyzing and using more complex hidden Markov probability models (we will discuss such HMMs in Section 8).

When evidence is entered into the observable states and assuming m discrete states per hidden variable, the computational complexity of solving the inference problem via the JLO algorithm is $O(Nm^2)$ (the same complexity as the standard F-B procedure).

Note that the obvious structural equivalence between PIN structures and HMM(1,1) has been noted before by Buntine (1994), Frasconi and Bengio (1994), and Lucke (1995) among others; however, this is the first publication of equivalence of specific inference algorithms as far as we are aware.

6.2 Equivalence of Dawid's Propagation Algorithm for Identifying MAP Assignments and the Viterbi Algorithm. Consider that one wishes to calculate $\hat{f}(u^h, e) = \max_{x_1, \ldots, x_K} p(x_1, \ldots, x_K, e)$ and also to identify a set of values of the unobserved variables that achieve this maximum, where K is the number of unobserved (hidden) variables. This calculation can be achieved using a local propagation algorithm on the junction tree with two modifications to the standard JLO inference algorithm. This algorithm is due to Dawid (1992a); this is the most general algorithm from a set of related methods.

First, during a flow, the marginalization of the separator is replaced by

$$\hat{b}_S(x_S) = \max_{C \backslash S} a_C(x_C), \tag{6.2}$$

where C is the originating clique for the flow. The definition for $\lambda_S(x_S)$ is also changed in the obvious manner.

Second, marginalization within a clique is replaced by maximization:

$$\hat{f}_C = \max_{u\backslash x_C} p(\mathbf{u}) . \tag{6.3}$$

Given these two changes, it can be shown that if the same propagation operations are carried out as described earlier, the resulting representation $\hat{K}_f$ at equilibrium is such that the potential function on each clique C is

$$\hat{f}(x_C) = \max_{u^h\backslash x_C} p(x_C^h, e, \{\mathbf{u}^h \backslash x_C\}), \tag{6.4}$$

where x_C^h denotes a value assignment of the hidden (unobserved) variables in clique C. Thus, once the $\hat{K}_f$ representation is obtained, one can locally identify the values of X_C^h, which maximize the full joint probability as

$$\hat{x}_C^h = \arg_{x_C^h} \hat{f}(x_C) . \tag{6.5}$$

In the probabilistic expert systems literature, this procedure is known as generating the most probable explanation (MPE) given the observed evidence (Pearl 1988).

The HMM(1,1) MAP problem consists of being given a set of values for the observable variables, $e = \{O_1 = o_1, O_2 = o_2, \dots, O_N = o_N\}$, and inferring

$$\max_{h_1,\dots,h_N} p(h_1, \dots, h_N, e) \tag{6.6}$$

or the set of arguments that achieve this maximum. Since Dawid's algorithm is applicable to any junction tree, it can be directly applied to the HMM(1,1) junction tree in Figure 5b. In Appendix B it is shown that Dawid's algorithm, when applied to HMM(1,1), is exactly equivalent to the standard Viterbi algorithm. Once again the equivalence is not surprising: Dawid's method and the Viterbi algorithm are both direct applications of dynamic programming to the MAP problem. However, once again, the important point is that Dawid's algorithm is specified for the general case of arbitrary PIN structures and can thus be directly applied to more complex HMMs than HMM(1,1) (such as those discussed later in Section 8).

7 Inference and MAP Algorithms for UPINs

In Section 5 we described the JLO algorithm for local inference given a DPIN. For UPINs the procedure is very similar except for two changes to the overall algorithm: the moralization step is not necessary, and initialization of the junction tree is less trivial. In Section 5.2 we described how to go from a specification of conditional probabilities in a directed graph to an initial potential function representation on the cliques in the junction tree. To utilize undirected links in the model specification process requires new machinery to perform the initialization step. In particular we wish to compile the model into the standard form of a product of potentials on the cliques of a triangulated graph (cf. equation 3.1):

$$P(\mathbf{u}) = \prod_{C \in V_C} a_C(x_C) .$$

Once this initialization step has been achieved, the JLO propagation procedure proceeds as before.

Consider the chordless cycle shown in Figure 4b. Suppose that we parameterize the probability distribution on this graph by specifying pairwise marginals on the four pairs of neighboring nodes. We wish to convert such a local specification into a globally consistent joint probability distribution, that is, a marginal representation. An algorithm known as iterative proportional fitting (IPF) is available to perform this conversion. Classically, IPF proceeds as follows (Bishop et al. 1973): Suppose for simplicity that all of the random variables are discrete (a gaussian version of IPF is also available, Whittaker 1990) such that the joint distribution can be represented as a table. The table is initialized with equal values in all of the cells. For each marginal in turn, the table is then rescaled by multiplying every cell by the ratio of the desired marginal to the corresponding marginal in the current table. The algorithm visits each marginal in turn, iterating over the set of marginals. If the set of marginals is consistent with a single joint distribution, the algorithm is guaranteed to converge to the joint distribution. Once the joint is available, the potentials in equation 3.1 can be obtained (in principle) by marginalization.

Although IPF solves the initialization problem in principle, it is inefficient. Jiroušek and Přeučil (1995) developed an efficient version of IPF that avoids the need for both storing the joint distribution as a table and explicit marginalization of the joint to obtain the clique potentials. Jiroušek's version of IPF represents the evolving joint distribution directly in terms of junction tree potentials. The algorithm proceeds as follows: Let $\mathcal{I}$ be a set of subsets of V. For each $I \in \mathcal{I}$, let $q(x_I)$ denote the desired marginal on the subset I. Let the joint distribution be represented as a product over junction tree potentials (see equation 3.1), where each a_C is initialized to an arbitrary constant. Visit each $I \in \mathcal{I}$ in turn, updating the corresponding clique potential a_C (i.e, that potential a_C for which $I \subseteq C$) as follows:

$$a_C^*(x_C) = a_C(x_C) \frac{q(x_I)}{p(x_I)} .$$

The marginal $p(x_I)$ is obtained via the JLO algorithm, using the current set of clique potentials. Intelligent choices can be made for the order in which to visit the marginals to minimize the amount of propagation needed to compute $p(x_I)$. This algorithm is simply an efficient way of organizing the IPF calculations and inherits the latter's guarantees of convergence.

Note that the Jiřousek and Přeučil algorithm requires a triangulation step in order to form the junction tree used in the calculation of $p(x_I)$. In the worst case, triangulation can yield a highly connected graph, in which case the Jiřousek and Přeučil algorithm reduces to classical IPF. For sparse graphs, however, when the maximum clique is much smaller than the entire graph, the algorithm should be substantially more efficient than classical IPF. Moreover, the triangulation algorithm itself need only be run once as a preprocessing step (as is the case for the JLO algorithm).

8 More Complex HMMs for Speech Modeling

Although HMMs have provided an exceedingly useful framework for the modeling of speech signals, it is also true that the simple HMM(1,1) model underlying the standard framework has strong limitations as a model of speech. Real speech is generated by a set of coupled dynamical systems (lips, tongue, glottis, lungs, air columns, etc.), each obeying particular dynamical laws. This coupled physical process is not well modeled by the unstructured state transition matrix of HMM(1,1). Moreover, the first-order Markov properties of HMM(1,1) are not well suited to modeling the ubiquitous coarticulation effects that occur in speech, particularly coarticulatory effects that extend across several phonemes (Kent and Minifie 1977). A variety of techniques have been developed to surmount these basic weaknesses of the HMM(1,1) model, including mixture modeling of emission probabilities, triphone modeling, and discriminative training. All of these methods, however, leave intact the basic probabilistic structure of HMM(1,1) as expressed by its PIN structure.

In this section we describe several extensions of HMM(1,1) that assume additional probabilistic structure beyond that assumed by HMM(1,1). PINs provide a key tool in the study of these more complex models. The role of PINs is twofold: they provide a concise description of the probabilistic dependencies assumed by a particular model, and they provide a general algorithm for computing likelihoods. This second property is particularly important because the existence of the JLO algorithm frees us from having to derive particular recursive algorithms on a case-by-case basis.

The first model that we consider can be viewed as a coupling of two HMM(1,1) chains (Saul and Jordan, 1995). Such a model can be useful in general sensor fusion problems, for example, in the fusion of an audio signal with a video signal in lipreading. Because different sensory signals generally have different bandwidths, it may be useful to couple separate Markov models that are developed specifically for each of the individual signals. The alternative is to force the problem into an HMM(1,1) framework by either oversampling the slower signal, which requires additional parameters and leads to a high-variance estimator, or downsampling the faster signal, which generally oversmoothes the data and yields a biased estimator. Consider the HMM(1,2) structure shown in Figure 8a. This model involves two HMM(1,1) backbones that are coupled together by undirected links between the state variables. Let $H_i^{(1)}$ and $O_i^{(1)}$ denote the ith state and ith output of the "fast" chain, respectively, and let $H_i^{(2)}$ and $O_i^{(2)}$ denote the ith state and ith output of the "slow" chain. Suppose that the fast chain is sampled τ times as often as the slow chain. Then $H_{i'}^{(1)}$ is connected to $H_i^{(2)}$ for i' equal to $\tau(i-1)+1$. Given this value for i', the Markov model for the coupled chain implies the following conditional independencies for the state variables:

$$\{H_{i'}^{(1)}, H_i^{(2)}\} \perp \{H_1^{(1)}, O_1^{(1)}, H_1^{(2)}, O_1^{(2)}, \dots, H_{i'-2}^{(1)}, O_{i'-2}^{(1)}, H_{i-2}^{(2)}, O_{i-2}^{(2)},$$
$$O_{i'-1}^{(1)}, O_{i-1}^{(2)}\} \mid \{H_{i'-1}^{(1)}, H_{i-1}^{(2)}\}, \tag{8.1}$$

as well as the following conditional independencies for the output variables:

$$\{O_{i'}^{(1)}, O_i^{(2)}\} \perp \{H_1^{(1)}, O_1^{(1)}, H_1^{(2)}, O_1^{(2)}, \dots, H_{i'-1}^{(1)}, O_{i'-1}^{(1)},$$
$$H_{i-1}^{(2)}, O_{i-1}^{(2)}\} \mid \{H_{i'}^{(1)}, H_i^{(2)}\}. \tag{8.2}$$

Additional conditional independencies can be read off the UPIN structure (see Figure 8a).

As is readily seen in Figure 8a, the HMM(1,2) graph is not triangulated; thus, the HMM(1,2) probability model is not decomposable. However, the graph can be readily triangulated to form a decomposable cover for the HMM(1,2) probability model (see Section 3.1.2). The JLO algorithm provides an efficient algorithm for calculating likelihoods in this graph. This can be seen in Figure 8b, where we show a triangulation of the HMM(1,2) graph. The triangulation adds $O(N_h)$ links to the graph (where N_h is the number of hidden nodes in the graph) and creates a junction tree in which each clique is a cluster of three state variables from the underlying UPIN structure. Assuming m values for each state variable in each chain, we obtain an algorithm whose time complexity is $O(N_h m^3)$. This can be compared to the naive approach of transforming the HMM(1,2) model to a Cartesian product HMM(1,1) model, which not only has the disadvantage of requiring subsampling or oversampling but also has a time complexity of $O(N_h m^4)$.

Directed graph semantics can also play an important role in constructing interesting variations on the HMM theme. Consider Figure 9a, which shows an HMM(1,2) model in which a single output stream is coupled to a pair of underlying state sequences. In a speech modeling application, such a structure might be used to capture the fact that a given acoustic pattern can have multiple underlying articulatory causes. For example, equivalent shifts in

(a)

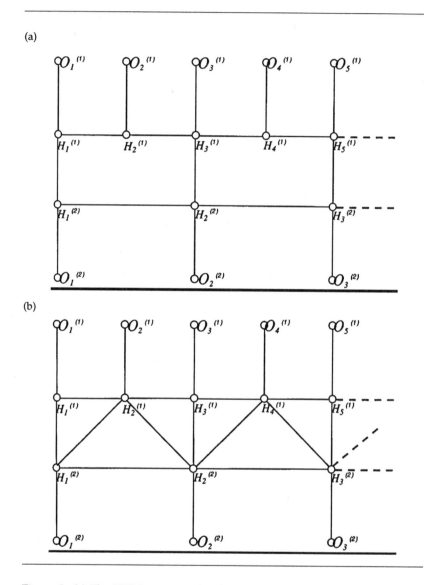

(b)

Figure 8: (a) The UPIN structure for the HMM(1,2) model with $\tau = 2$. (b) A triangulation of this UPIN structure.

formant frequencies can be caused by lip rounding or tongue raising; such phenomena are generically refered to as "trading relations" in the speech psychophysics literature (Lindblom 1990; Perkell *et al.* 1993). Once a particular acoustic pattern is observed, the causes become dependent; thus, for example, evidence that the lips are rounded would act to discount inferences that the tongue has been raised. These inferences propagate forward and backward in time and couple the chains. Formally, these induced dependencies are accounted for by the links added between the state sequences during the moralization of the graph (see Figure 9b). This figure shows that the underlying calculations for this model are closely related to those of the earlier HMM(1,2), but the model specification is very different in the two cases.

Saul and Jordan (1996) have proposed a second extension of the HMM(1,1) model that is motivated by the desire to provide a more effective model of coarticulation (see also Stolorz 1994). In this model, shown in Figure 10, coarticulatory influences are modeled by additional links between output variables and states along an HMM(1,1) backbone. One approach to performing calculations in this model is to treat it as a Kth-order Markov chain and transform it into an HMM(1,1) model by defining higher-order state variables. A graphical modeling approach is more flexible. It is possible, for example, to introduce links between states and outputs K time steps apart without introducing links for the intervening time intervals. More generally, the graphical modeling approach to the HMM(K,1) model allows the specification of different interaction matrices at different time scales; this is awkward in the Kth-order Markov chain formalism.

The HMM(3,1) graph is triangulated as is, and thus the time complexity of the JLO algorithm is $O(N_h m^3)$. In general an HMM(K,1) graph creates cliques of size $O(m^K)$, and the JLO algorithm runs in time $O(N_h m^K)$.

As these examples suggest, the graphical modeling framework provides a useful framework for exploring extensions of HMMs. The examples also make clear, however, that the graphical algorithms are no panacea. The m^K complexity of HMM(K,1) will be prohibitive for large K. Also, the generalization of HMM(1,2) to HMM(1,K) (couplings of K chains) is intractable. Recent research has therefore focused on approximate algorithms for inference in such structures; see Saul and Jordan (1996) for HMM(K,1) and Ghahramani and Jordan (1996) and Williams and Hinton (1990) for HMM(1,K). These authors have developed an approximation methodology based on mean-field theory from statistical physics. While discussion of mean-field algorithms is beyond the scope of this article, it is worth noting that the graphical modeling framework plays a useful role in the development of these approximations. Essentially the mean-field approach involves creating a simplified graph for which tractable algorithms are available, and minimizing a probabilistic distance between the tractable graph and the intractable graph. The JLO algorithm is called as a subroutine on the tractable graph during the minimization process.

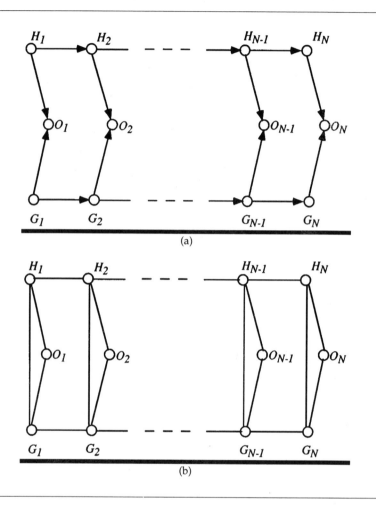

Figure 9: (a) The DPIN structure for HMM(1,2) with a single observable sequence coupled to a pair of underlying state sequences. (b) The moralization of this DPIN structure.

9 Learning and PINs

Until now, we have assumed that the parameters and structure of a PIN are known with certainty. In this section, we drop this assumption and discuss methods for learning about the parameters and structure of a PIN.

The basic idea behind the techniques that we discuss is that there is a true joint probability distribution described by some PIN structure and parameters, but we are uncertain about this structure and its parameters. We

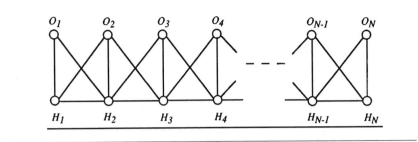

Figure 10: The UPIN structure for HMM(3,1).

are unable to observe the true joint distribution directly, but we are able to observe a set of *patterns* $\mathbf{u}_1, \ldots, \mathbf{u}_M$ that is a random sample from this true distribution. These patterns are independent and identically distributed (i.i.d.) according to the true distribution (note that in a typical HMM learning problem, each of the $\mathbf{u}_i$ consist of a sequence of observed data). We use these data to learn about the structure and parameters that encode the true distribution.

9.1 Parameter Estimation for PINs. First, let us consider the situation where we know the PIN structure S of the true distribution with certainty but are uncertain about the parameters of S.

In keeping with the rest of the article, let us assume that all variables in U are discrete. Furthermore, for purposes of illustration, let us assume that S is an ADG. Let x_i^k and $pa(X_i)^j$ denote the kth value of variable X_i and jth configuration of variables $pa(X_i)$ in S, respectively ($j = 1, \ldots, q_i$, $k = 1, \ldots, r_i$). As we have just discussed, we assume that each conditional probability $p(x_i^k|pa(X_i)^j)$ is an uncertain parameter, and for convenience we represent this parameter as θ_{ijk}. We use $\boldsymbol{\theta}_{ij}$ to denote the vector of parameters $(\theta_{ij1}, \ldots, \theta_{ijr_i})$ and $\boldsymbol{\theta}_s$ to denote the vector of all parameters for S. Note that $\sum_{k=1}^{r_i} \theta_{ijk} = 1$ for every i and j.

One method for learning about the parameters $\boldsymbol{\theta}_s$ is the Bayesian approach. We treat the parameters $\boldsymbol{\theta}_s$ as random variables, assign these parameters a prior distribution $p(\boldsymbol{\theta}_s|S)$, and update this prior distribution with data $D = (\mathbf{u}_1, \ldots, \mathbf{u}_M)$ according to Bayes' rule:

$$p(\boldsymbol{\theta}_s \mid D, S) = c \cdot p(\boldsymbol{\theta}_s \mid S)\, p(D \mid \boldsymbol{\theta}_s, S), \qquad (9.1)$$

where c is a normalization constant that does not depend on $\boldsymbol{\theta}_s$. Because the patterns in D are a random sample, equation 9.1 simplifies to

$$p(\boldsymbol{\theta}_s \mid D, S) = c \cdot p(\boldsymbol{\theta}_s \mid S) \prod_{l=1}^{M} p(\mathbf{u}_l \mid \boldsymbol{\theta}_s, S). \qquad (9.2)$$

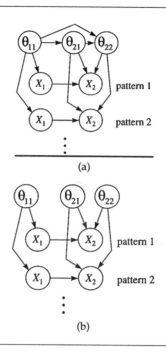

Figure 11: A Bayesian network structure for a two-binary-variable domain $\{X_1, X_2\}$ showing (a) conditional independencies associated with the random sample assumption and (b) the added assumption of parameter independence. In both parts of the figure, it is assumed that the network structure $X_1 \rightarrow X_2$ is generating the patterns.

Given some prediction of interest that depends on θ_s and S—say, $f(\theta_s, S)$— we can use the posterior distribution of θ_s to compute an expected prediction:

$$E(f(\theta_s, S) \mid D, S) = \int f(\theta_s, S) \, p(\theta_s \mid D, S) \, d\theta_s . \qquad (9.3)$$

Associated with our assumption that the data D are a random sample from structure S with uncertain parameters θ_s is a set of conditional independence assertions. Not surprisingly, some of these assumptions can be represented as a (directed) PIN that includes both the possible observations and the parameters as variables. Figure 11a shows these assumptions for the case where $\mathbf{U} = \{X_1, X_2\}$ and S is the structure with a directed edge from X_1 to X_2.

Under certain additional assumptions, described, for example, in Spiegelhalter and Lauritzen (1990), the evaluation of equation 9.2 is straightforward. In particular, if each pattern $\mathbf{u}_l$ is complete (i.e., every variable is observed), we have

$$p(\mathbf{u}_l \mid \boldsymbol{\theta}_s, S) = \prod_{i=1}^{N} \prod_{j=1}^{q_i} \prod_{k=1}^{r_i} \theta_{ijk}^{\delta_{ijkl}}, \tag{9.4}$$

where δ_{ijkl} is equal to one if $X_i = x_i^k$ and $pa(X_i) = pa(X_i)^j$ in pattern C_l and zero otherwise. Combining equations 9.2 and 9.4, we obtain

$$p(\boldsymbol{\theta}_s \mid D, S) = c \cdot p(\boldsymbol{\theta}_s \mid S) \prod_{i=1}^{N} \prod_{j=1}^{q_i} \prod_{k=1}^{r_i} \theta_{ijk}^{N_{ijk}}, \tag{9.5}$$

where N_{ijk} is the number of patterns in which $X_i = x_i^k$ and $pa(X_i) = pa(X_i)^j$. The N_{ijk} are the sufficient statistics for the random sample D. If we assume that the parameter vectors $\boldsymbol{\theta}_{ij}, i = 1, \ldots, n, j = 1, \ldots, q_i$ are mutually independent, an assumption we call parameter independence, then we get the additional simplification

$$p(\boldsymbol{\theta}_s \mid D, S) = c \prod_{i=1}^{N} \prod_{j=1}^{q_i} p(\boldsymbol{\theta}_{ij} \mid S) \prod_{k=1}^{r_i} \theta_{ijk}^{N_{ijk}}. \tag{9.6}$$

The assumption of parameter independence for our two-variable example is illustrated in Figure 11b. Thus, given complete data and parameter independence, each parameter vector $\boldsymbol{\theta}_{ij}$ can be updated independently. The update is particularly simple if each parameter vector has a conjugate distribution. For a discrete variable with discrete parents, the natural conjugate distribution is the Dirichlet,

$$p(\boldsymbol{\theta}_{ij} \mid S) \propto \prod_{k=1}^{r_i} \theta_{ijk}^{\alpha_{ijk}-1},$$

in which case equation 9.6 becomes

$$p(\boldsymbol{\theta}_s \mid D, S) = c \prod_{i=1}^{N} \prod_{j=1}^{q_i} \prod_{k=1}^{r_i} \theta_{ijk}^{N_{ijk}+\alpha_{ijk}-1}. \tag{9.7}$$

Other conjugate distributions include the normal Wishart distribution for the parameters of gaussian codebooks and the Dirichlet distribution for the mixing coefficients of gaussian-mixture codebooks (DeGroot 1970; Buntine 1994; Heckerman and Geiger 1995). Heckerman and Geiger (1995) describe a simple method for assessing these priors. These priors have also been used for learning parameters in standard HMMs (e.g., Gauvain and Lee 1994).

Parameter independence is usually not assumed in general for HMM structures. For example, in the HMM(1,1) model, a standard assumption is that $p(H_i|H_{i-1}) = p(H_j|H_{j-1})$ and $p(O_i|H_i) = p(O_j|H_j)$ for all appropriate i and j. Fortunately, parameter equalities such as these are easily handled in the framework above (see Thiesson 1995 for a detailed discussion).

In addition, the assumption that patterns are complete is clearly inappropriate for HMM structures in general, where some of the variables are hidden from observation. When data are missing, the exact evaluation of the posterior $p(\theta_s|D, S)$ is typically intractable, so we turn to approximations. Accurate but slow approximations are based on Monte Carlo sampling (e.g., Neal 1993). An approximation that is less accurate but more efficient is one based on the observation that, under certain conditions, the quantity $p(\theta_s|S) \cdot p(D|\theta_s, S)$ converges to a multivariate gaussian distribution as the sample size increases (see, e.g., Kass *et al.* 1988; MacKay, 1992a, 1992b).

Less accurate but more efficient approximations are based on the observation that the gaussian distribution converges to a delta function centered at the maximum a posteriori (MAP) and eventually the maximum likelihood (ML) value of θ_s. For the standard HMM(1,1) model discussed in this article, where either discrete, gaussian, or gaussian-mixture codebooks are used, an ML or MAP estimate is a well-known efficient approximation (Poritz 1988; Rabiner 1989).

MAP and ML estimates can be found using traditional techniques such as gradient descent and expectation-maximization (EM) (Dempster *et al.*, 1977). The EM algorithm can be applied efficiently whenever the likelihood function has sufficient statistics that are of fixed dimension for any data set. The EM algorithm finds a local maximum by initializing the parameters θ_s (e.g., at random or by some clustering algorithm) and repeating E and M steps to convergence. In the E step, we compute the expected sufficient statistic for each of the parameters, given D and the current values for θ_s. In particular, if all variables are discrete and parameter independence is assumed to hold, and all priors are Dirichlet, we obtain

$$E(N_{ijk} \mid D, \theta_s, S) = \sum_{l=1}^{M} p(x_i^k, pa(X_i)^j \mid \mathbf{u}_l, \theta_s, S).$$

An important feature of the EM algorithm applied to PINs under these assumptions is that each term in the sum can be computed using the JLO algorithm. The JLO algorithm may also be used when some parameters are equal and when the likelihoods of some variables are gaussian or gaussian-mixture distributions (Lauritzen and Wermuth 1989). In the M step, we use the expected sufficient statistics as if they were actual sufficient statistics and set the new values of θ_s to be the MAP or ML values given these statistics. Again, if all variables are discrete, parameter independence is assumed to hold, and all priors are Dirichlet, the ML is given by

$$\theta_{ijk} = \frac{E(N_{ijk} \mid D, \boldsymbol{\theta}_s, S)}{\sum_{k=1}^{r_i} E(N_{ijk} \mid D, \boldsymbol{\theta}_s, S)},$$

and the MAP is given by

$$\theta_{ijk} = \frac{E(N_{ijk} \mid D, \boldsymbol{\theta}_s, S) + \alpha_{ijk} - 1}{\sum_{k=1}^{r_i} (E(N_{ijk} \mid D, \boldsymbol{\theta}_s, S) + \alpha_{ijk} - 1)}.$$

9.2 Model Selection and Averaging for PINs. Now let us assume that we are uncertain not only about the parameters of a PIN but also about the true structure of a PIN. For example, we may know that the true structure is an HMM(K, J) structure, but we may be uncertain about the values of K and J.

One solution to this problem is Bayesian model averaging. In this approach, we view each possible PIN structure (without its parameters) as a model. We assign prior probabilities $p(S)$ to different models, and compute their posterior probabilities given data:

$$p(S \mid D) \propto p(S) \, p(D \mid S) = p(S) \int p(D \mid \boldsymbol{\theta}, S) \, p(\boldsymbol{\theta} \mid S) \, d\boldsymbol{\theta}. \qquad (9.8)$$

As indicated in equation 9.8, we compute $p(D|S)$ by averaging the likelihood of the data over the parameters of S. In addition to computing the posterior probabilities of models, we estimate the parameters of each model either by computing the distribution $p(\boldsymbol{\theta}|D, S)$ or using a gaussian, MAP, or ML approximation for this distribution. We then make a prediction of interest based on each model separately, as in equation 9.3, and compute the weighted average of these predictions using the posterior probabilities of models as weights.

One complication with this approach is that when data are missing—for example, when some variables are hidden—the exact computation of the integral in equation 9.8 is usually intractable. As discussed in the previous section, Monte Carlo and gaussian approximations may be used. One simple form of a gaussian approximation is the Bayesian information criterion (BIC) described by Schwarz (1978),

$$\log p(D \mid S) \approx \log p(D \mid \hat{\boldsymbol{\theta}}_s, S) - \frac{d}{2} \log M,$$

where $\hat{\boldsymbol{\theta}}_s$ is the ML estimate, M is the number of patterns in D, and d is the dimension of S—typically, the number of parameters of S. The first term of this "score" for S rewards how well the data fit S, whereas the second term punishes model complexity. Note that this score does not depend on the parameter prior, and thus can be applied easily.[3] For examples of applications of BIC in the context of PINs and other statistical models, see Raftery (1995).

The BIC score is the additive inverse of Rissanen's (1987) minimum description length (MDL). Other scores, which can be viewed as approximations to the marginal likelihood, are hypothesis testing (Raftery 1995) and cross validation (Dawid 1992b). Buntine (in press) provides a comprehensive review of scores for model selection and model averaging in the context of PINs.

Another complication with Bayesian model averaging is that there may be so many possible models that averaging becomes intractable. In this case, we select one or a handful of structures with high relative posterior probabilities and make our predictions with this limited set of models. This approach is called model selection. The trick here is finding a model or models with high posterior probabilities. Detailed discussions of search methods for model selection among PINs are given by, among others, Madigan and Raftery (1994), Heckerman *et al.* (1995), and Spirtes and Meek (1995). When the true model is some HMM(K, J) structure, we may have additional prior knowledge that strongly constrains the possible values of K and J. Here, exhaustive model search is likely to be practical.

10 Summary

Probabilistic independence networks provide a useful framework for both the analysis and application of multivariate probability models when there is considerable structure in the model in the form of conditional independence. The graphical modeling approach both clarifies the independence semantics of the model and yields efficient computational algorithms for probabilistic inference. This article has shown that it is useful to cast HMM structures in a graphical model framework. In particular, the well-known F-B and Viterbi algorithms were shown to be special cases of more general algorithms from the graphical modeling literature. Furthermore, more complex HMM structures, beyond the traditional first-order model, can be analyzed profitably and directly using generally applicable graphical modeling techniques.

Appendix A: The Forward-Backward Algorithm for HMM(1,1) Is a Special Case of the JLO Algorithm

Consider the junction tree for HMM(1,1) as shown in Figure 5b. Let the final clique in the chain containing (H_{N-1}, H_N) be the root clique. Thus, a

---

[3] One caveat: The BIC score is derived under the assumption that the parameter prior is positive throughout its domain.

nonredundant schedule consists of first recursively passing flows from each (O_i, H_i) and (H_{i-2}, H_{i-1}) to each (H_{i-1}, H_i) in the appropriate sequence (the "collect" phase), and then distributing flows out in the reverse direction from the root clique. If we are interested only in calculating the likelihood of e given the model, then the distribute phase is not necessary since we can simply marginalize over the local variables in the root clique to obtain $p(e)$. (Subscripts on potential functions and update factors indicate which variables have been used in deriving that potential or update factor; e.g., f_{O_1} indicates that this potential has been updated based on information about O_1 but not using information about any other variables.)

Assume that the junction tree has been initialized so that the potential function for each clique and separator is the local marginal. Given the observed evidence e, each individual piece of evidence $O = o_i^*$ is entered into its clique (O_i, H_i) such that each clique marginal becomes $f_{O_i}^*(h_i, o_i) = p(h_i, o_i^*)$ after entering the evidence (as in equation 5.8).

Consider the portion of the junction tree in Figure 12, and in particular the flow between (O_i, H_i) and (H_{i-1}, H_i). By definition the potential on the separator H_i is updated to

$$f_{O_i}^*(h_i) = \sum_{o_i} f^*(h_i, o_i) = p(h_i, o_i^*). \tag{A.1}$$

The update factor from this separator flowing into clique (H_{i-1}, H_i) is then

$$\lambda_{O_i}(h_i) = \frac{p(h_i, o_i^*)}{p(h_i)} = p(o_i^* \mid h_i). \tag{A.2}$$

This update factor is "absorbed" into (H_{i-1}, H_i) as follows:

$$f_{O_i}^*(h_{i-1}, h_i) = p(h_{i-1}, h_i)\lambda_{O_i}(h_i) = p(h_{i-1}, h_i)p(o_i^* \mid h_i). \tag{A.3}$$

Now consider the flow from clique (H_{i-2}, H_{i-1}) to clique (H_{i-1}, H_i). Let $\Phi_{i,j} = \{O_i, \ldots, O_j\}$ denote a set of consecutive observable variables and $\phi_{i,j}^* = \{o_i^*, \ldots, o_j^*\}$ denote a set of observed values for these variables, $1 \le i < j \le N$. Assume that the potential on the separator H_{i-1} has been updated to

$$f_{\Phi_{1,i-1}}^*(h_{i-1}) = p^*(h_{i-1}, \phi_{1,i-1}^*) \tag{A.4}$$

by earlier flows in the schedule. Thus, the update factor on separator H_{i-1} becomes

$$\lambda_{\Phi_{1,i-1}}(h_{i-1}) = \frac{p^*(h_{i-1}, \phi_{1,i-1}^*)}{p(h_{i-1})}, \tag{A.5}$$

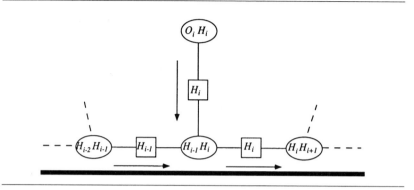

Figure 12: Local message passing in the HMM(1,1) junction tree during the collect phase of a left-to-right schedule. Ovals indicate cliques, boxes indicate separators, and arrows indicate flows.

and this gets absorbed into clique (H_{i-1}, H_i) to produce

$$
\begin{aligned}
f^*_{\Phi_{1,i}}(h_{i-1}, h_i) &= f^*_{O_i}(h_{i-1}, h_i)\lambda_{\Phi_{1,i-1}}(h_{i-1}) \\
&= p(h_{i-1}, h_i)p(o^*_i \mid h_i)\frac{p^*(h_{i-1}, \phi^*_{1,i-1})}{p(h_{i-1})} \\
&= p(o^*_i \mid h_i)p(h_i \mid h_{i-1})p^*(h_{i-1}, \phi^*_{1,i-1}) .
\end{aligned}
\tag{A.6}
$$

Finally, we can calculate the new potential on the separator for the flow from clique (H_{i-1}, H_i) to (H_i, H_{i+1}):

$$
f^*_{\Phi_{1,i}}(h_i) = \sum_{h_{i-1}} f^*_{\Phi_{1,i}}(h_{i-1}, h_i)
\tag{A.7}
$$

$$
= p(o^*_i \mid h_i) \sum_{h_{i-1}} p(h_i \mid h_{i-1})p^*(h_{i-1}, \phi^*_{1,i-1})
\tag{A.8}
$$

$$
= p(o^*_i \mid h_i) \sum_{h_{i-1}} p(h_i \mid h_{i-1})f^*_{\Phi_{1,i-1}}(h_{i-1}) .
\tag{A.9}
$$

Proceeding recursively in this manner, one finally obtains at the root clique

$$
f^*_{\Phi_{1,N}}(h_{N-1}, h_N) = p(h_{N-1}, h_N, \phi^*_{1,N})
\tag{A.10}
$$

from which one can get the likelihood of the evidence,

$$
p(e) = p(\phi^*_{1,N}) = \sum_{h_{N-1}, h_N} f^*_{\Phi_{1,N}}(h_{N-1}, h_N).
\tag{A.11}
$$

We note that equation A.9 directly corresponds to the recursive equation (equation 20 in Rabiner 1989) for the α variables used in the forward phase of the F-B algorithm, the standard HMM(1,1) inference algorithm. In particular, using a "left-to-right" schedule, the updated potential functions on the separators between the hidden cliques, the $f^*_{\Phi_{1,i}}(h_i)$ functions, are exactly the α variables. Thus, when applied to HMM(1,1), the JLO algorithm produces exactly the same local recursive calculations as the forward phase of the F-B algorithm.

One can also show an equivalence between the backward phase of the F-B algorithm and the JLO inference algorithm. Let the "leftmost" clique in the chain, (H_1, H_2), be the root clique, and define a schedule such that the flows go from right to left. Figure 13 shows a local portion of the clique tree and the associated flows. Consider that the potential on clique (H_i, H_{i+1}) has been updated already by earlier flows from the right. Thus, by definition,

$$f^*_{\Phi_{i+1,N}}(h_i, h_{i+1}) = p(h_i, h_{i+1}, \phi^*_{i+1,N}). \tag{A.12}$$

The potential on the separator between (H_i, H_{i+1}) and (H_{i-1}, H_i) is calculated as

$$f^*_{\Phi_{i+1,N}}(h_i) = \sum_{h_{i+1}} p(h_i, h_{i+1}, \phi^*_{i+1,N}) \tag{A.13}$$

$$= p(h_i) \sum_{h_{i+1}} p(h_{i+1} \mid h_i) p(o^*_{i+1} \mid h_{i+1}) p(\phi^*_{i+2,N} \mid h_{i+1}) \tag{A.14}$$

(by virtue of the various conditional independence relations in HMM(1,1))

$$= p(h_i) \sum_{h_{i+1}} p(h_{i+1} \mid h_i) p(o^*_{i+1} \mid h_{i+1}) \frac{p(\phi^*_{i+2,N}, h_{i+1})}{p(h_{i+1})} \tag{A.15}$$

$$= p(h_i) \sum_{h_{i+1}} p(h_i \mid h_{i+1}) p(o^*_{i+1} \mid h_{i+1}) \frac{f^*_{\Phi_{i+2,N}}(h_{i+1})}{p(h_{i+1})}. \tag{A.16}$$

Defining the update factor on this separator yields

$$\lambda^*_{\Phi_{i+1,N}}(h_i) = \frac{f^*_{\Phi_{i+2,N}}(h_i)}{p(h_i)} \tag{A.17}$$

$$= \sum_{h_{i+1}} p(h_i \mid h_{i+1}) p(o^*_{i+1} \mid h_{i+1}) \frac{f^*_{\Phi_{i+2,N}}(h_{i+1})}{p(h_{i+1})} \tag{A.18}$$

$$= \sum_{h_{i+1}} p(h_i \mid h_{i+1}) p(o^*_{i+1} \mid h_{i+1}) \lambda^*_{\Phi_{i+2,N}}(h_{i+1}). \tag{A.19}$$

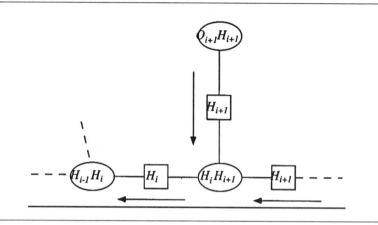

Figure 13: Local message passing in the HMM(1,1) junction tree during the collect phase of a right-to-left schedule. Ovals indicate cliques, boxes indicate separators, and arrows indicate flows.

This set of recursive equations in λ corresponds exactly to the recursive equation (equation 25 in Rabiner 1989) for the β variables in the backward phase of the F-B algorithm. In fact, the update factors λ on the separators are exactly the β variables. Thus, we have shown that the JLO inference algorithm recreates the F-B algorithm for the special case of the HMM(1,1) probability model.

Appendix B: The Viterbi Algorithm for HMM(1,1) Is a Special Case of Dawid's Algorithm. As with the inference problem, let the final clique in the chain containing (H_{N-1}, H_N) be the root clique and use the same schedule: first a left-to-right collection phase into the root clique, followed by a right-to-left distribution phase out from the root clique. Again it is assumed that the junction tree has been initialized so that the potential functions are the local marginals, and the observable evidence e has been entered into the cliques in the same manner as described for the inference algorithm.

We refer again to Figure 12. The sequence of flow and absorption operations is identical to that of the inference algorithm with the exception that marginalization operations are replaced by maximization. Thus, the potential on the separator between (O_i, H_i) and (H_{i-1}, H_i) is initially updated to

$$\hat{f}_{O_i}(h_i) = \max_{o_i} p(h_i, o_i) = p(h_i, o_i^*). \tag{B.1}$$

The update factor for this separator is

$$\lambda_{O_i}(h_i) = \frac{p(h_i, o_i^*)}{p(h_i)} = p(o_i^* \mid h_i), \tag{B.2}$$

and after absorption into the clique (H_{i-1}, H_i) one gets

$$\hat{f}_{O_i}(h_{i-1}, h_i) = p(h_{i-1}, h_i)p(o_i^* \mid h_i). \tag{B.3}$$

Now consider the flow from clique (H_{i-2}, H_{i-1}) to (H_{i-1}, H_i). Let $H_{i,j} = \{H_i, \ldots, H_j\}$ denote a set of consecutive observable variables and $h_{i,j}^* = \{h_i^*, \ldots, h_j^*\}$, denote the observed values for these variables, $1 \le i < j \le N$. Assume that the potential on separator H_{i-1} has been updated to

$$\hat{f}_{\Phi_{1,i-1}}(h_{i-1}) = \max_{h_{1,i-2}} p(h_{i-1}, h_{1,i-2}, \phi_{1,i-1}^*) \tag{B.4}$$

by earlier flows in the schedule. Thus, the update factor for separator H_{i-1} becomes

$$\lambda_{\Phi_{1,i-1}}(h_{i-1}) = \frac{\max_{h_{1,i-2}} p(h_{i-1}, h_{1,i-2}, \phi_{1,i-1}^*)}{p(h_{i-1})}, \tag{B.5}$$

and this gets absorbed into clique (H_{i-1}, H_i) to produce

$$\hat{f}_{\Phi_{1,i}}(h_{i-1}, h_i) = \hat{f}_{O_i}(h_{i-1}, h_i)\lambda_{\Phi_{1,i-1}}(h_{i-1}) \tag{B.6}$$

$$= p(h_{i-1}, h_i)p(o_i^* \mid h_i)\frac{\max_{h_{1,i-2}} p(h_{i-1}, h_{1,i-2}, \phi_{1,i-1}^*)}{p(h_{i-1})}. \tag{B.7}$$

We can now obtain the new potential on the separator for the flow from clique (H_{i-1}, H_i) to (H_i, H_{i+1}),

$$\hat{f}_{\Phi_{1,i}}(h_i) = \max_{h_{i-1}} \hat{f}_{\Phi_{1,i}}(h_{i-1}, h_i) \tag{B.8}$$

$$= p(o_i^* \mid h_i) \max_{h_{i-1}}\{p(h_i \mid h_{i-1}) \max_{h_{1,i-2}} p(h_{i-1}, h_{1,i-2}, \phi_{1,i-1}^*)\} \tag{B.9}$$

$$= p(o_i^* \mid h_i) \max_{h_{1,i-1}}\{p(h_i \mid h_{i-1})p(h_{i-1}, h_{1,i-2}, \phi_{1,i-1}^*)\} \tag{B.10}$$

$$= \max_{h_{1,i-1}} p(h_i, h_{1,i-1}, \phi_{1,i}^*), \tag{B.11}$$

which is the result one expects for the updated potential at this clique. Thus, we can express the separator potential $\hat{f}_{\Phi_{1,i}}(h_i)$ recursively (via equation B.10) as

$$\hat{f}_{\Phi_{1,i}}(h_i) = p(o_i^* \mid h_i) \max_{h_{i-1}}\{p(h_i \mid h_{i-1})\hat{f}_{\Phi_{1,i-1}}(h_{i-1})\}. \tag{B.12}$$

This is the same recursive equation as used in the δ variables in the Viterbi algorithm (equation 33a in Rabiner 1989): the separator potentials in Dawid's algorithm using a left-to-right schedule are exactly the same as the δ's used in the Viterbi method for solving the MAP problem in HMM(1,1).

Proceeding recursively in this manner, one finally obtains at the root clique

$$\hat{f}_{\Phi_{1,N}}(h_{N-1}, h_N) = \max_{h_{1,N-2}} p(h_{N-1}, h_N, h_{N-2}, \phi^*_{1,N}), \tag{B.13}$$

from which one can get the likelihood of the evidence given the most likely state of the hidden variables:

$$\hat{f}(e) = \max_{h_{N-1}, h_N} \hat{f}_{\Phi_{1,N}}(h_{N-1}, h_N) \tag{B.14}$$

$$= \max_{h_{1,N}} p(h_{1,N}, \phi^*_{1,N}). \tag{B.15}$$

Identification of the values of the hidden variables that maximize the evidence likelihood can be carried out in the standard manner as in the Viterbi method, namely, by keeping a pointer at each clique along the flow in the forward direction back to the previous clique and then backtracking along this list of pointers from the root clique after the collection phase is complete. An alternative approach is to use the distribute phase of the Dawid algorithm. This has the same effect: Once the distribution flows are completed, each local clique can calculate both the maximum value of the evidence likelihood given the hidden variables and the values of the hidden variables in this maximum that are local to that particular clique.

Acknowledgments

MIJ gratefully acknowledges discussions with Steffen Lauritzen on the application of the IPF algorithm to UPINs. The research described in this article was carried out in part by the Jet Propulsion Laboratory, California Institute of Technology, under a contract with the National Aeronautics and Space Administration.

References

Baum, L. E., and Petrie, T. 1966. Statistical inference for probabilistic functions of finite state Markov chains. *Ann. Math. Stat.* **37**, 1554–1563.

Bishop, Y. M. M., Fienberg, S. E., and Holland, P. W. 1973. *Discrete Multivariate Analysis: Theory and Practice*. MIT Press, Cambridge, MA.

Buntine, W. 1994. Operations for learning with graphical models. *Journal of Artificial Intelligence Research* **2**, 159–225.

Buntine, W. In press. A guide to the literature on learning probabilistic networks from data. *IEEE Transactions on Knowledge and Data Engineering*.

Dawid, A. P. 1992a. Applications of a general propagation algorithm for probabilistic expert systems. *Statistics and Computing* **2**, 25–36.

Dawid, A. P. 1992b. Prequential analysis, stochastic complexity, and Bayesian inference (with discussion). In *Bayesian Statistics 4*, J. M. Bernardo, J. Berger, A. P. Dawid, and A. F. M. Smith, eds., pp. 109–125. Oxford University Press, London.

DeGroot, M. 1970. *Optimal Statistical Decisions*. McGraw-Hill, New York.

Dempster, A., Laird, N., and Rubin, D. 1977. Maximum likelihood from incomplete data via the EM algorithm. *Journal of the Royal Statistical Society, Series B* **39**, 1–38.

Elliott, R. J., Aggoun, L., and Moore, J. B. 1995. *Hidden Markov Models: Estimation and Control*. Springer-Verlag, New York.

Frasconi, P., and Bengio, Y. 1994. An EM approach to grammatical inference: Input/output HMMs. In *Proceedings of the 12th IAPR Intl. Conf. on Pattern Recognition*, pp. 289–294. IEEE Computer Society Press, Los Altimos, CA.

Gauvain, J., and Lee, C. 1994. Maximum *a posteriori* estimation for multivariate Gaussian mixture observations of Markov chains. *IEEE Trans. Sig. Audio Proc.* **2**, 291–298.

Geman, S., and Geman, D. 1984. Stochastic relaxation, Gibbs distributions, and the Bayesian restoration of images. *IEEE Trans. Patt. Anal. Mach. Intell.* **6**, 721–741.

Ghahramani, Z., and Jordan, M. I. 1996. Factorial hidden Markov models. In *Advances in Neural Information Processing Systems 8*, D. S. Touretzky, M. C. Mozer, and M. E. Hasselmo, eds., pp. 472–478. MIT Press, Cambridge, MA.

Heckerman, D., and Geiger, D. 1995. *Likelihoods and Priors for Bayesian Networks*. MSR-TR-95-54. Microsoft Corporation, Redmond, WA.

Heckerman, D., Geiger, D., and Chickering, D. 1995. Learning Bayesian networks: The combination of knowledge and statistical data. *Machine Learning* **20**, 197–243.

Hinton, G. E., and Sejnowski, T. J. 1986. Learning and relearning in Boltzmann machines. In *Parallel Distributed Processing: Explorations in the Microstructure of Cognition*, D. E. Rumelhart, J. L. McClelland, and the PDP Research Group, eds., vol. 1, chap. 7. MIT Press, Cambridge, MA.

Huang, X. D., Ariki, Y., and Jack, M. A. 1990. *Hidden Markov Models for Speech Recognition*. Edinburgh University Press, Edinburgh.

Isham, V. 1981. An introduction to spatial point processes and Markov random fields. *International Statistical Review* **49**, 21–43.

Itzykson, C., and Drouffé, J-M. 1991. *Statistical Field Theory*. Cambridge University Press, Cambridge.

Jensen, F. V., Lauritzen, S. L., and Olesen, K. G. 1990. Bayesian updating in recursive graphical models by local computations. *Computational Statistical Quarterly* **4**, 269–282.

Jiřousek, R., and Přeučil, S. 1995. On the effective implementation of the iterative proportional fitting procedure. *Computational Statistics and Data Analysis* **19**, 177–189.

Kass, R., Tierney, L., and Kadane, J. 1988. Asymptotics in Bayesian computation. In *Bayesian Statistics 3*, J. Bernardo, M. DeGroot, D. Lindley, and A. Smith, eds., pp. 261–278. Oxford University Press, Oxford.

Kent, R. D., and Minifie, F. D. 1977. Coarticulation in recent speech production models. *Journal of Phonetics* **5**, 115–117.

Lauritzen, S. L., and Spiegelhalter, D. J. 1988. Local computations with probabilities on graphical structures and their application to expert systems (with discussion). *J. Roy. Statist. Soc. Ser. B*. **50**, 157–224.

Lauritzen, S. L., Dawid, A. P., Larsen, B. N., and Leimer, H. G. 1990. Independence properties of directed Markov fields. *Networks* **20**, 491–505.

Lauritzen, S., and Wermuth, N. 1989. Graphical models for associations between variables, some of which are qualitative and some quantitative. *Annals of Statistics* **17**, 31–57.

Lindblom, B. 1990. Explaining phonetic variation: A sketch of the H&H theory. In *Speech Production and Speech Modeling*, W. J. Hardcastle and A. Marchal, eds., pp. 403–440. Kluwer, Dordrecht.

Lucke, H. 1995. Bayesian belief networks as a tool for stochastic parsing. *Speech Communication* **16**, 89–118.

MacKay, D. J. C. 1992a. Bayesian interpolation. *Neural Computation* **4**, 415–447.

MacKay, D. J. C. 1992b. A practical Bayesian framework for backpropagation networks. *Neural Computation* **4**, 448–472.

Madigan, D., and Raftery, A. E. 1994. Model selection and accounting for model uncertainty in graphical models using Occam's window. *J. Am. Stat. Assoc.* **89**, 1535–1546.

Modestino, J., and Zhang, J. 1992. A Markov random field model-based approach to image segmentation. *IEEE Trans. Patt. Anal. Mach. Int.* **14**(6), 606–615.

Morgenstern, I., and Binder, K. 1983. Magnetic correlations in two-dimensional spin-glasses. *Physical Review B* **28**, 5216.

Neal, R. 1993. *Probabilistic inference using Markov chain Monte Carlo methods*. CRG-TR-93-1. Department of Computer Science, University of Toronto.

Pearl, J. 1988. *Probabilistic Reasoning in Intelligent Systems: Networks of Plausible Inference*. Morgan Kaufmann, San Mateo, CA.

Pearl, J., Geiger, D., and Verma, T. 1990. The logic of influence diagrams. In *Influence Diagrams, Belief Nets, and Decision Analysis*, R. M. Oliver and J. Q. Smith, eds., pp. 67–83. John Wiley, Chichester, UK.

Perkell, J. S., Matthies, M. L., Svirsky, M. A., and Jordan, M. I. 1993. Trading relations between tongue-body raising and lip rounding in production of the vowel /u/: A pilot motor equivalence study. *Journal of the Acoustical Society of America* **93**, 2948–2961.

Poritz, A. M. 1988. Hidden Markov models: A guided tour. In *Proceedings of the IEEE International Conference on Acoustics, Speech and Signal Processing*, 1:7–13, IEEE Press, New York.

Rabiner, L. 1989. A tutorial on hidden Markov models and selected applications in speech recognition. *Proceedings of the IEEE* **77**, 257–285.

Raftery, A. 1995. Bayesian model selection in social research (with discussion). In *Sociological Methodology*, P. Marsden, ed., pp. 111–196. Blackwell, Cambridge, MA.

Rissanen, J. 1987. Stochastic complexity (with discussion). *Journal of the Royal Statistical Society, Series B* **49**, 223–239, 253–265.

Saul, L. K., and Jordan, M. I. 1995. Boltzmann chains and hidden Markov models. In *Advances in Neural Information Processing Systems 7*, G. Tesauro, D. S. Touretzky, and T. K. Leen, eds., pp. 435–442. MIT Press, Cambridge, MA.

Saul, L. K., and Jordan, M. I. 1996. Exploiting tractable substructures in intractable networks. In *Advances in Neural Information Processing Systems 8*, D. S. Touretzky, M. C. Mozer, and M. E. Hasselmo, eds., pp. 486–492. MIT Press, Cambridge, MA.

Schwarz, G. 1978. Estimating the dimension of a model. *Annals of Statistics* **6**, 461–464.

Shachter, R. D., Anderson, S. K., and Szolovits, P. 1994. Global conditioning for probabilistic inference in belief networks. In *Proceedings of the Uncertainty in AI Conference 1994*, pp. 514–522. Morgan Kaufmann, San Mateo, CA.

Spiegelhalter, D. J., Dawid, A. P., Hutchinson, T. A., and Cowell, R. G. 1991. Probabilistic expert systems and graphical modelling: A case study in drug safety. *Phil. Trans. R. Soc. Lond. A* **337**, 387–405.

Spiegelhalter, D. J., and Lauritzen, S. L. 1990. Sequential updating of conditional probabilities on directed graphical structures. *Networks* **20**, 579–605.

Spirtes, P., and Meek, C. 1995. Learning Bayesian networks with discrete variables from data. In *Proceedings of First International Conference on Knowledge Discovery and Data Mining*, pp. 294–299. AAAI Press, Menlo Park, CA.

Stolorz, P. 1994. Recursive approaches to the statistical physics of lattice proteins. In *Proc. 27th Hawaii Intl. Conf. on System Sciences*, L. Hunter, ed., 5:316–325.

Swendsen, R. H., and Wang, J-S. 1987. Nonuniversal critical dynamics in Monte Carlo simulations. *Physical Review Letters* **58**.

Thiesson, B. 1995. *Score and information for recursive exponential models with incomplete data*. Tech. rep. Institute of Electronic Systems, Aalborg University, Aalborg, Denmark.

Vandermeulen, D., Verbeeck, R., Berben, L., Delaere, D., Suetens, P., and Marchal, G. 1994. Continuous voxel classification by stochastic relaxation: Theory and application to MR imaging and MR angiography. *Image and Vision Computing* **12**(9), 559–572.

Whittaker, J. 1990. *Graphical Models in Applied Multivariate Statistics*. John Wiley, Chichester, UK.

Williams, C., and Hinton, G. E. 1990. Mean field networks that learn to discriminate temporally distorted strings. In *Proc. Connectionist Models Summer School*, pp. 18–22. Morgan Kaufmann, San Mateo, CA.

2

Learning and Relearning in Boltzmann Machines

G. E. Hinton
T. J. Sejnowski

Many of the chapters in *Parallel Distributed Processing: Explorations in the Microstructure of Cognition, Volume 1: Foundations* make use of the ability of a parallel network to perform cooperative searches for good solutions to problems. The basic idea is simple: The weights on the connections between processing units encode knowledge about how things normally fit together in some domain and the initial states or external inputs to a subset of the units encode some fragments of a structure within the domain. These fragments constitute a problem: What is the whole structure from which they probably came? The network computes a "good solution" to the problem by repeatedly updating the states of units that represent possible other parts of the structure until the network eventually settles into a stable state of activity that represents the solution.

One field in which this style of computation seems particularly appropriate is vision (Ballard, Hinton, & Sejnowski, 1983). A visual system must be able to solve large constraint-satisfaction problems rapidly in order to interpret a two-dimensional intensity image in terms of the depths and orientations of the three-dimensional surfaces in the world that gave rise to that image. In general, the information in the image is not sufficient to specify the three-dimensional surfaces unless the interpretive process makes use of additional plausible constraints about the kinds of structures that typically appear. Neighboring pieces of an image, for example, usually depict fragments of surface that have similar depths, similar surface orientations, and the same reflectance. The most plausible interpretation of an image is the one that satisfies constraints of this kind as well as possible, and the human visual system stores enough plausible constraints and is good enough at applying them that it can arrive at the correct interpretation of most normal images.

The computation may be performed by an iterative search which starts with a poor interpretation and progressively improves it by reducing a cost function that measures the extent to which the current interpretation violates the plausible constraints. Suppose, for example, that each unit stands for a small three-dimensional surface fragment, and the state of the unit indicates the current bet about whether that surface fragment is part of the best three-dimensional interpretation. Plausible constraints about the nature of surfaces can then be encoded by the pairwise interactions between processing elements. For example, two units that stand for neighboring surface fragments of similar depth and surface orientation can be mutually excitatory to encode the constraints that each of these hypotheses tends to support the other (because objects tend to have continuous surfaces).

Relaxation Searches _____

The general idea of using parallel networks to perform relaxation searches that simultaneously satisfy multiple constraints is appealing. It might even provide a successor to telephone exchanges, holograms, or communities of agents as a metaphor for the style of computation in cerebral cortex. But some tough technical questions have to be answered before this style of computation can be accepted as either efficient or plausible:

- Will the network settle down or will it oscillate or wander aimlessly?

- What does the network compute by settling down? We need some characterization of the computation that the network performs other than the network itself. Ideally we would like to be able to say what *ought* to be computed (Marr, 1982) and then to show that a network can be made to compute it.

- How long does the network take to settle on a solution? If thousands of iterations are required the method becomes implausible as a model of how the cortex solves constraint-satisfaction problems.

- How much information does each unit need to convey to its neighbors? In many relaxation schemes the units communicate accurate real values to one another on each iteration. Again this is implausible if the units are intended to be like cortical neurons which communicate using all-or-none spikes. To send a real-value, accurate to within 5%, using firing rates requires about 100 ms which is about the time allowed for the whole iterative process to settle down.

- How are the weights that encode the knowledge acquired? For models of low-level vision it is possible for a programmer to decide on the weights, and evolution might do the same for the earliest stages of biological visual systems. But if the same kind of constraint-satisfaction searches are to be used for higher level functions like shape recognition or content-addressable memory, there must be some learning procedure that automatically encodes properties of the domain into the weights.

This chapter is mainly concerned with the last of these questions, but the learning procedure we present is an unexpected consequence of our attempt to answer the other questions, so we shall start with them.

Relaxation, Optimization, and Weak Constraints. One way of ensuring that a relaxation search is computing something sensible (and will eventually settle down) is to show that it is solving an optimization problem by progressively reducing the value of a cost function. Each possible state of activity of the network has an associated cost, and the rule used for updating activity levels is chosen so that this cost keeps falling. The cost function must be chosen so that low-cost states represent good solutions to problems in the domain.

Many optimization problems can be cast in a framework known as linear programming. There are some variables which take on real values and there are linear equality and inequality constraints between variables. Each combination of values for the variables has an associated cost which is the sum over all the variables of the current value times a cost-coefficient. The aim is to find a combination of values that satisfies all the constraints and minimizes the cost function. If the variables are further constrained to take on only the values 1 or 0 the problem is called zero-one programming. Hinton (1977) has shown that certain zero-one programming problems can be implemented as relaxation searches in parallel networks. This allows networks to find good solutions to problems in which there are discrete hypotheses that are true or false. Even though the allowable solutions all assign values of 1 or 0 to the hypotheses, the relaxation process works by passing through intermediate states in which hypothesis units have real-valued activity levels lying between 1 and 0. Each constraint is enforced by a feedback loop that measures the amount by which the current values violate the constraint and tries to alter the values of the variables to reduce this violation.

Linear programming and its variants make a sharp distinction between constraints (which *must* be satisfied) and costs. A solution which achieves a very low cost by violating one or two of the constraints is simply not allowed. In many domains, the distinction between constraints and costs is not so clear-cut. In vision, for example, it is usually helpful to use the constraint that neighboring pieces of surface are at similar depths because surfaces are mostly continuous and are rarely parallel to the line of sight. But this is not an absolute constraint. It doesn't apply at the edge of an object. So a visual system needs to be able to generate interpretations that violate this constraint if it can satisfy many other constraints by doing so. Constraints like these have been called "weak" constraints (Blake, 1983) and it is possible to formulate optimization problems in which all the constraints are weak and there is no distinction between constraints and costs. The optimal solution is then the one which minimizes the total constraint violation where different constraints are given different strengths depending on how reliable they are. Another way of saying this is that all the constraints have associated plausibilities, and the most plausible solution is the one which fits these plausible constraints as well as possible.

Some relaxation schemes dispense with separate feedback loops for the constraints and implement weak constraints directly in the excitatory and inhibitory interactions between units. We would like these networks to settle into states in which a few units are fully active and the rest are inactive. Such states constitute clean "digital" interpretations. To prevent the network from hedging its bets by settling into a state where many units are slightly active, it is usually necessary to use a strongly nonlinear decision rule, and this also speeds convergence. However, the strong nonlinearities that are needed to force the network to make a decision also cause it to converge on different states on different occasions: Even with the same external inputs, the final state depends on the initial state of the net. This has led many people (Hopfield, 1982; Rosenfeld, Hummel, & Zucker, 1976) to assume that the particular problem to be solved should be encoded by the initial state of the network rather than by sustained external input to some of its units.

Hummel and Zucker (1983) and Hopfield (1982) have shown that some relaxation schemes have an associated "potential" or cost function and that the states to which the network converges are local minima of this function. This means that the networks are performing optimization of a well-defined function. Unfortunately, there is no guarantee that the network will find the best minimum. One possibility is to redefine the problem as finding the local minimum which is closest to the initial state. This is useful if the minima are used to represent "items" in a memory, and the initial states are queries to memory which may contain missing or erroneous information. The network simply finds the minimum that best fits the query. This idea was used by Hopfield (1982) who introduced an interesting kind of network in which the units were always in one of two states.[1] Hopfield showed that if the units are symmetrically connected (i.e., the weight from unit i to unit j exactly equals the weight from unit j to unit i) and if they are updated one at a time, each update reduces (or at worst does not increase) the value of a cost function which he called "energy" because of the analogy with physical systems. Consequently, repeated iterations are guaranteed to find an energy minimum. The global energy of the system is defined as

$$E = - \sum_{i<j} w_{ij}s_i s_j + \sum_i \theta_i s_i \qquad (1)$$

where w_{ij} is the strength of connection (synaptic weight) from the jth to the ith unit, s_i is the state of the ith unit (0 or 1), and θ_i is a threshold.

The updating rule is to switch each unit into whichever of its two states yields the lower total energy given the current states of the other units. Because the connections are symmetrical, the difference between the energy of the whole system with the kth hypothesis false and its energy with the kth hypothesis true can be determined locally by the kth unit, and is just

$$\Delta E_k = \sum_i w_{ki}s_i - \theta_k. \qquad (2)$$

---

[1]Hopfield used the states 1 and −1 because his model was derived from physical systems called spin glasses in which spins are either "up" or "down." Provided the units have thresholds, models that use 1 and −1 can be translated into models that use 1 and 0 and have different thresholds.

Therefore, the rule for minimizing the energy contributed by a unit is to adopt the true state if its total input from the other units exceeds its threshold. This is the familiar rule for binary threshold units.

Using Probabilistic Decisions to Escape from Local Minima. At about the same time that Hopfield showed how parallel networks of this kind could be used to access memories that were stored as local minima, Kirkpatrick, working at IBM, introduced an interesting new search technique for solving hard optimization problems on conventional computers.

One standard technique is to use gradient descent: The values of the variables in the problem are modified in whatever direction reduces the cost function (energy). For hard problems, gradient descent gets stuck at *local* minima that are not globally optimal. This is an inevitable consequence of only allowing downhill moves. If jumps to higher energy states occasionally occur, it is possible to break out of local minima, but it is not obvious how the system will then behave and it is far from clear when uphill steps should be allowed.

Kirkpatrick, Gelatt, and Vecchi (1983) used another physical analogy to guide the use of occasional uphill steps. To find a very low energy state of a metal, the best strategy is to melt it and then to slowly reduce its temperature. This process is called annealing, and so they named their search method "simulated annealing." We give a simple intuitive account here.

One way of seeing why thermal noise is helpful is to consider the energy landscape shown in Figure 1. Let us suppose that a ball-bearing starts at a randomly chosen point on the landscape. If it always goes downhill (and has no inertia), it will have an even chance of ending up at A or B because both minima have the same width and so the initial random point is equally likely to lie in either minimum. If we shake the whole system, we are more likely to shake the ball-bearing from A to B than vice versa because the energy barrier is lower from the A side. If the shaking is gentle, a transition from A to B will be many times as probable as a transition from B to A, but both transitions will be very rare. So although gentle shaking will ultimately lead to a very high probability of being in B rather than A, it will take a very long time before this happens. On the other hand, if the shaking is violent, the ball-bearing will cross the barrier frequently and so the ultimate probability ratio will be approached rapidly, but this ratio will not be very good: With violent shaking it is almost as easy to cross the barrier in the wrong direction (from B to A) as in the right direction. A good compromise is to start by shaking hard and gradually shake more and more gently. This ensures that at some stage the noise level passes through the best possible compromise between the absolute probability of a transition and the ratio of the probabilities of good and bad transitions. It also means that at the end, the ball-bearing stays right at the bottom of the chosen minimum.

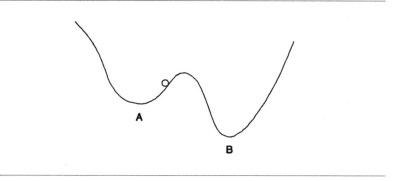

Figure 1: A simple energy landscape containing two local minima separated by an energy barrier. Shaking can be used to allow the state of the network (represented here by a ball-bearing) to escape from local minima.

This view of why annealing helps is not the whole story. Figure 1 is misleading because all the states have been laid out in one dimension. Complex systems have high-dimensional state spaces, and so the barrier between two low-lying states is typically massively degenerate: The number of ways of getting from one low-lying state to another is an exponential function of the height of the barrier one is willing to cross. This means that a rise in the level of thermal noise opens up an enormous variety of paths for escaping from a local minimum and even though each path by itself is unlikely, it is highly probable that the system will cross the barrier. We conjecture that simulated annealing will only work well in domains where the energy barriers are highly degenerate.

Applying Simulated Annealing to Hopfield Nets. There is a simple modification of Hopfield's updating rule that allows parallel networks to implement simulated annealing. If the energy gap between the 1 and 0 states of the kth unit is ΔE_k then, regardless of the previous state set, $s_k = 1$ with probability

$$p_k = \frac{1}{(1 + e^{-\Delta E_k/T})} \tag{3}$$

where T is a parameter which acts like the temperature of a physical system. This local decision rule ensures that in thermal equilibrium the relative probability of two global states is determined solely by their energy difference, and follows a Boltzmann distribution:

$$\frac{P_\alpha}{P_\beta} = e^{-(E_\alpha - E_\beta)/T} \tag{4}$$

where P_α is the probability of being in the αth global state, and E_α is the energy of that state.

At low temperatures there is a strong bias in favor of states with low energy, but the time required to reach equilibrium may be long. At higher temperatures the bias is not so favorable, but equilibrium is reached faster. The fastest way to reach equilibrium at a given temperature is generally to use simulated annealing: Start with a higher temperature and gradually reduce it.

The idea of implementing constraints as interactions between stochastic processing elements was proposed by Moussouris (1974) who discussed the identity between Boltzmann distributions and Markov random fields. The idea of using simulated annealing to find low energy states in parallel networks has been investigated independently by several different groups. S. Geman and D. Geman (1984) established limits on the allowable speed of the annealing schedule and showed that simulated annealing can be very effective for removing noise from images. Hinton and Sejnowski (1983b) showed how the use of binary stochastic elements could solve some problems that plague other relaxation techniques, in particular the problem of learning the weights. Smolensky (1983) has been investigating a similar scheme which he calls "harmony theory." Smolensky's harmony is equivalent to our energy (with a sign reversal).

Pattern Completion. One way of using a parallel network is to treat it as a pattern completion device. A subset of the units are "clamped" into their on or off states and the weights in the network then complete the pattern by determining the states of the remaining units. There are strong limitations on the sets of binary vectors that can be learned if the network has one unit for each component of the vector. These limits can be transcended by using extra units whose states do not correspond to components in the vectors to be learned. The weights of connections to these extra units can be used to represent complex interactions that cannot be expressed as pairwise correlations between the components of the vectors. We call these extra units *hidden units* (by analogy with hidden Markov processes) and we call the units that are used to specify the patterns to be learned the *visible units*. The visible units are the interface between the network and the environment that specifies vectors for it to learn or asks it to complete a partial vector. The hidden units are where the network can build its own internal representations.

Sometimes, we would like to be able to complete a pattern from any sufficiently large part of it without knowing in advance which part will be given and which part must be completed. Other times we know in advance which parts will be given as input and which parts will have to be completed as output. So there are two different completion paradigms. In the first, any of the visible units might be part of the required output. In the second, there is a distinguished subset of the visible units, called the input units, which are always clamped by the environment, so the network never needs to determine the states of these units.

Easy and Hard Learning ⎯⎯⎯⎯⎯⎯⎯⎯⎯⎯⎯⎯⎯⎯⎯⎯⎯⎯⎯⎯⎯⎯

Consider a network which is allowed to run freely, using the probabilistic decision rule in Equation 3, without having any of its units clamped by the environment. When the network reaches thermal equilibrium, the probability of finding it in any particular global state depends only on the energy of that state (Equation 4). We can therefore control the probabilities of global states by controlling their energies. If each weight only contributed to the energy of a single global state, this would be straightforward, but changing a weight will actually change the energies of many different states so it is not immediately obvious how a weight-change will affect the probability of a particular global state. Fortunately, if we run the network until it reaches thermal equilibrium, Equations 3 and 4 allow us to derive the way in which the probability of each global state changes as a weight is changed:

$$\frac{\partial \ln P_\alpha^-}{\partial w_{ij}} = \frac{1}{T}\left(s_i^\alpha s_j^\alpha - \sum_\beta P_\beta^- s_i^\beta s_j^\beta \right) \tag{5}$$

where s_i^α is the binary state of the ith unit in the αth global state and P_α^- is the probability, at thermal equilibrium, of global state α of the network when none of the visible units are clamped (the lack of clamping is denoted by the superscript $^-$). Equation 5 shows that the effect of a weight on the log probability of a global state can be computed from purely local information because it only involves the behavior of the two units that the weight connects (the second term is just the probability of finding the ith and jth units on together). This makes it easy to manipulate the probabilities of global states provided the desired probabilities are known (see Hinton & Sejnowski, 1983a, for details).

Unfortunately, it is normally unreasonable to expect the environment or a teacher to specify the required probabilities of entire global states of the network. The task that the network must perform is defined in terms of the states of the visible units, and so the environment or teacher only has direct access to the states of these units. The difficult learning problem is to decide how to use the hidden units to help achieve the requiredbehavior of the visible units. A learning rule which assumes that the network is instructed from outside on how to use *all* of its units is of limited interest because it evades the main problem which is to discover appropriate representations for a given task among the hidden units.

In statistical terms, there are many kinds of statistical structure implicit in a large ensemble of environmental vectors. The separate probability of each visible unit being active is the first-order structure and can be captured by the thresholds of the visible units. The $v^2/2$ pairwise correlations between the v visible units constitute the second-order structure and this can be captured by the weights between pairs of units.[2] All structure higher than second-order cannot be captured by pairwise weights *between the visible units*. A simple example may help to clarify this crucial point.

Suppose that the ensemble consists of the vectors: (1 1 0), (1 0 1), (0 1 1), and (0 0 0), each with a probability of 0.25. There is clearly some structure here because four of the eight possible 3-bit vectors never occur. However, the structure is entirely third-order. The first-order probabilities are all 0.5, and the second-order correlations are all 0, so if we consider only these statistics, this ensemble is indistinguishable from the ensemble in which all eight vectors occur equiprobably.

The Widrow-Hoff rule or perceptron convergence procedure (Rosenblatt, 1962) is a learning rule which is designed to capture second-order structure and it therefore fails miserably on the example just given. If the first two bits are treated as an input and the last bit is treated as the required output, the ensemble corresponds to the function "exclusive-or" which is one of the examples used by Minsky and Papert (1969) to show the strong limitations of one-layer perceptrons. The Widrow-Hoff rule can do easy learning, but it cannot do the kind of hard learning that involves deciding how to use extra units whose behavior is not directly specified by the task.

It is tempting to think that networks with pairwise connections can never capture higher than second-order statistics. There is one sense in which this is true and another in which it is false. By introducing extra units which are not part of the definition of the original ensemble, it is possible to express the third-order structure of the original ensemble in the second-order structure of the larger set of units. In the example given above, we can add a fourth component to get the ensemble {(1101), (1010), (0110), (0000)}. It is now possible to use the thresholds and weights between all four units to express the third-order structure in the first three components. A more familiar way of saying this is that we introduce an extra "feature detector" which in this example detects the case when the first two units are both on. We can then make each of the first two units excite the third unit, and use strong inhibition from the feature detector to overrule this excitation when *both* of the first two units are on. The difficult problem in introducing the extra unit was deciding when it should be on and when it should be off—deciding what feature it should detect.[3]

One way of thinking about the higher order structure of an ensemble of environmental vectors is that it implicitly specifies good sets of underlying features that can be used to model the structure of the environ-

---

[2]Factor analysis confines itself to capturing as much of the second-order structure as possible in a few underlying "factors." It ignores all higher order structure which is where much of the interesting information lies for all but the most simple ensembles of vectors.

[3]In this example there are six different ways of using the extra unit to solve the task.

ment. In common-sense terms, the weights in the network should be chosen so that the hidden units represent significant underlying features that bear strong, regular relationships to each other and to the states of the visible units. The hard learning problem is to figure out what these features are, i.e., to find a set of weights which turn the hidden units into useful feature detectors that explicitly represent properties of the environment which are only implicitly present as higher order statistics in the ensemble of environmental vectors.

Maximum Likelihood Models. Another view of learning is that the weights in the network constitute a generative model of the environment—we would like to find a set of weights so that when the network is running freely, the patterns of activity that occur over the visible units are the same as they would be if the environment was clamping them. The number of units in the network and their interconnectivity define a space of possible models of the environment, and any particular set of weights defines a particular model within this space. The learning problem is to find a combination of weights that gives a good model given the limitations imposed by the architecture of the network and the way it runs.

More formally, we would like a way of finding the combination of weights that is most likely to have produced the observed ensemble of environmental vectors. This is called a *maximum likelihood* model and there is a large literature within statistics on maximum likelihood estimation. The learning procedure we describe actually has a close relationship to a method called Expectation and Maximization (EM) (Dempster, Laird, & Rubin, 1976). EM is used by statisticians for estimating missing parameters. It represents probability distributions by using parameters like our weights that are exponentially related to probabilities, rather than using probabilities themselves. The EM algorithm is closely related to an earlier algorithm invented by Baum that manipulates probabilities directly. Baum's algorithm has been used successfully for speech recognition (Bahl, Jelinek, & Mercer, 1983). It estimates the parameters of a hidden Markov chain—a transition network which has a fixed structure but variable probabilities on the arcs and variable probabilities of emitting a particular output symbol as it arrives at each internal node. Given an ensemble of strings of symbols and a fixed-topology transition network, the algorithm finds the combination of transition probabilities and output probabilities that is most likely to have produced these strings (actually it only finds a local maximum).

Maximum likelihood methods work by adjusting the parameters to increase the probability that the generative model will produce the observed data. Baum's algorithm and EM are able to estimate new values for the probabilities (or weights) that are guaranteed to be better than the previous values. Our algorithm simply estimates the gradient of the log likelihood with respect to a weight, and so the magnitude of the weight change must be decided using additional criteria. Our algorithm, however, has the advantage that it is easy to implement in a parallel network of neuron-like units.

The idea of a stochastic generative model is attractive because it provides a clean quantitative way of comparing alternative representational schemes. The problem of saying which of two representational schemes is best appears to be intractable. Many sensible rules of thumb are available, but these are generally pulled out of thin air and justified by commonsense and practical experience. They lack a firm mathematical foundation. If we confine ourselves to a space of allowable stochastic models, we can then get a simple Bayesian measure of the quality of a representational scheme: How likely is the observed ensemble of environmental vectors given the representational scheme? In our networks, representations are patterns of activity in the units, and the representational scheme therefore corresponds to the set of weights that determines when those patterns are active.

The Boltzmann Machine Learning Algorithm

If we make certain assumptions it is possible to derive a measure of how effectively the weights in the network are being used for modeling the structure of the environment, and it is also possible to show how the weights should be changed to progressively improve this measure. We assume that the environment clamps a particular vector over the visible units and it keeps it there long enough for the network to reach thermal equilibrium with this vector as a boundary condition (i.e., to "interpret" it). We also assume (unrealistically) that the there is no structure in the sequential order of the environmentally clamped vectors. This means that the complete structure of the ensemble of environmental vectors can be specified by giving the probability, $P^+(V_\alpha)$, of each of the 2^v vectors over the v visible units. Notice that the $P^+(V_\alpha)$ do not depend on the weights in the network because the environment clamps the visible units.

A particular set of weights can be said to constitute a perfect model of the structure of the environment if it leads to exactly the same probability distribution of visible vectors when the network is running freely *with no units being clamped by the environment*. Because of the stochastic behavior of the units, the network will wander through a variety of states even with no environmental input and it will therefore generate a probability distribution, $P^-(V_\alpha)$, over all 2^v visible vectors. This distribution can be compared with the environmental distribution, $P^+(V_\alpha)$. In general, it will not be possible to exactly match the 2^v environmental probabilities using the weights among the v visible and h hidden units because there are at most $(v + h - 1)(v + h)/2$ symmetrical weights and $(v + h)$ thresholds. However, it may be possible to do very well if the environment contains regularities that can be expressed in the weights. An information theoretic measure (Kullback, 1959) of the distance between the environmental and free-running probability distributions is given by:

$$G = \sum_{\alpha} P^+(V_\alpha) \ln \frac{P^+(V_\alpha)}{P^-(V_\alpha)} \tag{6}$$

where $P^+(V_\alpha)$ is the probability of the αth state of the visible units in *phase$^+$* when their states are determined by the environment, and $P^-(V_\alpha)$ is the corresponding probability in *phase$^-$* when the network is running freely with no environmental input.

G is never negative and is only zero if the distributions are identical. G is actually the distance in bits *from* the free running distribution *to* the environmental distribution.[4] It is sometimes called the asymmetric divergence or information gain. The measure is not symmetric with respect to the two distributions. This seems odd but is actually very reasonable. When trying to approximate a probability distribution, it is more important to get the probabilities correct for events that happen frequently than for rare events. So the match between the actual and predicted probabilities of an event should be weighted by the actual probability as in Equation 6.

It is possible to improve the network's model of the structure of its environment by changing the weights so as to reduce G.[5] To perform gradient descent in G, we need to know how G will change when a weight is changed. But changing a single weight changes the energies of one quarter of all the global states of the network, and it changes the probabilities of all the states in ways that depend on *all* the other weights in the network. Consider, for example, the very simple network shown in Figure 2. If we want the two units at the ends of the chain to be either both on or both off, how should we change the weight $w_{3,4}$? It clearly depends on the signs of remote weights like $w_{1,2}$ because we need to have an even number of inhibitory weights in the chain.[6] So the partial derivative of G with respect to one weight depends on all the other weights and minimizing G appears to be a difficult computational problem that requires nonlocal information.

Fortunately, all the information that is required about the other weights in order to change w_{ij} appropriately shows up in the behavior of the ith and jth units at thermal equilibrium. In addition to performing a search for low energy states of the network, the process of reaching thermal equilibrium ensures that the joint activity of any two units contains all the information required for changing the weight between them in order to give the network a better model of its environment. The joint activity implicitly encodes information about all the other weights in the network. The Appendix shows that

---

[4]If we use base 2 logarithms.

[5]Peter Brown (personal communication) has pointed out that minimizing G is equivalent to maximizing the log of the likelihood of generating the environmental probability distribution when the network is running freely at equilibrium.

[6]The thresholds must also be adjusted appropriately.

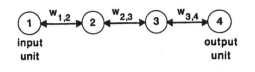

Figure 2: A very simple network with one input unit, one output unit, and two hidden units. The task is to make the output unit adopt the same state as the input unit. The difficulty is that the correct value for weight $w_{3,4}$ depends on remote information like the value of weight $w_{1,2}$.

$$\frac{\partial G}{\partial w_{ij}} = -\frac{1}{T}[p_{ij}^+ - p_{ij}^-] \qquad (7)$$

where p_{ij}^+ is the probability, averaged over all environmental inputs and measured at equilibrium, that the ith and jth units are both on when the network is being driven by the environment, and p_{ij}^- is the corresponding probability when the network is free running. One surprising feature of Equation 7 is that it does not matter whether the weight is between two visible units, two hidden units, or one of each. The same rule applies for the gradient of G.

Unlearning. Crick and Mitchison (1983) have suggested that a form of reverse learning might occur during REM sleep in mammals. Their proposal was based on the assumption that parasitic modes develop in large networks that hinder the distributed storage and retrieval of information. The mechanism that Crick and Mitchison propose is based on

More or less random stimulation of the forebrain by the brain stem that will tend to stimulate the inappropriate modes of brain activity ... and especially those which are too prone to be set off by random noise rather than by highly structured specific signals. (p. 112)

During this state of random excitation and free running they postulate that changes occur at synapses to decrease the probability of the spurious states.

A simulation of reverse learning was performed by Hopfield, Feinstein, and Palmer (1983) who independently had been studying ways to improve the associative storage capacity of simple networks of binary processors (Hopfield, 1982). In their algorithm an input is presented to the network as an initial condition, and the system evolves by falling into a nearby local energy minimum. However, not all local energy minima represent stored information. In creating the desired minima, they accidentally create other spurious minima, and to eliminate these they use "unlearning": The learning procedure is applied with reverse sign to the states found after starting from random initial conditions.

Following this procedure, the performance of the system in accessing stored states was found to be improved.

There is an interesting relationship between the reverse learning proposed by Crick and Mitchison and Hopfield et al. and the form of the learning algorithm which we derived by considering how to minimize an information theory measure of the discrepancy between the environmental structure and the network's internal model (Hinton & Sejnowski, 1983b). The two phases of our learning algorithm resemble the learning and unlearning procedures: Positive Hebbian learning occurs in $phase^+$ during which information in the environment is captured by the weights; during $phase^-$ the system randomly samples states according to their Boltzmann distribution and Hebbian learning occurs with a negative coefficient.

However, these two phases need not be implemented in the manner suggested by Crick and Mitchison. For example, during $phase^-$ the average co-occurrences could be computed without making any changes to the weights. These averages could then be used as a baseline for making changes during $phase^+$; that is, the co-occurrences during $phase^+$ could be computed and the baseline subtracted before each permanent weight change. Thus, an alternative but equivalent proposal for the function of dream sleep is to recalibrate the baseline for plasticity—the break-even point which determines whether a synaptic weight is incremented or decremented. This would be safer than making permanent weight decrements to synaptic weights during sleep and solves the problem of deciding how much "unlearning" to do.

Our learning algorithm refines Crick and Mitchison's interpretation of why two phases are needed. Consider a hidden unit deep within the network: How should its connections with other units be changed to best capture regularity present in the environment? If it does not receive direct input from the environment, the hidden unit has no way to determine whether the information it receives from neighboring units is ultimately caused by structure in the environment or is entirely a result of the other weights. This can lead to a "folie a deux" where two parts of the network each construct a model of the other and ignore the external environment. The contribution of internal and external sources can be separated by comparing the co-occurrences in $phase^+$ with similar information that is collected in the absence of environmental input. $phase^-$ thus acts as a control condition. Because of the special properties of equilibrium it is possible to subtract off this purely internal contribution and use the difference to update the weights. Thus, the role of the two phases is to make the system maximally responsive to regularities present in the environment and to prevent the system from using its capacity to model internally-generated regularities.

Ways in Which the Learning Algorithm Can Fail. The ability to discover the partial derivative of G by observing p_{ij}^+ and p_{ij}^- does not completely determine the learning algorithm. It is still necessary to decide how much to change each weight, how long to collect co-occurrence statistics before changing the weight, how many weights to change at a time, and what temperature schedule to use during the annealing searches. For very simple networks in very simple environments, it is possible to discover reasonable values for these parameters by trial and error. For more complex and interesting cases, serious difficulties arise because it is very easy to violate the assumptions on which the mathematical results are based (Derthick, 1984).

The first difficulty is that there is nothing to prevent the learning algorithm from generating very large weights which create such high energy barriers that the network cannot reach equilibrium in the allotted time. Once this happens, the statistics that are collected will not be the equilibrium statistics required for Equation 7 to hold and so all bets are off. We have observed this happening for a number of different networks. They start off learning quite well and then the weights become too large and the network "goes sour"—its performance deteriorates dramatically.

One way to ensure that the network gets close to equilibrium is to keep the weights small. Pearlmutter (personal communication) has shown that the learning works much better if, in addition to the weight changes caused by the learning, every weight continually decays towards a value of zero, with the speed of the decay being proportional to the absolute magnitude of the weight. This keeps the weights small and eventually leads to a relatively stable situation in which the decay rate of a weight is balanced by the partial derivative of G with respect to the weight. This has the satisfactory property that the absolute magnitude of a weight shows how important it is for modeling the environmental structure.

The use of weight-decay has several other consequences which are not so desirable. Because the weights stay small, the network cannot construct very deep minima in the energy landscape and so it cannot make the probability ratios for similar global states be very different. This means that it is bound to give a significant number of errors in modeling environments where very similar vectors have very different probabilities. Better *performance* can be achieved by annealing the network to a lower final temperature (which is equivalent to making all the weights larger), but this will make the *learning* worse for two separate reasons. First, with less errors there is less to drive the learning because it relies on the difference between the *phase*$^+$ and *phase*$^-$ statistics. Second, it will be harder to reach thermal equilibrium at this lower temperature and so the co-occurrence statistics will be unreliable. One way of getting good statistics to drive the learning and also getting very few overt errors is to measure the co-occurrence statistics at a temperature higher than the final one.

Another way of ensuring that the network approaches equilibrium is to eliminate deep, narrow minima that are often not found by the annealing process. Derthick (1984) has shown that this can be done using a longer gentler annealing schedule in *phase⁻*. This means that the network is more likely to occupy the hard-to-find minima in *phase⁻* than in *phase⁺*, and so these minima will get filled in because the learning rule raises the energies of states that are occupied more in *phase⁻* than in *phase⁺*.

An Example of Hard Learning

A simple example which can only be solved by capturing the higher order statistical structure in the ensemble of input vectors is the "shifter" problem. The visible units are divided into three groups. Group V_1 is a one-dimensional array of 8 units, each of which is clamped on or off at random with a probability of 0.3 of being on. Group V_2 also contains 8 units and their states are determined by shifting and copying the states of the units in group V_1. The only shifts allowed are one to the left, one to the right, or no shift. Wrap-around is used so that when there is a right shift, the state of the right-most unit in V_1 determines the state of the left-most unit in V_2. The three possible shifts are chosen at random with equal probabilities. Group V_3 contains three units to represent the three possible shifts, so at any one time one of them is clamped on and the others are clamped off.

The problem is to learn the structure that relates the states of the three groups. One facet of this problem is to "recognize" the shift—i.e., to complete a partial input vector in which the states of V_1 and V_2 are clamped but the units in V_3 are left free. It is fairly easy to see why this problem cannot possibly be solved by just adding together a lot of pairwise interactions between units in V_1, V_2, and V_3. If you know that a particular unit in V_1 is on, it tells you nothing whatsoever about what the shift is. It is only by finding *combinations* of active units in V_1 and V_2 that it is possible to predict the shift, so the information required is of at least third-order. This means that extra hidden units are required to perform the task.

The obvious way to recognize the shift is to have extra units which detect informative features such as an active unit in V_1 and an active unit one place to the right in V_2 and then support the unit V_3 that represents a right shift. The empirical question is whether the learning algorithm is capable of turning some hidden units into feature detectors of this kind, and whether it will generate a set of detectors that work well together rather than duplicating the same detector. The set of weights that minimizes G defines the *optimal* set of detectors but it is not at all obvious what these detectors are, nor is it obvious that the learning algorithm is capable of finding a good set.

Figure 3 shows the result of running a version of the Boltzmann machine learning procedure. Of the 24 hidden units, 5 seem to be doing very little but the remainder are sensible looking detectors and most of them have become spatially localized. One type of detector which occurs several times consists of two large negative weights, one above the other, flanked by smaller excitatory weights on each side. This is a more discriminating detector of no-shift than simply having two positive weights, one above the other. It interesting to note that the various instances of this feature type all have different locations in V_1 and V_2, even though the hidden units are not connected to each other. The pressure for the feature detectors to be different from each other comes from the gradient of G, rather than from the kind of lateral inhibition among the feature detectors that is used in "competitive learning" paradigms (Fukushima, 1980; Rumelhart & Zipser, 1985).

The Training Procedure. The training procedure alternated between two phases. In $phase^+$, all the units in V_1, V_2, and V_3 were clamped into states representing a pair of 8-bit vectors and their relative shift. The hidden units were then allowed to change their states until the system approached thermal equilibrium at a temperature of 10. The annealing schedule is described below. After annealing, the network was assumed to be close to thermal equilibrium and it was then run for a further 10 iterations during which time the frequency with which each pair of connected units were both on was measured. This was repeated 20 times with different clamped vectors and the co-occurrence statistics were averaged over all 20 runs to yield an estimate, for each connection, of p_{ij}^+ in Equation 7. In $phase^-$, none of the units were clamped and the network was annealed in the same way. The network was then run for a further 10 iterations and the co-occurrence statistics were collected for all connected pairs of units. This was repeated 20 times and the co-occurrence statistics were averaged to yield an estimate of p_{ij}^-.

The entire set of 40 annealings that were used to estimate p_{ij}^+ and p_{ij}^- was called a sweep. After each sweep, every weight was incremented by $5(p_{ij}^+ - p_{ij}^-)$. In addition, every weight had its absolute magnitude decreased by 0.0005 times its absolute magnitude. This weight decay prevented the weights from becoming too large and it also helped to resuscitate hidden units which had predominantly negative or predominantly positive weights. Such units spend all their time in the same state and therefore convey no information. The $phase^+$ and $phase^-$ statistics are identical for these units, and so the weight decay gradually erodes their weights until they come back to life (units with all zero weights come on half the time).

The Annealing Schedule. The annealing schedule spent the following number of iterations at the following temperatures: 2 at 40, 2 at 35, 2 at 30, 2 at 25, 2 at 20, 2 at 15, 2 at 12, 2 at 10. One iteration is defined as the number of random probes required so that each unit is probed one time on average. When it is probed, a unit uses its energy gap to decide which of its two states to adopt using the stochastic decision rule in Equation 3. Since each unit gets to see the most recent states of all the other units, an iteration cannot be regarded as a single parallel step. A truly parallel asynchronous system must tolerate time delays. Units must decide on

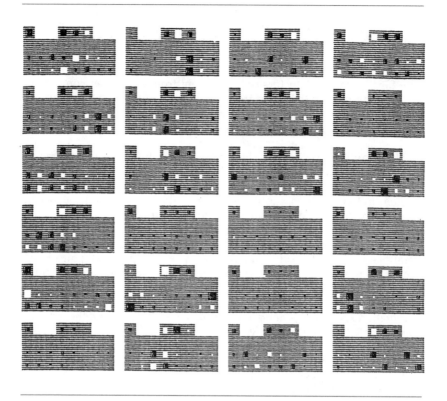

Figure 3: The weights of the 24 hidden units in the shifter network. Each large region corresponds to a unit. Within this region the black rectangles represent negative weights and the white rectangles represent positive ones. The size of a rectangle represents the magnitude of the weight. The two rows of weights at the bottom of each unit are its connections to the two groups of input units, V_1 and V_2. These weights therefore represent the "receptive field" of the hidden unit. The three weights in the middle of the top row of each unit are its connections to the three output units that represent shift-left, no-shift, and shift-right. The solitary weight at the top left of each unit is its threshold. Each hidden unit is directly connected to all 16 input units and all 3 output units. In this example, the hidden units are not connected to each other. The top-left unit has weights that are easy to understand: Its optimal stimulus is activity in the fourth unit of V_1 and the fifth unit of V_2, and it votes for shift-right. It has negative weights to make it less likely to come on when there is an alternative explanation for why its two favorite input units are active.

their new states without being aware of very recent changes in the states of other units. It can be shown (Sejnowski, Hinton, Kienker, & Schumacher, 1985) that first-order time delays act like added temperature and can therefore be tolerated by networks of this kind.

The Performance of the Shifter Network. The shifter network is encouraging because it is a clear example of the kind of learning of higher order structure that was beyond the capability of perceptrons, but it also illustrates several weaknesses in the current approach.

- The learning was very slow. It required 9000 learning sweeps, each of which involved reaching equilibrium 20 times in $phase^+$ with vectors clamped on V_1, V_2, and V_3, and 20 times in $phase^-$ with no units clamped. Even for low-level perceptual learning, this seems excessively slow.

- The weights are fairly clearly not optimal because of the 5 hidden units that appear to do nothing useful. Also, the performance is far from perfect. When the states of the units in V_1 and V_2 are clamped and the network is annealed gently to half the final temperature used during learning, the units in V_3 quite frequently adopt the wrong states. If the number of *on* units in V_1 is 1, 2, 3, 4, 5, 6, 7, the percentage of correctly recognized shifts is 50%, 71%, 81%, 86%, 89%, 82%, and 66% respectively. The wide variation in the number of active units in V_1 naturally makes the task harder to learn than if a constant proportion of the units were active. Also, some of the input patterns are ambiguous. When all the units in V_1 and V_2 are off, the network can do no better than chance.

Achieving Reliable Computation with Unreliable Hardware _____

Conventional computers only work if all their individual components work perfectly, so as systems become larger they become more and more unreliable. Current computer technology uses extremely reliable components and error-correcting memories to achieve overall reliability. The brain appears to have much less reliable components, and so it must use much more error-correction. It is conceivable that the brain uses the kinds of representations that would be appropriate given reliable hardware and then superimposes redundancy to compensate for its unreliable hardware.

The reliability issue is typically treated as a tedious residual problem to be dealt with after the main decisions about the form of the computation have been made. A more direct approach is to treat reliability as a serious design constraint from the outset and to choose a basic style of computation that does not require reliable components. Ideally, we want a system in which *none* of the individual components are critical to the ability of the whole system to meet its requirements. In other words, we want some high-level description of the behavior of the system to remain valid even when the low-level descriptions of the behavior of some of the individual components change. This is only possible if the high-level description is related to the low level descriptions in a particular way: Every robust high-level property must be implemented by the combined effect of many local components, and no single component must be crucial for the realization of the high-level property. This makes distributed representations a natural choice when designing a damage-resistant system.

Distributed representations tend to behave robustly because they have an internal coherence which leads to an automatic "clean-up" effect. This effect can be seen in the patterns of activity that occur within a group of units and also in the interactions between groups. If a group of units, A, has a number of distinct and well-defined energy minima then these minima will remain even if a few units are removed or a little noise is added to many of the connections within A. The damage may distort the minima slightly and it may also change their relative probabilities, but minor damage will not alter the gross topography of the energy landscape, so it will not affect higher level descriptions that depend only on this gross topography.

Even if the patterns of activity in A are slightly changed, this will often have *no* effect on the patterns caused in other groups of units. If the weights between groups of units have been fixed so that a particular pattern in A regularly causes a particular pattern in B, a small variation in the input coming from A will typically make no difference to the pattern that gets selected in B, because this pattern has its own internal coherence, and if the input from A is sufficiently accurate to select approximately the right pattern, the interactions among the elements in B will ensure that the details are right.

Damage resistance can be achieved by using a simple kind of representation in which there are many identical copies of each type of unit and each macroscopic item is encoded by activity in all the units of one type. In the undamaged system all these copies behave identically and a lot of capacity is therefore wasted. If we use distributed representations in which each unit may be used for representing many different items we can achieve comparable resistance to damage without wasting capacity. Because all the units behave differently from each other, the undamaged system can implement many fine distinctions in the fine detail of the energy landscape. At the macroscopic level, these fine distinctions will appear as somewhat unreliable probabilistic tendencies and will be very sensitive to minor damage.

The fine details in the current energy landscape may contain the seeds of future changes in the gross topography. If learning novel distinctions involves the progressive strengthening of regularities that are initially tentative and unreliable, then it follows that learning may well suffer considerably when physical damage washes out these minor regularities. However, the simulations described below do not bear on this interesting issue.

An Example of the Effects of Damage

To show the effects of damage on a network, it is necessary to choose a task for the network to perform. Since we are mainly concerned with properties that are fairly domain-independent, the details of the task are not especially relevant here. We were interested in networks that can learn an *arbitrary* mapping between items in two different domains, and we use that network to investigate the effects of damage. As we shall see, the fact that the task involves purely arbitrary associations makes it easier to interpret some of the interesting transfer effects that occur when a network relearns after sustaining major damage.

The Network. The network consisted of three groups or layers of units. The *grapheme* group was used to represent the letters in a three-letter word. It contained 30 units and was subdivided into three groups of 10 units each. Each subgroup was dedicated to one of the three letter positions within a word, and it represented one of the 10 possible letters in that position by having a single active unit for that letter. The three-letter grapheme strings were not English words. They were chosen randomly, subject to the constraint that each of the 10 possible graphemes in each position had to be used at least once. The *sememe* group was used to encode the semantic features of the "word."[7] It contained 30 units, one for each possible semantic feature. The semantic features to be associated with a word were chosen randomly, with each feature having a probability of 0.2 of being chosen for each word. There were connections between all pairs of units in the sememe group to allow the network to learn familiar combinations of semantic features. There were no direct connections between the grapheme and sememe groups. Instead, there was an intermediate layer of 20 units, each of which was connected to all the units in both the grapheme and the sememe groups. Figure 4 is an artist's impression of the network. It uses English letters and words to convey the functions of the units in the various layers. Most of the connections are missing.

The Training Procedure. The network was trained to associate each of 20 patterns of activity in the grapheme units with an arbitrarily related pattern in the sememe units. As before, the training procedure alternated between two phases. In *phase*$^+$ all the grapheme and sememe units were clamped in states that represented the physical form and the meaning of a single word, and the intermediate units were allowed to change their states until the system approached thermal equilibrium at a temperature of 10. The annealing schedule was: 2 at 30, 2 at 26, 2 at 22, 2 at 20, 2 at 18, 2 at 16, 2 at 15, 2 at 14, 2 at 13, 4 at 12, 4 at 11, 8 at 10. After annealing, the network was assumed to be close to thermal equilibrium

---

[7]The representation of meaning is clearly more complicated than just a set of features, so the use of the word "semantic" here should not be taken too literally.

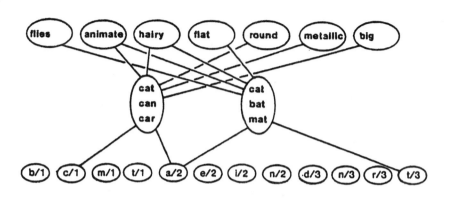

Figure 4: Part of the network used for associating three-letter words with sets of semantic features. English words are used in this figure to help convey the functional roles of the units. In the actual simulation, the letter-strings and semantic features were chosen randomly.

and it was then run for a further 5 iterations during which time the frequency with which each pair of connected units were both on was measured. This was repeated twice for each of the 20 possible grapheme/sememe associations and the co-occurrence statistics were averaged over all 40 annealings to yield an estimate, for each connection, of p_{ij}^+. In *phase⁻*, only the grapheme units were clamped and the network settled to equilibrium (using the same schedule as before) and thus decided for itself what sememe units should be active. The network was then run for a further 5 iterations and the co-occurrence statistics were collected for all connected pairs of units. This was repeated twice for each of the 20 grapheme strings and the co-occurrence statistics were averaged to yield an estimate of p_{ij}^-. Each learning sweep thus involved a total of 80 annealings.

After each sweep, every weight was either incremented or decremented by 1, with the sign of the change being determined by the sign of $p_{ij}^+ - p_{ij}^-$.[8] In addition, some of the weights had their absolute magnitude decreased by 1. For each weight, the probability of this happening was 0.0005 times the absolute magnitude of the weight.

We found that the network performed better if there was a preliminary learning stage which just involved the sememe units. In this stage, the intermediate units were not yet connected. During *phase⁺* the required patterns were clamped on the sememe units and p_{ij}^+ was mea-

---

[8]See Hinton, Sejnowski, and Ackley (1984) for a discussion of the advantages of discrete weight increments over the more obvious steepest descent technique in which the weight increment is proportional to $p_{ij}^+ - p_{ij}^-$.

sured (annealing was not required because all the units involved were clamped). During *phase⁻* no units were clamped and the network was allowed to reach equilibrium 20 times using the annealing schedule given above. After annealing, p_{ij}^- was estimated from the co-occurrences as before, except that only 20 *phase⁻* annealings were used instead of 40. There were 300 sweeps of this learning stage and they resulted in weights between pairs of sememe units that were sufficient to give the sememe group an energy landscape with 20 strong minima corresponding to the 20 possible "word meanings." This helped subsequent learning considerably, because it reduced the tendency for the intermediate units to be recruited for the job of modeling the structure *among* the sememe units. They were therefore free to model the structure *between* the grapheme units and the sememe units.[9] The results described here were obtained using the preliminary learning stage and so they correspond to learning to associate grapheme strings with "meanings" that are already familiar.

The Performance of the Network. Using the same annealing schedule as was used during learning, the network can be tested by clamping a grapheme string and looking at the resulting activities of the sememe units. After 5000 learning sweeps, it gets the semantic features exactly correct 99.3% of the time. A performance level of 99.9% can be achieved by using a "careful" annealing schedule that spends twice as long at each temperature and goes down to half the final temperature.

The Effect of Local Damage. The learning procedure generates weights which cause each of the units in the intermediate layer to be used for many different words. This kind of distributed representation should be more tolerant of local damage than the more obvious method of using one intermediate unit per word. We were particularly interested in the pattern of errors produced by local damage. If the connections between sememe units are left intact, they should be able to "clean up" patterns of activity that are close to familiar ones. So the network should still produce perfect output even if the input to the sememe units is slightly disrupted. If the disruption is more severe, the clean-up effect may actually produce a *different* familiar meaning that happens to share the few semantic features that were correctly activated by the intermediate layer.

To test these predictions we removed each of the intermediate units in turn, leaving the other 19 intact. We tested the network 25 times on each of the 20 words with each of the 20 units removed. In all 10,000 tests, using the careful annealing schedule, it made 140 errors (98.6% correct). Many errors consisted of the correct set of semantic features with one or

---

[9]There was no need to have a similar stage for learning the structure among the grapheme units because in the main stage of learning the grapheme units are always clamped and so there is no tendency for the network to try to model the structure among them.

two extra or missing features, but 83 of the errors consisted of the precise meaning of some other grapheme string. An analysis of these 83 errors showed that the hamming distance between the correct meanings and the erroneous ones had a mean of 9.34 and a standard deviation of 1.27 which is significantly lower ($p < .01$) than the complete set of hamming distances which had a mean of 10.30 and a standard deviation of 2.41. We also looked at the hamming distances between the grapheme strings that the network was given as input and the grapheme strings that corresponded to the erroneous familiar meanings. The mean was 3.95 and the standard deviation was 0.62 which is significantly lower ($p < .01$) than the complete set which had mean 5.53 and standard deviation 0.87. (A hamming distance of 4 means that the strings have one letter in common.)

In summary, when a single unit is removed from the intermediate layer, the network still performs well. The majority of its errors consist of producing exactly the meaning of some other grapheme string, and the erroneous meanings tend to be similar to the correct one and to be associated with a grapheme string that has one letter in common with the string used as input.

The Speed of Relearning. The original learning was very slow. Each item had to be presented 5000 times to eliminate almost all the errors. One reason for the slowness is the shape of the G-surface in weight-space. It tends to have long diagonal ravines which can be characterized in the following way: In the direction of steepest descent, the surface slopes steeply down for a short distance and then steeply up again (like the cross-section of a ravine).[10] In most other directions the surface slopes gently upwards. In a relatively narrow cone of directions, the surface slopes gently down with very low curvature. This narrow cone corresponds to the floor of the ravine and to get a low value of G (which is the definition of good performance) the learning must follow the floor of the ravine without going up the sides. This is particularly hard in a high-dimensional space. Unless the gradient of the surface is measured very accurately, a step in the direction of the *estimated* gradient will have a component along the floor of the ravine and a component up one of the many sides of the ravine. Because the sides are much steeper than the floor, the result of the step will be to raise the value of G which makes performance worse. Once out of the bottom of the ravine, almost all the measurable gradient will be down towards the floor of the ravine instead of along the ravine. As a result, the path followed in weight space tends to consist of an irregular sloshing across the ravine with only a small amount of forward progress. We are investigating ways of ameliorating this difficulty, but it is a well-known problem of gradient descent techniques in high-dimensional spaces, and it may be unavoidable.

---

[10]The surface is never very steep. Its gradient parallel to any weight axis must always lie between 1 and -1 because it is the difference of two probabilities.

The ravine problem leads to a very interesting prediction about relearning when random noise is added to the weights. The original learning takes the weights a considerable distance along a ravine which is slow and difficult because most directions in weight space are up the sides of the ravine. When a lot of random noise is added, there will typically be a small component along the ravine and a large component up the sides. Performance will therefore get much worse (because height in this space *means* poor performance), but relearning will be fast because the network can get back most of its performance by simply descending to the floor of the ravine (which is easy) without making progress along the ravine (which is hard).

The same phenomenon can be understood by considering the energy landscape rather than the weight-space (recall that one point in weight-space constitutes a whole energy landscape). Good performance requires a rather precise balance between the relative depths of the 20 energy minima and it also requires that all the 20 minima have considerably lower energy than other parts of the energy landscape. The balance between the minima in energy-space is the cross-section of the ravine in weight-space (see Figure 5) and the depth of all the minima compared with the rest of the energy landscape corresponds to the direction along the ravine. Random noise upsets the precise balance between the various minima without significantly affecting the gross topography of the energy landscape. Relearning can then restore most of the performance by restoring the balance between the existing minima.

The simulation behaved as predicted. The mean absolute value of the weights connecting the intermediate units to the other two groups was 21.5. These weights were first perturbed by adding uniform random noise in the range -2 to $+2$. This had surprisingly little effect, reducing the performance using the normal annealing schedule from 99.3% to 98.0%. This shows that the network is robust against slight noise in the weights. To cause significant deterioration, uniform random noise between -22 and $+22$ was added. On average, this perturbs each weight by about half its magnitude which was enough to reduce normal performance to 64.3% correct. Figure 6 shows the course of the relearning and compares it with the speed of the original learning when performance was at this level. It also shows that other kinds of damage produce very similar relearning curves.

Spontaneous Recovery of Unrehearsed Items. When it learns the associations, the network uses distributed representations among the intermediate units. This means that many of the weights are involved in encoding several different associations, and each association is encoded in many weights. If a weight is changed, it will affect several different energy minima and all of them will require the same change in the weight to restore them to their previous depths. So, in relearning any one of the associations, there should be a positive transfer effect which tends to restore the others. This effect is actually rather weak and is

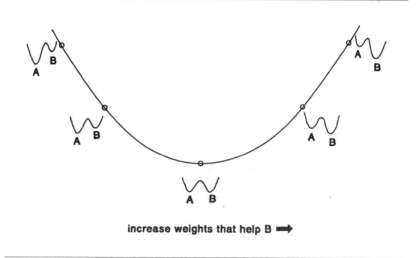

increase weights that help B ➡

Figure 5: One cross-section of a ravine in weight-space. Each point in weight space corresponds to a whole energy landscape. To indicate this, we show how a very simple landscape changes as the weights are changed. Movement to the right along the x-axis corresponds to increasing the weights between pairs of units that are both on in state B and not both on in state A. This increases the depth of A. If the task requires that A and B have about the same depth, an imbalance between them will lower the performance and thus raise G.

easily masked so it can only be seen clearly if we retrain the network on most of the original associations and watch what happens to the remaining few. As predicted, these showed a marked improvement even though they were only randomly related to the associations on which the network was retrained.

We took exactly the same perturbed network as before (uniform random noise between +22 and −22 added to the connections to and from the intermediate units) and retrained it on 18 of the associations for 30 learning sweeps. The two associations that were not retrained were selected to be ones where the network made frequent minor errors even when the careful annealing schedule was used. As a result of the retraining, the performance on these two items rose from 30/100 correct to 90/100 correct with the careful schedule, but the few errors that remained tended to be completely wrong answers rather than minor perturbations of the correct answer. We repeated the experiment selecting two associations for which the error rate was high and the errors were typically large. Retraining on the other 18 associations caused an improvement from 17/100 correct to 98/100 correct. Despite these impressive improvements, the effect disappeared when we retrained on only 15 of the associations. The remaining 5 actually got slightly worse.

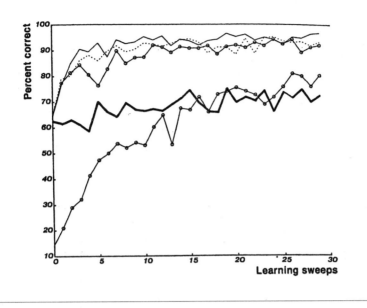

Figure 6: The recovery of performance after various types of damage. Each data-point represents 500 tests (25 with each word). The heavy line is a section of the original learning curve after a considerable number of learning sweeps. It shows that in the original learning, performance increases by less than 10% in 30 learning sweeps. All the other lines show recovery after damaging a net that had very good performance (99.3% correct). The lines with open circles show the rapid recovery after 20% or 50% of the weights to the hidden units have been set to zero (but allowed to relearn). The dashed line shows recovery after 5 of the 20 hidden units have been permanently ablated. The remaining line is the case when uniform random noise between −22 and +22 is added to all the connections to the hidden units. In all cases, a successful trial was defined as one in which the network produced *exactly* the correct semantic features when given the graphemic input.

It is clear that the fraction of the associations which needs to be retrained to cause improvement in the remainder depends on how distributed the representations are, but more analysis is required to characterize this relationship properly.

The spontaneous recovery of unrehearsed items seems paradoxical because the set of 20 associations was randomly generated and so there is no way of generalizing from the 18 associations on which the network is retrained to the remaining two. During the original learning, however, the weights capture regularities in the whole set of associations. In this example, the regularities are spurious but the network doesn't know that—it just finds whatever regularities it can and expresses the associations in terms of them. Now, consider two different regularities that are equally strong among 18 of the associations. If one regularity also holds for the remaining two associations and the other doesn't, the first regularity is more likely to be captured by the weights. During retraining, the learning procedure restores the weights to the values needed to express the regularities it originally chose to capture and it therefore tends to restore the remaining associations.

It would be interesting to see if any of the neuro-psychological data on the effects of brain damage could be interpreted in terms of the kinds of qualitative effects exhibited by the simulation when it is damaged and relearns. However, we have not made any serious attempt to fit the simulation to particular data.

Conclusion

We have presented three ideas:

- Networks of symmetrically connected, binary units can escape from local minima during a relaxation search by using a stochastic decision rule.

- The process of reaching thermal equilibrium in a network of stochastic units propagates exactly the information needed to do credit assignment. This makes possible a *local* learning rule which can modify the weights so as to create new and useful feature detectors. The learning rule only needs to observe how often two units are both active (at thermal equilibrium) in two different phases. It can then change the weight between the units to make the spontaneous behavior of the network in one phase mimic the behavior that is forced on it in the other phase.

- The learning rule tends to construct distributed representations which are resistant to minor damage and exhibit rapid relearning after major damage. The relearning process can bring back associations that are not practiced during the relearning and are only randomly related to the associations that are practiced.

These three ideas can be assessed separately. In particular, resistance to damage, rapid relearning, and spontaneous recovery of unrehearsed items can be exhibited by other kinds of parallel network that use distributed representations. The use of stochastic units, annealing search, and the two-phase learning algorithm are not crucial for these properties, though they are a convenient testbed in which to investigate them. Hogg and Huberman (1984) have demonstrated self-repair effects in nonstochastic, layered networks similar to those used by Fukushima (1980).

We have left many loose ends, some of which are discussed elsewhere. Sejnowski and Hinton (in press) give a detailed example of a search problem where annealing helps, and they also discuss the relationship between these networks and the mammalian cortex. Ackley, Hinton, and Sejnowski (1985) give a different example of learning in which the network constructs efficient internal codes for communicating information across narrow bandwidth channels. At present, the learning algorithm is too slow to be tested properly on large networks and future progress hinges on being able to speed it up.

Acknowledgments

This research was supported by grants from the System Development Foundation. We thank David Ackley, Peter Brown, Francis Crick, Mark Derthick, Scott Fahlman, Stuart Geman, John Hopfield, Paul Kienker, Jay McClelland, Barak Pearlmutter, David Rumelhart, Tim Shallice, and Paul Smolensky for helpful discussions.

Appendix: Derivation of the Learning Algorithm

When a network is free-running at equilibrium the probability distribution over the visible units is given by

$$P^-(V_\alpha) = \sum_\beta P^-(V_\alpha \wedge H_\beta) = \frac{\sum_\beta e^{-E_{\alpha\beta}/T}}{\sum_{\lambda\mu} e^{-E_{\lambda\mu}/T}} \tag{8}$$

where V_α is a vector of the states of the visible units, H_β is a vector of states of the hidden units, and $E_{\alpha\beta}$ is the energy of the system in state $V_\alpha \wedge H_\beta$

$$E_{\alpha\beta} = -\sum_{i<j} w_{ij} s_i^{\alpha\beta} s_j^{\alpha\beta}.$$

Hence,

$$\frac{\partial e^{-E_{\alpha\beta}/T}}{\partial w_{ij}} = \frac{1}{T} s_i^{\alpha\beta} s_j^{\alpha\beta} e^{-E_{\alpha\beta}/T}.$$

Differentiating (8) then yields

$$\frac{\partial P^-(V_\alpha)}{\partial w_{ij}} = \frac{\frac{1}{T}\sum_\beta e^{-E_{\alpha\beta}/T} s_i^{\alpha\beta} s_j^{\alpha\beta}}{\sum_{\alpha\beta} e^{-E_{\alpha\beta}/T}} - \frac{\sum_\beta e^{-E_{\alpha\beta}/T} \frac{1}{T}\sum_{\lambda\mu} e^{-E_{\lambda\mu}/T} s_i^{\lambda\mu} s_j^{\lambda\mu}}{\left(\sum_{\lambda\mu} e^{-E_{\lambda\mu}/T}\right)^2}$$

$$= \frac{1}{T}\left[\sum_\beta P^-(V_\alpha \wedge H_\beta) s_i^{\alpha\beta} s_j^{\alpha\beta} - P^-(V_\alpha)\sum_{\lambda\mu} P^-(V_\lambda \wedge H_\mu) s_i^{\lambda\mu} s_j^{\lambda\mu}\right].$$

This derivative is used to compute the gradient of the G-measure

$$G = \sum_\alpha P^+(V_\alpha) \ln \frac{P^+(V_\alpha)}{P^-(V_\alpha)}$$

where $P^+(V_\alpha)$ is the clamped probability distribution over the visible units and is independent of w_{ij}. So

$$\frac{\partial G}{\partial w_{ij}} = -\sum_\alpha \frac{P^+(V_\alpha)}{P^-(V_\alpha)} \frac{\partial P^-(V_\alpha)}{\partial w_{ij}}$$

$$= -\frac{1}{T} \left[\sum_\alpha \frac{P^+(V_\alpha)}{P^-(V_\alpha)} \sum_\beta P^-(V_\alpha \wedge H_\beta) s_i^{\alpha\beta} s_j^{\alpha\beta} \right.$$

$$\left. - \sum_\alpha \frac{P^+(V_\alpha)}{P^-(V_\alpha)} P^-(V_\alpha) \sum_{\lambda\mu} P^-(V_\lambda \wedge H_\mu) s_i^{\lambda\mu} s_j^{\lambda\mu} \right].$$

Now,

$$P^+(V_\alpha \wedge H_\beta) = P^+(H_\beta|V_\alpha) P^+(V_\alpha),$$

$$P^-(V_\alpha \wedge H_\beta) = P^-(H_\beta|V_\alpha) P^-(V_\alpha),$$

and

$$P^-(H_\beta|V_\alpha) = P^+(H_\beta|V_\alpha). \tag{9}$$

Equation 9 holds because the probability of a hidden state given some visible state must be the same in equilibrium whether the visible units were clamped in that state or arrived there by free-running. Hence,

$$P^-(V_\alpha \wedge H_\beta) \frac{P^+(V_\alpha)}{P^-(V_\alpha)} = P^+(V_\alpha \wedge H_\beta).$$

Also,

$$\sum_\alpha P^+(V_\alpha) = 1.$$

Therefore,

$$\frac{\partial G}{\partial w_{ij}} = -\frac{1}{T} [p_{ij}^+ - p_{ij}^-]$$

where

$$p_{ij}^+ \equiv \sum_{\alpha\beta} P^+(V_\alpha \wedge H_\beta) s_i^{\alpha\beta} s_j^{\alpha\beta}$$

and

$$p_{ij}^- \equiv \sum_{\lambda\mu} P^-(V_\lambda \wedge H_\mu) s_i^{\lambda\mu} s_j^{\lambda\mu}.$$

The Boltzmann machine learning algorithm can also be formulated as an input-output model. The visible units are divided into an input set I and an output set O, and an environment specifies a set of conditional probabilities of the form $P^+(O_\beta|I_\alpha)$. During $phase^+$ the environment clamps both the input and output units, and the p_{ij}^+s are estimated. During $phase^-$ the input units are clamped and the output units and hidden units free-run, and the p_{ij}^-s are estimated. The appropriate G measure in this case is

$$G = \sum_{\alpha\beta} P^+(I_\alpha \wedge O_\beta)\ln \frac{P^+(O_\beta|I_\alpha)}{P^-(O_\beta|I_\alpha)}.$$

Similar mathematics apply in this formulation and $\partial G/\partial w_{ij}$ is the same as before.

References

Ackley, D. H., Hinton, G. E., & Sejnowski, T. J. (1985). A learning algorithm for Boltzmann machines. *Cognitive Science, 9*, 147–169.

Bahl, L. R., Jelinek, F., & Mercer, R. L. (1983). A maximum likelihood approach to continuous speech recognition. *IEEE Transactions on Pattern Analysis and Machine Intelligence, 5*, 179–190.

Ballard, D. H., Hinton, G. E., & Sejnowski, T. J. (1983). Parallel visual computation. *Nature, 306*, 21–26.

Blake, A. (1983). The least disturbance principle and weak constraints. *Pattern Recognition Letters, 1*, 393–399.

Crick, F., & Mitchison, G. (1983). The function of dream sleep. *Nature, 304*, 111–114.

Dempster, A. P., Laird, N. M., & Rubin, D. B. (1976). Maximum likelihood from incomplete data via the EM algorithm. *Proceedings of the Royal Statistical Society*, 1–38.

Derthick, M. (1984). *Variations on the Boltzmann machine learning algorithm* (Tech. Rep. No. CMU-CS-84-120). Pittsburgh: Carnegie-Mellon University, Department of Computer Science.

Fukushima, K. (1980). Neocognitron: A self-organizing neural network model for a mechanism of pattern recognition unaffected by shift in position. *Biological Cybernetics, 36*, 193–202.

Geman, S., & Geman, D. (1984). Stochastic relaxation, Gibbs distributions, and the Bayesian restoration of images. *IEEE Transactions on Pattern Analysis and Machine Intelligence, 6*, 721–741.

Hinton, G. E. (1977). *Relaxation and its role in vision*. Unpublished doctoral dissertation, University of Edinburgh.

Hinton, G. E., & Sejnowski, T. J. (1983a). Analyzing cooperative computation. *Proceedings of the Fifth Annual Conference of the Cognitive Science Society*.

Hinton, G. E., & Sejnowski, T. J. (1983b). Optimal perceptual inference. *Proceedings of the IEEE Computer Society Conference on Computer Vision and Pattern Recognition*, 448–453.

Hinton, G. E., Sejnowski, T. J., & Ackley, D. H. (1984). *Boltzmann machines: Constraint satisfaction networks that learn* (Tech. Rep. No. CMU-CS-84-119). Pittsburgh, PA: Carnegie-Mellon University, Department of Computer Science.

Hogg, T., & Huberman, B. A. (1984). Understanding biological computation. *Proceedings of the National Academy of Sciences, USA, 81*, 6871–6874.

Hopfield, J. J. (1982). Neural networks and physical systems with emergent collective computational abilities. *Proceedings of the National Academy of Sciences, USA, 79*, 2554–2558.

Hopfield, J. J., Feinstein, D. I., & Palmer, R. G. (1983). "Unlearning" has a stabilizing effect in collective memories. *Nature, 304*, 158–159.

Hummel, R. A., & Zucker, S. W. (1983). On the foundations of relaxation labeling processes. *IEEE Transactions on Pattern Analysis and Machine Intelligence, 5*, 267–287.

Kirkpatrick, S., Gelatt, C. D. Jr., & Vecchi, M. P. (1983). Optimization by simulated annealing. *Science, 220*, 671–680.

Kullback, S. (1959). *Information theory and statistics.* New York: Wiley.

Marr, D. (1982). *Vision.* San Francisco: Freeman.

Minsky, M., & Papert, S. (1969). *Perceptrons.* Cambridge, MA: MIT Press.

Moussouris, J. (1974). Gibbs and Markov random systems with constraints. *Journal of Statistical Physics, 10*, 11–33.

Rosenblatt, F. (1962). *Principles of neurodynamics.* New York: Spartan.

Rosenfeld, A., Hummel, R. A., & Zucker, S. W. (1976). Scene labeling by relaxation operations. *IEEE Transactions on Systems, Man, and Cybernetics, 6*, 420–433.

Rumelhart, D. E., & Zipser, D. (1985). Feature discovery by competitive learning. *Cognitive Science, 9*, 75–112.

Sejnowski, T. J., & Hinton, G. E. (1987). Separating figure from ground with a Boltzmann machine. In M. A. Arbib & A. R. Hanson (Eds.), *Vision, brain, and cooperative computation* (pp. 703–724). Cambridge, MA: MIT Press/Bradford.

Sejnowski, T. J., Hinton, G. E., Kienker, P., & Schumacher, L. E. (1985). *Figure-ground separation by simulated annealing.* Unpublished manuscript.

Smolensky, P. (1983). Schema selection and stochastic inference in modular environments. *Proceedings of the National Conference on Artificial Intelligence AAAI-83*, 109–113.

3

Learning in Boltzmann Trees

Lawrence Saul
Department of Physics, Massachusetts Institute of Technology,
Cambridge, MA 02139 USA

Michael I. Jordan
Department of Brain and Cognitive Sciences, Massachusetts Institute of Technology,
Cambridge, MA 02139 USA

We introduce a large family of Boltzmann machines that can be trained by standard gradient descent. The networks can have one or more layers of hidden units, with tree-like connectivity. We show how to implement the supervised learning algorithm for these Boltzmann machines exactly, without resort to simulated or mean-field annealing. The stochastic averages that yield the gradients in weight space are computed by the technique of decimation. We present results on the problems of N-bit parity and the detection of hidden symmetries.

1 Introduction

Boltzmann machines (Ackley *et al.* 1985) have several compelling virtues. Unlike simple perceptrons, they can solve problems that are not linearly separable. The learning rule, simple and locally based, lends itself to massive parallelism. The theory of Boltzmann learning, moreover, has a solid foundation in statistical mechanics. Unfortunately, Boltzmann machines—as originally conceived—also have some serious drawbacks. In practice, they are relatively slow. Simulated annealing (Kirkpatrick *et al.* 1983), though effective, entails a great deal of computation. Finally, compared to backpropagation networks (Rumelhart *et al.* 1986), where weight updates are computed by the chain rule, Boltzmann machines lack a certain degree of exactitude. Monte Carlo estimates of stochastic averages (Binder and Heerman 1988) are not sufficiently accurate to permit further refinements to the learning rule, such as quasi-Newton or conjugate-gradient techniques (Press *et al.* 1986).

There have been efforts to overcome these difficulties. Peterson and Anderson (1987) introduced a mean-field version of the original Boltzmann learning rule. For many problems, this approximation works surprisingly well (Hinton 1989), so that mean-field Boltzmann machines learn much more quickly than their stochastic counterparts. Under certain circumstances, however, the approximation breaks down, and the

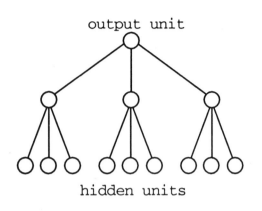

Figure 1: Boltzmann tree with two layers of hidden units. The input units (not shown) are fully connected to all the units in the tree.

mean-field learning rule works badly if at all (Galland 1993). Another approach (Hopfield 1987) is to focus on Boltzmann machines with architectures simple enough to permit exact computations. Learning then proceeds by straightforward gradient descent on the cost function (Yair and Gersho 1988), without the need for simulated or mean-field annealing. Hopfield (1987) wrote down the complete set of learning equations for a Boltzmann machine with one layer of noninterconnected hidden units. Freund and Haussler (1992) derived the analogous equations for the problem of unsupervised learning.

In this paper, we pursue this strategy further, concentrating on the case of supervised learning. We exhibit a large family of architectures for which it is possible to implement the Boltzmann learning rule in an exact way. The networks in this family have a hierarchical structure with tree-like connectivity. In general, they can have one or more layers of hidden units. We call them Boltzmann trees; an example is shown in Figure 1. We use a decimation technique from statistical physics to compute the averages in the Boltzmann learning rule. After describing the method, we give results on the problems of N-bit parity and the detection of hidden symmetries (Sejnowski *et al.* 1986). We also compare the performance of deterministic and true Boltzmann learning. Finally, we discuss a number of possible extensions to our work.

2 Boltzmann Machines

We briefly review the learning algorithm for the Boltzmann machine (Hertz *et al.* 1991). The Boltzmann machine is a recurrent network with binary units $S_i = \pm 1$ and symmetric weights $w_{ij} = w_{ji}$. Each configuration of units in the network represents a state of energy

$$\mathcal{H} = -\sum_{ij} w_{ij} S_i S_j \tag{2.1}$$

The network operates in a stochastic environment in which states of lower energy are favored. The units in the network change states with probability

$$P(S_i \rightarrow -S_i) = \frac{1}{1 + e^{\Delta \mathcal{H}/T}} \tag{2.2}$$

Once the network has equilibrated, the probability of finding it in a particular state obeys the Boltzmann distribution from statistical mechanics:

$$P = \frac{1}{Z} e^{-\mathcal{H}/T} \tag{2.3}$$

The partition function $Z = \sum e^{-\mathcal{H}/T}$ is the weighted sum over states needed to normalize the Boltzmann distribution. The temperature T determines the amount of noise in the network; as the temperature is decreased, the network is restricted to states of lower energy.

We consider a network with I input units, H hidden units, and O output units. The problem to be solved is one of supervised learning. Input patterns are selected from a training set with probability $P^*(I_\mu)$. Likewise, target outputs are drawn from a probability distribution $P^*(O_\nu | I_\mu)$. The goal is to teach the network the desired associations. Both the input and output patterns are binary. A particular example is said to be learned if after clamping the input units to the selected input pattern and waiting for the network to equilibrate, the output units are in the desired target states.

A suitable cost function for this supervised learning problem is

$$E = \sum_\mu P^*(I_\mu) \sum_\nu P^*(O_\nu | I_\mu) \ln \left[\frac{P^*(O_\nu | I_\mu)}{P(O_\nu | I_\mu)} \right] \tag{2.4}$$

where $P^*(O_\nu | I_\mu)$ and $P(O_\nu | I_\mu)$ are the desired and observed probabilities that the output units have pattern O_ν when the input units are clamped to pattern I_μ. The Boltzmann learning algorithm attempts to minimize this cost function by gradient descent. The calculation of the gradients in weight space is straightforward. The final result is the Boltzmann learning rule

$$\Delta w_{ij} = \frac{\eta}{T} \sum_\mu P^*(I_\mu) \left[\langle S_i S_j \rangle_{I,O}^\mu - \langle S_i S_j \rangle_I^\mu \right] \tag{2.5}$$

where brackets $\langle \cdots \rangle$ indicate expectation values over the Boltzmann distribution. The gradients in weight space depend on two sets of correlations—one in which the O output units are clamped to their desired targets, the other in which they are allowed to equilibrate. In both cases, the I input units are clamped to the pattern being learned. The differences in these correlations, averaged over the examples in the training set, yield the weight updates Δw_{ij}. An on-line version of Boltzmann learning is obtained by foregoing the average over input patterns and updating the weights after each example. Finally, the parameter η sets the learning rate.

The main drawback of Boltzmann learning is that, in most networks, it is not possible to compute the gradients in weight space directly. Instead, one must resort to estimating the correlations $\langle S_i S_j \rangle$ by Monte Carlo simulation (Binder *et al.* 1988). The method of simulated annealing (Kirkpatrick *et al.* 1983) leads to accurate estimates but has the disadvantage of being very computation-intensive. A mean-field version of the algorithm (Peterson and Anderson 1987) was proposed to speed up learning. It makes the approximation $\langle S_i S_j \rangle \approx \langle S_i \rangle \langle S_j \rangle$ in the learning rule and estimates the magnetizations $\langle S_i \rangle$ by solving a set of nonlinear equations. This is done by iteration, combined when necessary with an annealing process. So-called mean-field annealing can yield an order-of-magnitude improvement in convergence. Clearly, however, the ideal algorithm would be one that computes expectation values exactly and does not involve the added complication of annealing. In the next section, we investigate a large family of networks amenable to exact computations of this sort.

3 Boltzmann Trees

A Boltzmann tree is a Boltzmann machine whose hidden and output units have a special hierarchical organization. There are no restrictions on the input units, and, in general, we will assume them to be fully connected to the rest of the network. For convenience, we will focus on the case of one output unit; an example of such a Boltzmann tree is shown in Figure 1. Modifications to this basic architecture and the generalization to many output units will be discussed later.

The key technique to compute partition functions and expectation values in these trees is known as decimation (Eggarter 1974; Itzykson and Drouffe 1991). The idea behind decimation is the following. Consider three units connected in series, as shown in Figure 2a. Though not directly connected, the end units S_1 and S_2 have an effective iteration that is mediated by the middle one S. Define the temperature-rescaled weights $J_{ij} \equiv w_{ij}/T$. We claim that the combination of the two weights J_1 and J_2 in series has the same effect as a single weight J. Replacing the weights in this way, we have integrated out, or "decimated," the degree of freedom represented by the intermediate unit. To derive an expression for J, we require that the units S_1 and S_2 in both systems obey the same Boltzmann distribution. This will be true if

$$\sum_{S=\pm 1} e^{J_1 S_1 S + J_2 S S_2} = \sqrt{C} e^{J S_1 S_2} \tag{3.1}$$

where C is a constant prefactor, independent of S_1 and S_2. Enforcing equality for the possible values of $S_1 = \pm 1$ and $S_2 = \pm 1$, we obtain the constraints

$$\sqrt{C} e^{\pm J} = 2 \cosh(J_1 \pm J_2)$$

It is straightforward to eliminate C and solve for the effective weight J. Omitting the algebra, we find

$$\tanh J = \tanh J_1 \tanh J_2 \tag{3.2}$$

Choosing J in this way, we ensure that all expectation values involving S_1 and/or S_2 will be the same in both systems.

Decimation is a technique for combining weights "in series." The much simpler case of combining weights "in parallel" is illustrated in Figure 2b. In this case, the effective weight is simply the additive sum of J_1 and J_2, as can be seen by appealing to the energy function of the network, equation 2.1. Note that the rules for combining weights in series and in parallel are valid if either of the end units S_1 or S_2 happen to be clamped. They also hold locally for weight combinations that are embedded in larger networks. The rules have simple analogs in other types of networks (e.g., the law for combining resistors in electric circuits). Indeed, the strategy for exploiting these rules is a familiar one. Starting with a complicated network, we iterate the rules for combining weights until we have a simple network whose properties are easily computed. Clearly, the rules do not make all networks tractable; networks with full connectivity between hidden units, for example, cannot be systematically reduced. Hierarchical networks with tree-like connectivity, however, lend themselves naturally to these types of operations.

Let us see how we can use these rules to implement the Boltzmann learning rule in an exact way. Consider the two-layer Boltzmann tree in Figure 1. The effect of clamping the input units to a selected pattern is to add a bias to each of the units in the tree, as in Figure 3a. Note that these biases depend not only on the input weights, but also on the pattern distributed over the input units. Having clamped the input units, we must now compute expectation values. For concreteness, we consider the case where the output unit is allowed to equilibrate. Correlations between adjacent units are computed by decimating over the other units in the tree; the procedure is illustrated in Figure 3b for the lower leftmost hidden units. The final, reduced network consists of the two adjacent

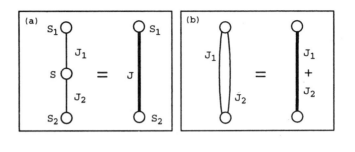

Figure 2: (a) Combining weights in series: the effective interaction between units S_1 and S_2 is the same as if they were directly connected by weight J, where $\tanh J = \tanh J_1 \tanh J_2$. (b) Combining weights in parallel: the effective weight is simply the additive sum. The same rules hold if either of the end units is clamped.

units with weight J and effective biases (h_1, h_2). A short calculation gives

$$\langle S_1 S_2 \rangle = \frac{e^J \cosh(h_1 + h_2) - e^{-J} \cosh(h_1 - h_2)}{e^J \cosh(h_1 + h_2) + e^{-J} \cosh(h_1 - h_2)} \tag{3.3}$$

The magnetization of a tree unit can be computed in much the same way. We combine weights in series and parallel until only the unit of interest remains, as in Figure 3c. In terms of the effective bias h, we then have the standard result

$$\langle S_1 \rangle = \tanh h \tag{3.4}$$

The rules for combining weights thus enable us to compute expectation values without enumerating the $2^{13} = 8192$ possible configurations of units in the tree. To compute the correlation $\langle S_1 S_2 \rangle$ for two adjacent units in the tree, one successively removes all "outside" fluctuating units until only units S_1 and S_2 remain. To compute the magnetization $\langle S_1 \rangle$, one removes unit S_2 as well.

Implementing these operations on a computer is relatively straightforward, due to the hierarchical organization of the output and hidden units. The entire set of correlations and magnetizations can be computed by making two recursive sweeps through the tree, storing effective weights as necessary to maximize the efficiency of the algorithm. Having to clamp the output unit to the desired target does not introduce any difficulties. In this case, the output unit merely contributes (along with the input units) to the bias on its derivative units. Again, we use recursive decimation to compute the relevant stochastic averages. We are thus able to implement the Boltzmann learning rule in an exact way.

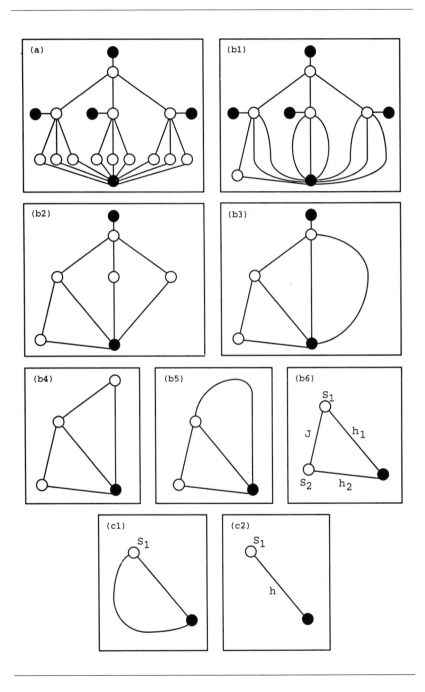

Table 1: Boltzmann Tree Performance on N-bit Parity.[a]

N	Hidden units	e_{max}	Success %	e_{avg}
2	1	50	97.2 (89.3)	25.8
3	1	250	96.1 (88.5)	42.1
4	3	1000	95.1 (69.2)	281.1
5	4	1000	92.9 (84.2)	150.0

[a]The results in parentheses are for mean-field learning.

4 Results

We tested Boltzmann trees on two familiar problems: N-bit parity and the detection of hidden symmetries (Sejnowski et al. 1986). We hope our results demonstrate not only the feasibility of the algorithm, but also the potential of exact Boltzmann learning. Table 1 shows our results on the N-bit parity problem, using Boltzmann trees with one layer of hidden units. In each case, we ran the algorithm 1000 times. All 2^N possible input patterns were included in the training set. A success indicates that the tree learned the parity function in less than e_{max} epochs. We also report the average number of epochs e_{avg} per successful trial; in these cases, training was stopped when $P(O^* \mid I_\mu) \geq 0.9$ for each of the 2^N inputs, with $O^* = \text{parity}(I_\mu)$. The results show Boltzmann trees to be competitive with standard backpropagation networks (Møller, 1993).

We also tested Boltzmann trees on the problem of detecting hidden symmetries. In the simplest version of this problem, the input patterns are square pixel arrays that have mirror symmetry about a fixed horizontal or vertical axis (but not both). We used a two-layer tree with the architecture shown in Figure 1 to detect these symmetries in 10×10 square arrays. The network learned to differentiate the two types of patterns from a training set of 2000 examples. After each epoch, we tested the network on a set of 200 unknown examples. The performance on these patterns measures the network's ability to generalize to unfamiliar inputs. The results, averaged over 100 separate trials, are shown in Figure 4. After 100 epochs, average performance was over 95% on the training set and over 85% on the test set.

Figure 3: *Facing page.* Reducing Boltzmann trees by combining weights in series and parallel. Solid circles represent clamped units. (a) Effect of clamping the input units to a selected pattern. (b) Computing the correlation between adjacent units. (c) Computing the magnetization of a single unit.

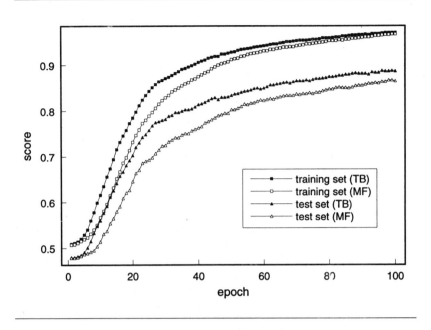

Figure 4: Results on the problem of detecting hidden symmetries for true Boltzmann (TB) and mean-field (MF) learning.

Finally, we investigated the use of the deterministic, or mean-field, learning rule (Peterson and Anderson 1987) in Boltzmann trees. We repeated our experiments, substituting $\langle S_i \rangle \langle S_j \rangle$ for $\langle S_i S_j \rangle$ in the update rule. Note that we computed the magnetizations $\langle S_i \rangle$ exactly using decimation. In fact, in most deterministic Boltzmann machines, one does not compute the magnetizations exactly, but estimates them within the mean-field approximation. Such networks therefore make two approximations—first, that $\langle S_i S_j \rangle \approx \langle S_i \rangle \langle S_j \rangle$ and second, that $\langle S_i \rangle \approx \tanh(\sum J_{ij} \langle S_j \rangle + h_i)$. Our results speak to the first of these approximations. At this level alone, we find that exact Boltzmann learning is perceptibly faster than mean-field learning. On one problem in particular, that of $N = 4$ parity (see Table I), the difference between the two learning schemes was quite pronounced.

5 Extensions

In conclusion, we mention several possible extensions to the work in this paper. Clearly, a number of techniques used in backpropagation networks, such as conjugate-gradient and quasi-Newton methods (Press *et al.* 1986), could also be used to accelerate learning in Boltzmann trees. In this paper, we have considered the basic architecture in which a single output unit sits atop a tree of one or more hidden layers. Depending on the problem, a variation on this architecture may be more appropriate. The network must have a hierarchical organization to remain tractable; within this framework, however, the algorithm permits countless arrangements of hidden and output units. In particular, a tree can have one or more output units, and these output units can be distributed in an arbitrary way throughout the tree. One can incorporate certain intralayer connections into the tree at the expense of introducing a slightly more complicated decimation rule, valid when the unit to be decimated is biased by a connection to an additional clamped unit. There are also decimation rules for q-state (Potts) units, with $q > 2$ (Itzykson and Drouffe 1991).

The algorithm for Boltzmann trees raises a number of interesting questions. Some of these involve familiar issues in neural network design—for instance, how to choose the number of hidden layers and units. We would also like to characterize the types of learning problems best suited to Boltzmann trees. A recent study by Galland (1993) suggests that mean-field learning has trouble in networks with several layers of hidden units and/or large numbers of output units. Boltzmann trees with exact Boltzmann learning may present a viable option for problems in which the basic assumption behind mean-field learning—that the units in the network can be treated independently—does not hold. We know of constructive algorithms (Frean 1990) for feedforward nets that yield tree-like solutions; an analogous construction for Boltzmann machines has obvious appeal, in view of the potential for exact computations. Finally, the tractability of Boltzmann trees is reminiscent of the tractability of tree-like belief networks, proposed by Pearl (1986, 1988); more sophisticated rules for computing probabilities in belief networks (Lauritzen and Spiegelhalter, 1988) may have useful counterparts in Boltzmann machines. These issues and others are left for further study.

Acknowledgments

The authors thank Mehran Kardar for useful discussions. This research was supported by the Office of Naval Research and by the MIT Center for Materials Science and Engineering through NSF Grant DMR-90-22933.

References

Ackley, D. H., Hinton, G. E., and Sejnowski, T. J. 1985. A learning algorithm for Boltzmann machines. *Cog. Sci.* **9**, 147–169.
Binder, K., and Heerman, D. W. 1988. *Monte Carlo Simulation in Statistical Mechanics.* Springer-Verlag, Berlin.

Eggarter, T. P. 1974. Cayley trees, the Ising problem, and the thermodynamic limit. *Phys. Rev. B* **9**, 2989–2992.

Frean, M. 1990. The upstart algorithm: A method for constructing and training feedforward neural networks. *Neural Comp.* **2**, 198–209.

Freund, Y., and Haussler, D. 1992. Unsupervised learning of distributions on binary vectors using two layer networks. In *Advances in Neural Information Processing Systems IV* (Denver 1992), J. E. Moody, S. J. Hanson, and R. P. Lippman, eds., pp. 912–919. Morgan Kaufmann, San Mateo, CA.

Galland, C. C. 1993. The limitations of deterministic Boltzmann machine learning. *Network: Comp. Neural Syst.* **4**, 355–379.

Hertz, J., Krogh, A., and Palmer, R. G. 1991. *Introduction to the Theory of Neural Computation.* Addison-Wesley, Redwood City.

Hinton, G. E. 1989. Deterministic Boltzmann learning performs steepest descent in weight space. *Neural Comp.* **1**, 143–150.

Hopfield, J. J. 1987. Learning algorithms and probability distributions in feedforward and feed-back networks. *Proc. Natl. Acad. Sci. U.S.A.* **84**, 8429–8433.

Itzykson, C., and Drouffe, J. 1991. *Statistical Field Theory.* Cambridge University Press, Cambridge.

Kirkpatrick, S., Gellatt Jr, C. D., and Vecchi, M. P. 1983. Optimization by simulated annealing. *Science* **220**, 671–680.

Lauritzen, S. L., and Spiegelhalter, D. J. 1988. Local computations with probabilities on graphical structures and their application to expert systems. *J. R. Stat. Soc. B* **50**, 157–224.

Møller, M. F. 1993. A scaled conjugate gradient algorithm for fast supervised learning. *Neural Networks* **6**, 525–533.

Pearl, J. 1986. Fusion, propagation, and structuring in belief networks. *Artif. Intelligence* **19**, 241–288.

Pearl, J. 1988. *Probabilistic Reasoning in Intelligent Systems.* Morgan Kaufmann, San Mateo, CA.

Peterson, C., and Anderson, J. R. 1987. A mean field theory learning algorithm for neural networks. *Complex Syst.* **1**, 995–1019.

Press, W. H., Flannery, B. P., Teukolsky, S. A., and Vetterling, W. T. 1986. *Numerical Recipes.* Cambridge University Press, Cambridge.

Rumelhart, D. E., Hinton, G. E., and Williams, R. J. 1986. Learning representations by back-propagating errors. *Nature (London)* **323**, 533–536.

Sejnowski, T. J., Kienker, P. K., and Hinton, G. E. 1986. Learning symmetry groups with hidden units. *Physica* **22D**, 260–275.

Yair, E., and Gersho, A. 1988. The Boltzmann perceptron network: A multilayered feed-forward network equivalent to the Boltzmann machine. In *Advances in Neural Information Processing Systems I* (Denver 1988), D. S. Touretzky, ed., pp. 116–123. Morgan Kaufmann, San Mateo, CA.

4

Deterministic Boltzmann Learning Performs Steepest Descent in Weight-Space

Geoffrey E. Hinton
Department of Computer Science, University of Toronto,
10 King's College Road, Toronto M5S 1A4, Canada

The Boltzmann machine learning procedure has been successfully applied in deterministic networks of analog units that use a mean field approximation to efficiently simulate a truly stochastic system (Peterson and Anderson 1987). This type of "deterministic Boltzmann machine" (DBM) learns much faster than the equivalent "stochastic Boltzmann machine" (SBM), but since the learning procedure for DBM's is only based on an analogy with SBM's, there is no existing proof that it performs gradient descent in any function, and it has only been justified by simulations. By using the appropriate interpretation for the way in which a DBM represents the probability of an output vector given an input vector, it is shown that the DBM performs steepest descent in the same function as the original SBM, except at rare discontinuities. A very simple way of forcing the weights to become symmetrical is also described, and this makes the DBM more biologically plausible than back-propagation (Werbos 1974; Parker 1985; Rumelhart et al. 1986).

1 Introduction

The promising results obtained by Peterson and Anderson (Peterson and Anderson 1987) using a DBM are hard to assess because they present no mathematical guarantee that the learning does gradient descent in any error function (except in the limiting case of a very large net with small random weights). It is quite conceivable that in a DBM the computed gradient might have a small systematic difference from the true gradient of the normal performance measure for each training case, and when these slightly incorrect gradients are added together over many cases their resultant might bear little relation to the resultant of the true casewise gradients (see Fig. 1).

2 The Learning Procedure for Stochastic Boltzmann Machines

A Boltzmann machine (Hinton and Sejnowski 1986) is a network of symmetrically connected binary units that asynchronously update their states according to a *stochastic* decision rule. The units have states of 1 or 0 and the probability that unit i adopts the state 1 is given by

$$p_i = \sigma(\frac{1}{T}\sum_j s_j w_{ij})$$ (2.1)

where s_j is the state of the jth unit, w_{ij} is the weight on the connection between the jth and the ith unit, T is the "temperature" and σ is a smooth non-linear function defined as

$$\sigma(x) = \frac{1}{1 + e^{-x}}$$ (2.2)

If the binary states of units are updated asynchronously and repeatedly using equation 2.1, the network will reach "thermal equilibrium" so that the relative probabilities of global configurations are determined by their energies according to the Boltzmann distribution:

$$\frac{P_\alpha}{P_\beta} = \frac{e^{-E_\alpha/T}}{e^{-E_\beta/T}}$$ (2.3)

where P_α is the probability of a global configuration and E_α is its energy defined by

$$E_\alpha = -\sum_{i<j} s_i^\alpha s_j^\alpha w_{ij}$$ (2.4)

where s_i^α is the binary state of unit i in the αth global configuration, and bias terms are ignored because they can always be treated as weights on connections from a permanently active unit.

At any given temperature, T, the Boltzmann distribution is the one that minimizes the Helmholtz free energy, F, of the distribution. F is defined by the equation

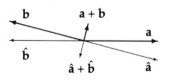

Figure 1: The true gradients of the performance measure are **a** and **b** for two training cases. Even fairly accurate estimates, **â** and **b̂**, can have a resultant that points in a very different direction.

$$F = \langle E \rangle - TH \tag{2.5}$$

where $\langle E \rangle$ is the expected value of the energy given the probability distribution over configurations and H is the entropy of the distribution. It can be shown that minima of F (which will be denoted by F^*) satisfy the equation

$$e^{-F^*/T} = \sum_\alpha e^{-E_\alpha/T} \tag{2.6}$$

In a stochastic Boltzmann machine, the probability of an output vector, O_β, given an input vector, I_α is represented by

$$P^-(O_\beta|I_\alpha) = \frac{e^{-F^*_{\alpha\beta}/T}}{e^{-F^*_\alpha/T}} \tag{2.7}$$

where $F^*_{\alpha\beta}$ is the minimum free energy with I_α and O_β clamped, and F^*_α is the minimum free energy with just I_α clamped. A very natural way to observe $P^-(O_\beta|I_\alpha)$ is to allow the network to reach thermal equilibrium with I_α clamped, and to observe the probability of O_β. The key to Boltzmann machine learning is the simple way in which a small change to a weight, w_{ij}, affects the free energy and hence the log probability of an output vector in a network at thermal equilibrium.

$$\frac{\partial F^*}{\partial w_{ij}} = -\langle s_i s_j \rangle \tag{2.8}$$

where $\langle s_i s_j \rangle$ is the expected value of $s_i s_j$ in the minimum free energy distribution. The simple relationship between weight changes and log probabilities of output vectors makes it easy to teach the network an input-output mapping. The network is "shown" the mapping that it is required to perform by clamping an input vector on the input units and clamping the required output vector on the output units (with the appropriate conditional probability). It is then allowed to reach thermal equilibrium at $T = 1$, and at equilibrium each connection measures how often the units it connects are simultaneously active. This is repeated for all input-output pairs so that each connection can measure $\langle s_i s_j \rangle^+$, the expected probability, averaged over all cases, that unit i and unit j are simultaneously active at thermal equilibrium when the input and output vectors are both clamped. The network must also be run in just the same way but without clamping the output units to measure $\langle s_i s_j \rangle^-$, the expected probability that both units are active at thermal equilibrium when the output vector is determined by the network. Each weight is then updated by

$$\Delta w_{ij} = \epsilon(\langle s_i s_j \rangle^+ - \langle s_i s_j \rangle^-) \tag{2.9}$$

It follows from equation 2.7 and equation 2.8 that if ϵ is sufficiently small this performs steepest descent in an information theoretic measure, G, of the difference between the behavior of the output units when they are clamped and their behavior when they are not clamped.

$$G = \sum_{\alpha,\beta} P^+(I_\alpha, O_\beta) \log \frac{P^+(O_\beta \mid I_\alpha)}{P^-(O_\beta \mid I_\alpha)} \tag{2.10}$$

where I_α is a state vector over the input units, O_β is a state vector over the output units, P^+ is a probability measured at thermal equilibrium when both the input and output units are clamped, and P^- is a probability measured when only the input units are clamped.

Stochastic Boltzmann machines learn slowly, partly because of the time required to reach thermal equilibrium and partly because the learning is driven by the *difference* between two noisy variables, so these variables must be sampled for a long time at thermal equilibrium to reduce the noise. If we could achieve the same simple relationships between log probabilities and weights in a deterministic system, learning would be much faster.

3 Mean field theory

Under certain conditions, a stochastic system can be approximated by a deterministic one by replacing the stochastic binary variables of equation 2.1 by deterministic real-valued variables that represent their mean values

$$p_i = \sigma(\frac{1}{T} \sum_j p_j w_{ij}) \tag{3.1}$$

We could now perform discrete, asynchronous updates of the p_i using equation 3.1 or we could use a synchronous, discrete time approximation of the set of differential equations

$$\frac{dp_i}{dt} = -p_i + \sigma(\frac{1}{T} \sum_j p_j w_{ij}) \tag{3.2}$$

We shall view the p_i as a representation of a probability distribution over all binary global configurations. Since many different distributions can give rise to the same mean values for the p_i we shall assume that the distribution being represented is the one that maximizes the entropy, subject to the constraints imposed on the mean values by the p_i. Equivalently, it is the distribution in which the p_i are treated as the mean values of *independent* stochastic binary variables. Using equation 2.5 we can calculate the free energy of the distribution represented by the state of a DBM (at $T = 1$).

$$F = -\sum_{i<j} p_i p_j w_{ij} + \sum_i [p_i \log(p_i) + (1 - p_i) \log(1 - p_i)] \qquad (3.3)$$

Although the dynamics of the system defined by equation 3.2 do not consist in following the gradient of F, it can be shown that it always moves in a direction that has a positive cosine with the gradient of $-F$ so it settles to one of the minima of F (Hopfield 1984).

Mean field systems are normally viewed as approximations to systems that really contain higher order statistics, but they can also be viewed as exact systems that are strongly limited in the probability distributions that they can represent because they use only N real values to represent distributions over 2^N binary states. Within the limits of their representational powers, they are an efficient way of manipulating these large but constrained probability distributions.

4 Deterministic Boltzmann machine learning ──────────────

In a DBM, we shall define the representation of $P^-(O_\beta|I_\alpha)$ exactly as in equation 2.7, but now $F^*_{\alpha\beta}$ and F^*_α will refer to the free energies of the particular minima that the network actually settles into. Unfortunately, in a DBM this representation is no longer equivalent to the obvious way of defining $P^-(O_\beta|I_\alpha)$ which is to clamp I_α on the input units, settle to a minimum of F_α, and interpret the values of the output units as a representation of a probability distribution over output vectors, using the maximum entropy assumption.

The reason for choosing the first definition rather than the second is this: Provided the stable states that the network settles to do not change radically when the weights are changed slightly, it can now be shown that the mean field version of the Boltzmann machine learning procedure changes each weight in proportion to the gradient of $\log P^-(O_\beta|I_\alpha)$, which is exactly what is required to perform steepest descent in the performance measure G defined in equation 2.10.

When w_{ij} is incremented by an infinitessimal amount $\epsilon p_i p_j$ two things happen to F^* (see Fig. 2). First, the mean energy of the probability distribution represented by the state of the DBM is decreased by $\epsilon p^2_i p^2_j$ and, to first order, the mean energy of all nearby states of the DBM is decreased by the same amount. Second, the values of the p_i at which F is minimized change slightly so the stable state moves slightly. But, to first order, this movement of the minimum has *no* effect on the value of F because we are at a stable state in which $\partial F/\partial p_i = 0$ for all i. Hence the effect of incrementing w_{ij} by $\epsilon p_i p_j$ is simply to create a new, nearby stable state which, to first order, has a free energy that is $\epsilon p^2_i p^2_j$ lower than the old stable state. So, assuming $T = 1$, if all weights are incremented by $\epsilon p^+_i p^+_j$ in the stable state that has I_α and O_β clamped and are decremented by $\epsilon p^-_i p^-_j$ in the stable state that has only I_α clamped we have, from equation 2.7

$$\Delta w_{ij} = \epsilon(p_i^+ p_j^+ - p_i^- p_j^-) = \epsilon \frac{\partial \log P^-(O_\beta | I_\alpha)}{\partial w_{ij}} \tag{4.1}$$

This ensures that by making ϵ sufficiently small the learning procedure can be made to approximate steepest descent in G arbitrarily closely.

The derivation above is invalid if, with the same boundary conditions, a small change in the weights causes the network to settle to a stable state with a very different free energy. This can happen with energy landscapes like the one shown in figure 3. A small weight change caused by some other training case can cause a free energy barrier that prevents the network finding the deeper minimum. In simulations that repeatedly sweep through a fixed set of training cases, it is easy to avoid this phenomenon by always starting the network at the stable state that was found using the same boundary conditions on the previous sweep. This has the added advantage of eliminating almost all the computation required to settle on a stable state, and thus making a settling almost as fast as a forward pass of the back-propagation procedure.

Unfortunately, starting from the previous best state does not eliminate the possibility that a small free-energy barrier will disappear and a much better state will then be found when the network is running with the output units unclamped. This can greatly increase the denominator in equation 2.7 and thus greatly decrease the network's representation of the probability of a correct output vector. It should also be noted that it is conceivable that, due to local minima in the free energy landscape, F_α^* may actually be higher than $F_{\alpha\beta}^*$, in which case the network's representation of $P^-(O_\beta | I_\alpha)$ will exceed 1. In practice this does not seem to be a problem, and DBM's compare very favorably with back-propagation in learning speed.

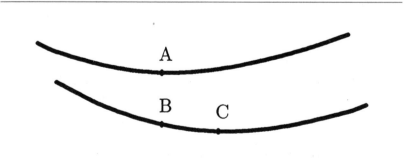

Figure 2: The effect of a small weight increment on a free energy minimum. To first order, the difference in free energy between A and C is equal to the difference between A and B. At a minimum, small changes in the distribution (sideways movements) have negligible effects on free energy, even though they may have significant (and opposite) effects on the energy and the entropy terms.

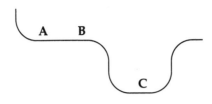

Figure 3: A small increase in the free energy of B can prevent a network from settling to the free energy minimum at C. So small changes in weights occasionally cause large changes in the final free energy.

5 Symmetry of the Weights

We have assumed that the weight of the connection from i to j is the same as the weight from j to i. If these weights are asymmetric, the learning procedure will automatically symmetrize them provided that, after each weight update, each weight is decayed slightly towards zero by an amount proportional to its magnitude. This favors "simple" networks that have small weights, and it also reduces the energy barriers that create local minima. Weight-decay always reduces the difference between w_{ij} and w_{ji}, and since the learning rule specifies weight changes that are exactly symmetrical in i and j, the two weights will always approach one another. Williams (1985) makes a similar argument about a different learning procedure. Thus the symmetry that is required to allow the network to compute its own error derivatives is easily achieved, whereas achieving symmetry between forward and backward weights in back-propagation networks requires much more complex schemes (Parker 1985).

6 Acknowledgments

I thank Christopher Longuet-Higgins, Conrad Galland, Scott Kirkpatrick, and Yann Le Cun for helpful comments. This research was supported by grants from the Ontario Information Technology Research Center, the National Science and Engineering Research Council of Canada, and DuPont. Geoffrey Hinton is a fellow of the Canadian Institute for Advanced Research.

References

Hinton, G.E. and T.J. Sejnowski. 1986. Learning and relearning in Boltz-
mann machines. *In:* Parallel Distributed Processing: Explorations in the
Microstructure of Cognition, Volume 1: Foundations, eds. D.E. Rumelhart,
J.L. McClelland, and the PDP group. Cambridge, MA: MIT Press.

Hopfield, J.J. 1984. Neurons with Graded Response Have Collective Computational Properties like Those of Two-state Neurons. *Proceedings of the National
Academy of Sciences U.S.A.* **81**, 3088–3092.

Parker, D.B. 1985. *Learning-logic.* Technical Report TR-47, Sloan School of Man-
agement, Massachusetts Institute of Technology, Cambridge, MA.

Peterson, C. and J.R. Anderson. 1987. A Mean Field Theory Learning Algorithm
for Neural Networks. *Complex Systems* **1**, 995–1019.

Rumelhart, D.E., G.E. Hinton, and R.J. Williams. 1986. Learning Representations by Back-propagating Errors. *Nature* **323**, 533–536.

Werbos, P.J. 1974. *Beyond Regression: New Tools for Prediction and Analysis in the
Behavioral Sciences.* PhD Thesis, Harvard University, Cambridge, MA.

Williams, R.J. 1985. *Feature Discovery through Error-correction Learning.* Technical
Report ICS-8501, Institute for Cognitive Science, University of California,
San Diego, La Jolla, CA.

5

Attractor Dynamics in Feedforward Neural Networks

Lawrence K. Saul
AT&T Labs—Research, Florham Park, NJ 07932, U.S.A.

Michael I. Jordan
University of California, Berkeley, CA 94720, U.S.A.

We study the probabilistic generative models parameterized by feedforward neural networks. An attractor dynamics for probabilistic inference in these models is derived from a mean field approximation for large, layered sigmoidal networks. Fixed points of the dynamics correspond to solutions of the mean field equations, which relate the statistics of each unit to those of its Markov blanket. We establish global convergence of the dynamics by providing a Lyapunov function and show that the dynamics generate the signals required for unsupervised learning. Our results for feedforward networks provide a counterpart to those of Cohen-Grossberg and Hopfield for symmetric networks.

1 Introduction

Attractor neural networks lend a computational purpose to continuous dynamical systems. Celebrated uses of these networks include the storage of associative memories (Amit, 1989), the reconstruction of noisy images (Koch, Marroquin, & Yuille, 1986), and the search for shortest paths in the traveling salesman problem (Hopfield & Tank, 1986). In all of these examples, a distributed computation is performed by an attractor dynamics and its flow to stable fixed points. These examples can also be formulated as problems in probabilistic reasoning; indeed, it is well known that symmetric neural networks can be analyzed as statistical mechanical ensembles or Markov random fields (MRFs).

Attractor neural networks and MRFs are connected by the idea of an energy surface. This connection has led to new algorithms for probabilistic inference in symmetric networks, a problem traditionally addressed by stochastic sampling procedures (Metropolis, Rosenbluth, Rosenbluth, Teller, & Teller, 1953; Geman & Geman, 1984). For example, in one of the first unsupervised learning algorithms for neural networks, Ackley, Hinton, and Sejnowski (1985) applied Gibbs sampling to estimate the statistics of binary MRFs. Known as Boltzmann machines, these networks relied on time-consuming Monte Carlo simulation and simulated annealing as an inner loop of their learning procedure. Subsequently, Peterson and Anderson

(1987) introduced a faster deterministic method for probabilistic inference. Their method, based on the so-called mean field approximation from statistical mechanics, transformed the binary-valued MRF into a network with continuous-valued units. The continuous network, endowed with dynamics given by the mean field equations, is itself an attractor network; in particular, it possesses a Lyapunov function (Cohen & Grossberg, 1983; Hopfield, 1984). Thus, one can perform approximate probabilistic inference in a binary MRF by relaxing a deterministic, continuous network.

In this article, we show that this linkage of attractor dynamics and probabilistic inference is not limited to symmetric networks or (equivalently) to models represented as undirected graphs. We investigate an attractor dynamics for feedforward networks, or directed acyclic graphs (DAGs); these are networks with directed edges but no directed loops. The probabilistic models represented by DAGs are known as Bayesian networks, and together with MRFs, they comprise the class of probabilistic models known as graphical models (Lauritzen, 1996). Like their undirected counterparts, Bayesian networks have been proposed as models of both artificial and biological intelligence (Pearl, 1988).

The units in Bayesian networks represent random variables, while the links represent assertions of conditional independence. These independence relations endow DAGs with a precise probabilistic semantics. Any joint distribution over a fixed, finite set of random variables can be represented by a Bayesian network, just as it can be represented by an MRF. What is compactly represented by one type of graphical model, however, may be quite clumsily represented by the other. MRFs arise naturally in statistical mechanics, where they describe the Gibbs distributions for systems in thermal equilibrium. Bayesian networks, on the other hand, are designed to model causal or generative processes; hidden Markov models, Kalman filters, soft-split decision trees—these are all examples of Bayesian networks.

The connection between Bayesian networks and neural network models of learning was pointed out by Neal (1992). Neal studied Bayesian networks whose units represented binary random variables and whose conditional probability tables were parameterized by sigmoid functions. He showed that these probabilistic networks have gradient-based learning rules that depend only on locally available information (Buntine, 1994; Binder, Koller, Russell, & Kanazawa, 1997). These observations led Dayan, Hinton, Neal, and Zemel (1995) and Hinton, Dayan, Frey, and Neal (1995) to propose the Helmholtz machine—a multilayered probabilistic network that learns hierarchical generative models of sensory inputs. Helmholtz machines were conceived not only as tools for statistical pattern recognition, but also as abstract models of top-down and bottom-up processing in the brain.

Following the work on Helmholtz machines, a number of researchers began to investigate unsupervised learning in large, layered Bayesian networks (Lewicki & Sejnowski, 1996; Saul, Jaakkola, & Jordan, 1996). As in undirected MRFs, probabilistic inference in these networks is generally intractable, and approximations are required. Saul et al. (1996) proposed a mean field approximation for these networks, analogous to the existing one for Boltzmann machines. Their approximation transformed the binary-valued network into a continuous-valued network whose statistics were described by a set of mean field equations. These equations related the statistics of each unit to a weighted sum of statistics from its Markov blanket (Pearl, 1988), a natural generalization of the notion of neighborhood in undirected MRFs. This earlier work did not, however, exhibit the solutions of these equations as fixed points of a simple continuous dynamical system. In particular, Saul et al. (1996) did not provide an attractor dynamics nor a Lyapunov function for their mean field equations.

In this article, we bring this sequence of ideas full circle by forging a link between attractor dynamics and probabilistic inference for directed networks. The link is achieved via mean field theory, just as in the undirected case. In particular, we describe an attractor dynamics whose stable fixed points correspond to solutions of the mean field equations. We also establish global convergence of these dynamics by providing a Lyapunov function. Our results thus provide an understanding of feedforward (Bayesian) networks that parallels the usual understanding of symmetric (MRF) networks. In both cases, we have a satisfying semantics for the set of allowed probability distributions; in both cases, we have a mean field theory that sidesteps the intractability of exact probabilistic inference; and in both cases, we have an attractor dynamics that transforms a discrete-valued network into a continuous dynamical system.

While this article builds on previous work, we have tried to keep it self-contained. The organization is as follows. In section 2, we introduce the probabilistic models represented by DAGs and review the problems of inference and learning. In section 3, we present the mean field theory for these networks: the mean field equations, the attractor dynamics, and the learning rule. In section 4, we describe some experiments on a database of handwritten digits and compare our results to known benchmarks. Finally, in section 5, we present our conclusions, as well as directions for future research.

2 Probabilistic DAGs

Consider a feedforward network—or equivalently, a directed acyclic graph—in which each unit represents a binary random variable $S_i \in \{0, 1\}$ and each link corresponds to a nonzero, real-valued weight, W_{ij}, to unit i from unit j. Thus, W_{ij} is a weight matrix whose zeros indicate missing links in the underlying DAG. Note that by assumption, W_{ij} is zero for $j \geq i$.

We can view this network as defining a probabilistic model in which missing links correspond to statements of conditional independence. In particular, suppose that the instantiations of the random variables S_i are generated by a causal process in which each unit is activated or inhibited (i.e., set to one or zero) depending on the values of its parents. This generative process is modeled by the joint distribution

$$P(S) = \prod_i P(S_i|S_1, S_2, \ldots, S_{i-1}) = \prod_i P(S_i|\pi_{S_i}), \tag{2.1}$$

where π_{S_i} denotes the parents of the ith unit. Equation 2.1 states that given the values of its parents, the ith unit is conditionally independent of its other ancestors in the graph. These qualitative statements of conditional independence are encoded by the structure of the graph and hold for arbitrary values of the weights W_{ij} attached to nonmissing links.

The quantitative predictions of the model are determined by the conditional distributions, $P(S_i|\pi_{S_i})$, in equation 2.1. In this article, we consider sigmoid networks for which

$$P(S_i = 1|\pi_{S_i}) = \sigma\left(\sum_j W_{ij}S_j\right), \tag{2.2}$$

where $\sigma(z) = [1 + e^{-z}]^{-1}$; thus the sign of W_{ij}, positive or negative, determines whether unit j excites or inhibits unit i in the generative process. Although we have not done so here, it is straightforward to include a bias term in the argument of the sigmoid function. Note that the weights in the network induce correlations between the units in the network, with higher-order correlations arising as information is propagated through one or more layers. The sigmoid nonlinearity ensures that the multilayer network does not have a single-layer equivalent. In what follows, we denote by $\sigma_i = \sigma(\sum_j W_{ij}S_j)$ the squashed weighted sum on the right-hand side of equation 2.2; this top-down signal, received by each unit from its parents, can also be regarded as a random variable in its own right.

Layered networks of this form (see Figure 1) were introduced as hierarchical generative models by Hinton et al. (1995). In typical applications, one imagines the units in the bottom layer to encode sensory data and the units in the top layers to encode different dimensions of variability. Thus, for example, in networks for image recognition, the bottom units might encode pixel values, while the top units encode higher-order features such as orientation and occlusion. The promise of these networks lies in their ability to parameterize hierarchical, nonlinear models of multiple interacting causes.

Effective use of these networks requires the ability to make probabilistic inferences. Essentially these are queries to ascertain likely values for certain units in the network, given values—or evidence—for other units. Let V denote the visible units for which values are known and H the hidden units for which values must be inferred. In principle, inferences can be made from the posterior distribution,

$$P(H|V) = \frac{P(H, V)}{P(V)}, \tag{2.3}$$

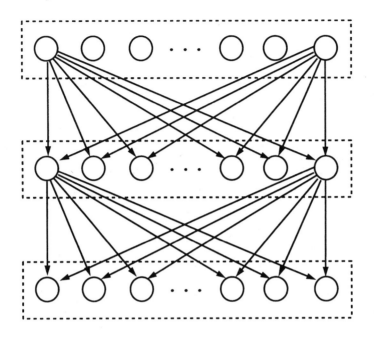

Figure 1: A layered Bayesian network parameterizes a hierarchical generative model for the data encoded by the units in its bottom layer.

where $P(H, V)$ is the joint distribution over hidden and visible units, as given by equation 2.1, and $P(V) = \sum_H P(H, V)$ is the marginal distribution obtained by summing over all configurations of hidden units. Exact probabilistic inference, however, is generally intractable in large Bayesian networks (Cooper, 1990). In particular, if there are many hidden units, then the sum to compute $P(V)$ involves an exponentially large number of terms. The same difficulty makes it impossible to compute statistics of the posterior distribution, $P(H|V)$.

Besides the problem of inference, one can also consider the problem of learning, or parameter estimation, in these networks. Unsupervised learning algorithms in probabilistic networks are designed to maximize the log-likelihood[1] of observed data. The likelihood of each data vector is given by the marginal distribution, $P(V) = \sum_H P(H, V)$. Local learning rules are derived by computing the gradients of the log-likelihood, $\ln P(V)$, with respect to the weights of the network (Neal, 1992; Binder et al., 1997). For each

---

[1] For simplicity of exposition, we do not consider forms of regularization (e.g., penalized likelihoods, cross-validation) that may be necessary to prevent overfitting.

data vector, this gives the on-line update:

$$\Delta W_{ij} \propto E\left[(S_i - \sigma_i)S_j\right],\tag{2.4}$$

where $E[\cdots]$ denotes an expectation with respect to the conditional distribution, $P(H|V)$, and $\sigma_i = \sigma(\sum_j W_{ij}S_j)$ is the top-down signal from the parents of the ith unit. Note that the update takes the form of a delta rule, with the top-down signal σ_i being matched to the target value provided by S_i. Intuitively, the learning rule adjusts the weights to bring each unit's expected value in line with an appropriate target value. These target values are specified explicitly by the evidence for the visible units in the network. For the other units in the network—the hidden units—appropriate target values must be computed by running an inference algorithm.

Generally in large, layered networks, we can compute neither the log-likelihood $\ln P(V)$ nor the statistics of $P(H|V)$ that appear in the learning rule, equation 2.4. A learning procedure can finesse these problems in two ways: (1) by optimizing the weights with respect to a more tractable cost function, or (2) by substituting approximate values for the statistics of the hidden units. As we shall see, both strategies are employed in the mean-field theory for these networks.

3 Mean Field Theory

Mean field theory is a general method from statistical mechanics for estimating the statistics of correlated random variables (Parisi, 1988). The name arises from physical models in which weighted sums of random variables, such as $\sum_j W_{ij}S_j$, are interpreted as local magnetic fields. Roughly speaking, under certain conditions, a central limit theorem may be applied to these sums, and a useful approximation is to ignore the fluctuations in these fields and replace them by their mean value—hence the name, "mean field" theory. More sophisticated versions of the approximation also exist, in which one incorporates the leading terms in an expansion about the mean.

The mean field approximation was originally developed for Gibbs distributions, as arise in MRFs. In this article we develop a mean field approximation for large, layered networks whose probabilistic semantics are given by equations 2.1 and 2.2. As in MRFs, our approximation exploits the averaging phenomena that occur at units whose conditional distributions, $P(S_i|\pi_{S_i})$, are parameterized in terms of weighted sums, such as $\sum_j W_{ij}S_j$. Addressing the twin issues of inference and learning, the approximation enables one to compute effective substitutes for the log-likelihood, $\ln P(V)$, and the statistics of the posterior distribution, $P(H|V)$.

The organization of this section is as follows. Section 3.1 describes the general approach behind the mean field approximation. Among its many interpretations, mean field theory can be viewed as a principled way of approximating an intractable probabilistic model by a tractable one. A variational principle chooses the parameters of the tractable model to minimize an entropic measure of error. The parameters of the tractable model are known as the mean field parameters, and they serve as placeholders for the true statistics of the posterior distribution, $P(H|V)$.

Our most important result for feedforward neural networks is a compact set of equations for determining the mean field parameters. These mean field equations relate the statistics of each unit to those of its Markov blanket. Section 3.2 gives a succinct statement of the mean field equations, along with a number of useful intuitions. A more detailed derivation is given in the appendix.

The mean field equations are a coupled set of nonlinear equations whose solutions cannot be expressed in closed form. Naturally, this raises the following concern: Have we merely replaced one intractable problem—that of calculating averages over the posterior distribution, $P(H|V)$—by an equally intractable one—that of solving the mean field equations? In section 3.3, we show how to solve the mean field equations using an attractor dynamics. This makes it quite straightforward to solve the mean field equations, typically at much less computational cost than (say) sampling the statistics of $P(H|V)$.

Finally, in section 3.4, we present a mean field learning algorithm for these networks. Weights are adapted by a regularized delta rule that depends only on locally available information. Interestingly, the attractor dynamics for solving the mean field equations generates precisely those signals required for unsupervised learning.

3.1 A Variational Principle. We now return to the problem of probabilistic inference in layered feedforward networks. Our goal is to obtain the statistics of the posterior distribution, $P(H|V)$, for some full or partial instantiation V of the units in the network. Since it is generally intractable to compute these statistics exactly, we adopt the following two-step approach: (1) introduce a parameterized family of simpler distributions whose statistics are easily computed; (2) approximate $P(H|V)$ by the member of this family that is "closest," as determined by some entropic measure of distance.

The starting point of the mean field approximation is to consider the family of factorial distributions:

$$Q(H|V) = \prod_{i \in H} \mu_i^{S_i} (1 - \mu_i)^{1-S_i}. \tag{3.1}$$

The parameters μ_i represent the mean values of the hidden units under the factorial distribution, $Q(H|V)$. Note that by design, most statistics of $Q(H|V)$ are easy to compute because the distribution is factorial.

We can measure the distance between the distribution $Q(H|V)$ in equation 3.1 and the true posterior distribution $P(H|V)$ by the Kullback-Leibler (KL) divergence:

$$KL(Q||P) = \sum_H Q(H|V) \ln \left[\frac{Q(H|V)}{P(H|V)} \right].$$ (3.2)

The KL divergence is strictly nonnegative, vanishing only if $Q(H|V) = P(H|V)$. The idea behind the mean field approximation is to find the parameters $\{\mu_i\}$ that minimize $KL(Q||P)$ and then to use the statistics of $Q(H|V)$ as a substitute for the statistics of $P(H|V)$. The first step of this calculation is to rewrite the posterior distribution $P(H|V)$ using equation 2.3, thus breaking the right-hand side of equation 3.1 into three terms:

$$KL(Q||P) = \sum_H Q(H|V) \ln Q(H|V)$$

$$- \sum_H Q(H|V) \ln P(H, V) + \ln P(V).$$ (3.3)

The first two terms on the right-hand side of this equation depend on properties of the approximate distribution, $Q(H|V)$. The first measures the (negative) entropy, and the second term measures the expected value of $\ln P(H, V)$. The last term in equation 3.3 is simply the log-likelihood of the evidence, which—importantly—does not depend on the statistics of $Q(H|V)$. Thus, this last term can be ignored when we minimize $KL(Q||P)$ with respect to the parameters $\{\mu_i\}$. It nevertheless has important consequences for learning, a subject to which we return in section 3.4.

3.2 Mean Field Equations. The first-order statistics of $Q(H|V)$ that minimize $KL(Q||P)$ naturally depend on the weights of the network, W_{ij}, and the evidence, V. This dependence is captured by the mean field equations, which are derived by evaluating and minimizing the right-hand side of equation 3.3. In this work, we make two simplifying assumptions to derive the mean field equations: first, that the weighted sum of inputs to each unit can be modeled by a gaussian distribution in large networks, and second, that certain intractable averages over $Q(H|V)$ can be approximated by the use of an additional variational principle. Details of these calculations are given in the appendix. In what follows, we present the mean field equations as a fait accompli so that we can emphasize the main intuitions that emerge from the approximation of $P(H|V)$ by $Q(H|V)$.

For sigmoid DAGs, the mean field approximation works by keeping track of two parameters, $\{\mu_i, \xi_i\}$, for each unit in the network. Although only the first of these appears explicitly in equation 3.1, it turns out that both are needed to evaluate and minimize the right-hand side of equation 3.3. Roughly speaking, these parameters are stored as approximations to the statistics of the true posterior distribution. In particular, $\mu_i \approx E[S_i|V]$ approximates each unit's posterior mean, while $\xi_i \approx E[\sigma_i|V]$ approximates the expected top-down signal in equation 2.2. In some trivial cases, these statistics can be computed exactly. For visible units, $E[S_i|V]$ is identically zero or one, as determined by the evidence, and for units with no parents, $E[\sigma_i|V]$ is constant, independent of the evidence. More generally, though, these statistics cannot be exactly computed, and the parameters $\{\mu_i, \xi_i\}$ represent approximate values.

The values of the mean field parameters $\{\mu_i, \xi_i\}$ are computed by solving a coupled set of nonlinear equations. For large, layered networks, these mean field equations are:

$$\mu_i = \sigma\left[\sum_j W_{ij}\mu_j + \sum_j W_{ji}(\mu_j - \xi_j) - \frac{1}{2}(1 - 2\mu_i)\sum_j W_{ji}^2\xi_j(1 - \xi_j)\right], \quad (3.4)$$

$$\xi_i = \sigma\left[\sum_j W_{ij}\mu_j + \frac{1}{2}(1 - 2\xi_i)\sum_j W_{ij}^2\mu_j(1 - \mu_j)\right]. \quad (3.5)$$

In certain cases, these equations may have multiple solutions. Roughly speaking, in these cases, each solution corresponds to the statistics of a different mode (or peak) of the posterior distribution.

The mean field equations couple the parameters of each unit to those of its parents and children. In layered networks, this amounts to a direct coupling between units in adjacent layers. The terms inside the brackets of equations 3.4 and 3.5 can be viewed as effective influences on each unit in the network. Let us examine these influences, concentrating for the moment on the leading-order terms linear in the weights, W_{ij}. In equation 3.4, we see that the parameter μ_i depends on the statistics of its Markov blanket (Pearl, 1988)—that is, on its parents through the weighted sum $\sum_j W_{ij}\mu_j$, on its children through the weighted sum $\sum_j W_{ji}\mu_j$, and on the parents of its children through the weighted sum $\sum_j W_{ji}\xi_j$. To some extent, the difference, $\sum_j W_{ji}(\mu_j - \xi_j)$, captures the effect of explaining away in which units in one layer are coupled by evidence in the layers below. In equation 3.5, we see that the parameter ξ_i depends on only the statistics of its parents, with the leading dependence coming through the weighted sum $\sum_j W_{ij}\mu_j$. Thus, we can interpret ξ_i as an approximation to the expected top-down signal, $E[\sigma_i|V]$. The quadratic terms in equations 3.4 and 3.5, proportional to W_{ij}^2, capture higher-order corrections to the dependencies already noted. For example, in equation 3.5, these terms cause any variance in the parents of unit i to push $\xi_i \approx E[\sigma_i|V]$ away from the extreme values of zero or one.

These directed probabilistic networks have twice as many mean field parameters as their undirected counterparts. For this we can offer the following intuition. Whereas the parameters μ_i are determined by top-down and bottom-up influences, the parameters ξ_i are determined only by top-down influences. The distinction—essentially one between parents and children—is meaningful only for directed graphical models.

3.3 Attractor Dynamics.
The mean field equations provide a self-consistent description of the statistics $\mu_i \approx E[S_i|V]$ and $\xi_i \approx E[\sigma_i|V]$ in terms of the corresponding statistics for the ith unit's Markov blanket. Except in special cases, however, the solutions to these equations cannot be expressed in closed form. Thus, in general, the values for the parameters $\{\mu_i, \xi_i\}$ must be found by numerically solving equations 3.4 and 3.5. This is greatly facilitated by expressing the solutions to these equations as fixed points of an attractor dynamics; we can then solve the mean field equations by integrating a set of differential equations. To this end, we associate with each unit the conjugate parameters:

$$g_i = \sum_j W_{ij}\mu_j + \sum_j W_{ji}(\mu_j - \xi_j) - \frac{1}{2}(1 - 2\mu_i)\sum_j W_{ji}^2\xi_j(1 - \xi_j), \quad (3.6)$$

$$h_i = \sum_j W_{ij}\mu_j + \frac{1}{2}(1 - 2\xi_i)\sum_j W_{ij}^2\mu_j(1 - \mu_j), \quad (3.7)$$

whose values are simply equal to the arguments of the sigmoid functions in the mean field equations. The variables g_i and h_i summarize the influences of the ith unit's Markov blanket. We consider the dynamics:

$$\tau_\mu\dot{\mu}_i = -[\mu_i - \sigma(g_i)], \quad (3.8)$$

$$\tau_h\dot{h}_i = +[\xi_i - \sigma(h_i)], \quad (3.9)$$

where τ_μ and τ_h are (positive) time constants and $\dot{\mu}_i$ and $\dot{h}_i$ are the time derivatives of μ_i and h_i. Note that equation 3.9 specifies the time derivative of h_i, not ξ_i. As we show below, however, this does not present any difficulty in integrating the dynamics.

By construction, the fixed points of this dynamics correspond to solutions of the mean field equations. To prove the stability of these fixed points, we introduce the Lyapunov function,

$$L = \sum_{ij}\left[-W_{ij}\mu_i\mu_j + \frac{1}{2}W_{ij}^2\xi_i^2\mu_j(1 - \mu_j)\right]$$

$$+ \sum_i\left[\int_0^{\mu_i}\sigma^{-1}(\mu)d\mu + \int_{-\infty}^{h_i}\sigma(h)dh\right], \quad (3.10)$$

where $\sigma^{-1}(\mu)$ is the inverse sigmoid function, that is, $\sigma^{-1}(\sigma(h)) = h$. The first and third terms in this Lyapunov function are identical to what Hopfield (1984) considered for symmetric networks; the others are peculiar to sigmoid DAGs. Consider the time derivative of this Lyapunov function under the dynamics of equations 3.8 and 3.9. Note that this dynamics does not correspond to a strict gradient descent in L, which would trivially give rise to a proof of convergence. With some straightforward algebra, however, one can show that

$$\dot{L} = -\sum_i \left\{ \left[\sigma^{-1}(\mu_i + \tau_\mu \dot{\mu}_i) - \sigma^{-1}(\mu_i) \right] \dot{\mu}_i + \tau_h \dot{h}_i^2 \right\} \leq 0, \qquad (3.11)$$

where the inequality follows from the observation that the sigmoid function is monotonically increasing. Thus, the function L always decreases under the attractor dynamics. As we discuss in the appendix, the flow to stable fixed points can be viewed as computing the approximate distribution, $Q(H|V)$, that best matches the true posterior distribution, $P(H|V)$.

In practice, one solves the mean field equations by discretizing the attractor dynamics in equations 3.8 and 3.9. We experimented with two simple schemes to compute updated values $\{\tilde{\mu}_i, \tilde{\xi}_i\}$ at time $t + \Delta t$ based on current values $\{\mu_i, \xi_i\}$ at time t. One of these was a first-order Euler method:

$$\tilde{\mu}_i = \mu_i + \dot{\mu}_i \Delta t, \qquad (3.12)$$

$$\tilde{\xi}_i = \frac{1}{2} - \left[\sum_j W_{ij}^2 \tilde{\mu}_j (1 - \tilde{\mu}_j) \right]^{-1} \left(h_i + \dot{h}_i \Delta t - \sum_j W_{ij} \tilde{\mu}_j \right), \qquad (3.13)$$

followed (when necessary) by clipping operations that projected $\{\mu_i, \xi_i\}$ into the interval $[0, 1]$. The other scheme we tried was a slight variant that sidestepped the division operation in equation 3.13. This was done by making additional use of the sigmoid squashing function, replacing equation 3.13 by

$$\tilde{\xi}_i = \sigma(h_i + \dot{h}_i \Delta t). \qquad (3.14)$$

This second method does not strictly reduce to the continuous attractor dynamics in the limit $\Delta t \rightarrow 0$; however, empirically it tended to converge more rapidly to solutions of the mean field equations. For this reason, and also because of its naturalness, we favored this method in practice. Figure 2 shows typical traces of L versus time for both methods. The traces were computed from one of the networks learned in section 4.

3.4 Mean Field Learning. The Lyapunov function in equation 3.10 has another interpretation that is important for unsupervised learning. Noting that the KL divergence between two distributions is strictly nonnegative, it

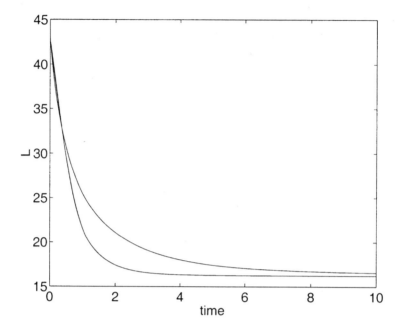

Figure 2: Typical convergence of the Lyapunov function, L, under the discretized attractor dynamics. The top curve shows the trace using equation 3.13 and the bottom curve using equation 3.14.

follows from equation 3.3 that

$$\ln P(V) \geq -\sum_H Q(H|V) \ln \left[\frac{Q(H|V)}{P(H, V)} \right]. \tag{3.15}$$

Equation 3.15 gives a lower bound on the log-likelihood of the evidence, $\ln P(V)$, in terms of an average over the tractable distribution, $Q(H|V)$. The lower bound on $\ln P(V)$ can be used as an objective function for unsupervised learning in generative models (Hinton et al., 1995). Whereas in tractable networks, one adapts the weights to maximize the log-likelihood $\ln P(V)$, as in equation 2.4, in intractable networks, one adapts the weights to maximize the lower bound.

In general, it is not possible to evaluate the right-hand side of equation 3.15 exactly; further approximations are required. In the appendix, we evaluate equation 3.15 assuming that the weighted sum of inputs to each unit has a gaussian distribution. We also make use of an additional variational principle to estimate intractable averages over $Q(H|V)$. Evaluating equation 3.15 in this way leads to the Lyapunov function in equation 3.10. With this interpretation, we can view equation 3.10 as a surrogate objective function for unsupervised learning. Thus, in addition to computing approximate statistics of the posterior distribution, $P(H|V)$, the attractor dynamics in equations 3.8 and 3.9 also computes a useful objective function. (Under certain limiting conditions, the Lyapunov function in equation 3.10 actually provides a lower bound on the log-likelihood, $\ln P(V) \geq -L$, as opposed to merely an estimate.)

Note the dual role of the Lyapunov function in the mean field approximation: the attractor dynamics minimizes L with respect to the mean field parameters $\{\mu_i, \xi_i\}$, while the learning rule minimizes L with respect to the weights W_{ij}. A useful picture is to imagine these two minimizations occurring on vastly different timescales, with the mean field parameters $\{\mu_i, \xi_i\}$ tracking changes in the evidence much more rapidly than the weights, W_{ij}. Put another way, short-term memories are stored by the mean field parameters and long-term memories by the weights.

We derive a mean field learning rule by computing the gradients of the Lyapunov function L with respect to the weights, W_{ij}. Applying the chain rule gives

$$\frac{dL}{dW_{ij}} = \frac{\partial L}{\partial W_{ij}} + \sum_k \frac{\partial L}{\partial \mu_k} \frac{\partial \mu_k}{\partial W_{ij}} + \sum_k \frac{\partial L}{\partial \xi_k} \frac{\partial \xi_k}{\partial W_{ij}}, \tag{3.16}$$

where the last two terms account for the fact that the mean field parameters depend implicitly on the weights through equations 3.4 and 3.5. (Here we have assumed that the attractor dynamics are allowed to converge fully before adapting the weights to new evidence.) We can simplify this expression by noting that the mean field equations describe fixed points at which $\partial L/\partial \mu_k = \partial L/\partial \xi_k = 0$; thus the last two terms in equation 3.16 vanish. Evaluating the first term in equation 3.16 gives rise to the on-line learning rule:

$$\Delta W_{ij} \propto \left[(\mu_i - \xi_i)\,\mu_j - W_{ij}\xi_i(1 - \xi_i)\mu_j(1 - \mu_j) \right]. \tag{3.17}$$

Comparing this learning rule to equation 2.4, we see that the mean field parameters fill in for the statistics of S_i and σ_i. This is, of course, what makes the learning algorithm tractable. Whereas the statistics of $P(H|V)$ cannot be efficiently computed, the parameters $\{\mu_i, \xi_i\}$ are found by solving the mean field equations.

Note that the right-most term of equation 3.7 has no counterpart in equation 2.4. This term, a regularizer induced by the mean field approximation, causes W_{ij} to be decayed according to the mean field statistics of σ_i and S_j. In particular, the weight decay is suppressed if either ξ_i or μ_j is saturated near zero or one; in effect, weights between highly correlated units are burned in to their current values.

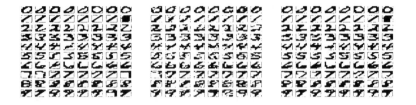

Figure 3: (Left) Actual images from the training set. (Middle) Images sampled from the generative models of trained networks. (Right) Images whose bottom halves were inferred from their top halves.

4 Experimental Results

We used a database of handwritten digits to evaluate the computational abilities of unsupervised neural networks represented by DAGs. The database consisted of 11,000 examples of handwritten digits compiled by the U.S. Postal Service Office of Advanced Technology. The examples were preprocessed to produce 8×8 binary images, as in Figure 3. For each digit, we divided the data into a training set of 700 examples and a test set of 400 examples. The partition of data into training and test sets was the same as used in previous studies (Hinton et al., 1995; Saul et al., 1996).

We used the mean field algorithm from the previous section to learn generative models of each digit class. The generative models were parameterized by three-layer networks with $8 \times 24 \times 64$ architectures. In 100 independent experiments,[2] we trained 10 networks, one for each digit class, and then used these networks to classify the images in the test set. The test images were labeled by whichever network returned the highest value of $-L$, used as a stand-in for the true log-likelihood, $\ln P(V)$. The mean classification error rate in these experiments was 4.4%, with a standard deviation of 0.2%. These results are considerably better than standard benchmarks on this database (Hinton et al., 1995), such as k-nearest neighbors (6.7%) and backpropagation (5.6%). They also improve slightly on results from the wake-sleep learning rule (4.8%) in Hemholtz machines (Hinton et al., 1995) and from an earlier version (4.6%) of the mean field learning rule (Saul et al., 1996).

---

[2] The experimental details were as follows. Each network was trained by five passes through the training examples. The weights were adapted using a fixed learning rate of 0.05. Mean field parameters were computed by 16 iterations of the discretized attractor dynamics, equations 3.12 and 3.14, with $\tau_\mu = \tau_h = 1$ and a step size of $\Delta t = 0.25$. The mean field parameters were initialized by a top-down pass through the network, setting $\xi_i = \sigma(\sum_j W_{ij}\xi_j)$ and $\mu_i = \xi_i$ for the hidden units. The weights W_{ij} were initialized by random draws from a gaussian distribution with zero mean and small variance.

The classification results show that the mean field networks have learned noisy but essentially accurate models of each digit class. This is confirmed visually by looking at images sampled from the generative model of each network (see Figure 3). The three columns in this figure show, from left to right, actual images from the training set, fantasies sampled from the generative models of trained networks, and images whose top halves were taken from those in the first column and whose bottom halves were inferred, or filled in, by the attractor dynamics. These last images show that probabilistic DAGs can function as associative memories in the same way as symmetric neural networks, such as the Hopfield model (1984).

5 Discussion

In this article we have extended the attractor paradigm of neural computation to feedforward networks parameterizing probabilistic generative models. The probabilistic semantics of these networks (Lauritzen, 1996; Neal, 1992; Pearl, 1988) differ in useful respects from those of symmetric neural networks, for which the attractor paradigm was first established (Cohen & Grossberg, 1983; Hopfield, 1982; Geman & Geman, 1984; Ackley et al., 1985; Peterson & Anderson, 1987). Borrowing ideas from statistical mechanics, we have derived a mean field theory for approximate probabilistic inference. We have also exhibited an attractor dynamics that converges to solutions of the mean field equations and that generates the signals required for unsupervised learning.

While learning and dynamics have been twin themes of neural network research since its inception, it often appears that the field is divided into two camps: one studying symmetric networks with energy functions, the other studying feedforward networks that do not involve iterative forms of relaxation. In our view, this split has prevented researchers from combining the benefits of both approaches to computation. We note that despite the strong convergence results available for symmetric networks, there have been few applications for these networks involving any significant element of learning. Likewise, despite the powerful learning abilities of feedforward networks, there have been few applications involving more complex forms of inference and decision making. In the remainder of this section, we discuss the many compelling reasons for combining these two approaches and suggest how this might be done using the ideas in this article.

Let us begin by considering feedforward networks. Many practical learning algorithms have been developed for feedforward networks, and numerous theoretical results are available to characterize their properties for approximation and estimation. The usual framework for feedforward networks is one of supervised learning, or function approximation. In particular, a network induces a functional relationship between x and y based on a training set consisting of (x, y) pairs. Subsequent x inputs can be used as queries, and the network interpolates or extrapolates to provide a response y.

Although useful and general, this framework also has limitations. In particular, it is not always the case that the form of future queries is known in advance of training, and indeed, as in the classical setting of associative memory, it can be useful to allow arbitrary components of the joint (x, y) vector to serve as queries. For example, in control and optimization applications, one would like to use y as a query and extract a corresponding x. In missing data problems, one would like to fill in components of the x vector given y or other components of x. In applications involving diagnosis, model critiquing, explanation, and sensitivity analysis, one would often like to find values of hidden units that correspond to particular input or output patterns. Finally, in problems with unlabeled examples, one would like to do some form of unsupervised learning. In our view, these manifold problems are best treated as general inference problems on the database of knowledge stored by the network. Moreover, as is suggested by the heuristic iterative techniques that have been employed to "invert" feedforward networks (Hoskins, Hwang, & Vagners, 1992; Jordan & Rumelhart, 1992), we expect issues in dynamical systems to become relevant when inference is performed in an "upstream" direction.

Even in the classical setting, where feedforward networks are used for function approximation, an inferential perspective can be useful. Consider two logistic hidden units with strong, positive connections to a logistic output unit. If the output unit has a target value of one, then we can exploit the fact that only one hidden unit suffices to activate the output unit. In particular, if we have additional evidence that (say) the first hidden unit is activated, perhaps via its connection to another output unit, then we can infer that the second hidden unit is not required to be activated, and thus can be used for other purposes. This explaining-away phenomenon reflects an induced correlation between the hidden units, and it is natural in many diagnostic settings involving hidden causes (Pearl, 1988). It and other induced correlations between hidden units can be exploited if we augment our view of feedforward network learning to include an "upstream" inferential component.

While classical feedforward networks are powerful learning machines and weak inference engines, the opposite can be said of symmetric neural networks. Properly configured, symmetric networks can perform inferences as complex as solving the traveling salesman problem (Hopfield & Tank, 1986), yet few have emerged in applications involving a significant element of learning. In our view, the reasons for this are twofold (Pearl, 1988). First, it is a general fact that undirected graphical models—of which symmetric neural networks, such as the Boltzmann machine, are a special case—are less modular than directed graphical models. In a directed model, units that are downstream from the queried and observed units can simply be deleted; they have no effect on the query. In undirected networks no such modularity generally exists; units are generally coupled via the partition function. Second, in a directed network, it is possible to use causal intuitions to understand representation and processing in the model. This can often be an overwhelming advantage. Moreover, if the domain being modeled has a natural causal structure, then it is natural to use a directed model that accords with the observed direction of causality.

We take two lessons from the previous successes of neural computation: (1) from the abilities of symmetric networks, that complex forms of inference require an element of iterative processing; and (2) from the abilities of feedforward networks, that the capacity to learn is greatly enhanced by the element of directionality. We believe that the formalism in this article combines the best aspects of symmetric and feedforward neural networks. The models we study are represented by directed acyclic graphs and thus have the natural advantages of modularity and causality that accrue to feedforward networks. Moreover, because they are endowed with probabilistic semantics, they also support complex types of inference and reasoning. This allows them to be applied to a broad range of problems involving diagnosis, explanation, control, optimization, and missing data. Our formalism also reconciles the problems of unsupervised and supervised learning in a manner reminiscent of the Boltzmann machine (Ackley et al., 1985). The supervised case simply emerges as the limiting case in which all of the input and output units are contained in the set of visible units. Finally, as in symmetric neural networks, approximate probabilistic inference is performed by relaxing a continuous dynamical system. Our formalism thus preserves the many compelling features of the attractor paradigm, including the guarantees of stability and convergence, the potential for massive parallelism, and the physical analogy of an energy surface.

We have contrasted the networks in this article to standard backpropagation networks, which do not make use of probabilistic semantics or attractor dynamics. Another representational difference is that the units in backpropagation networks take on continuous values, whereas the units in sigmoid Bayesian networks represent binary random variables. Our focus on binary random variables, as opposed to continuous ones, however, should not be construed as a fundamental limitation of our methods. Ideas from mean field theory can be applied to probabilistic models of continuous random variables, and such applications may be of interest for more sophisticated generative models (Hinton & Ghahramani, 1997).

Note that our analysis transforms a feedforward network into a recurrent network that possesses a Lyapunov function. This recurrent network (essentially equations 3.8 and 3.9 viewed as a recurrent network) is not a symmetric network, and its Lyapunov function does not follow directly from the theorems of Cohen and Grossberg (1983) and Hopfield (1984). We have derived the attractor dynamics for these networks by combining ideas from statistical mechanics with the probabilistic machinery of directed graphical models. Of course, one can also study recurrent networks that possess a Lyapunov function, independent of any underlying probabilistic formulation. In fact, Seung, Richardson, Lagarias, and Hopfield (1998) recently exhibited a Lyapunov function for excitatory-inhibitory neural networks with a mixture of symmetric and antisymmetric interactions. Interestingly, their Lyapunov function has a similar structure to the one in equation 3.10.

A general concern with dynamical approaches to computation involves the amount of time required to relax to equilibrium. Although we found empirically that this relaxation time was not long for the problem of recognizing handwritten digits (16 iterations of the discretized differential equations), the issue requires further attention. Beyond general numerical methods for speeding convergence, one obvious approach is to consider methods for providing better initial estimates of the mean field parameters. This general idea is suggestive of the Helmholtz machine of Hinton et al. (1995). The Helmholtz machine is a pair of feedforward networks, a top-down generative model that corresponds to the Bayesian network in Figure 1, and a bottom-up recognition model that computes the conditional statistics of the hidden units induced by the input vector. This latter network replaces the mean field equations in our approach. The recognition model is itself learned, essentially as a probabilistic inverse to the generative model. This approach obviates the need for the iterative solution of mean field equations. The trade-off for this simplicity is a lack of theoretical guarantees, and the fact that the recognition model cannot handle missing data or support certain types of reasoning, such as explaining away, that rely on the combination of top-down and bottom-up processing. One attractive idea, however, is to use a bottom-up recognition model to make initial guesses for the mean field parameters, then to use an attractor dynamics to refine these guesses.

Even without such enhancements, however, we believe that the attractor paradigm in directed graphical models is worthy of further investigation. Attractor neural networks have provided a viable approach to probabilistic inference in undirected graphical models (Peterson & Anderson, 1987), particularly when combined with deterministic annealing. We attribute the lack of learning-based applications for symmetric neural networks to their representational limitations for modeling causal processes (Pearl, 1988) and the peculiar instabilities arising from the sleep phase of Boltzmann learning (Neal, 1992; Galland, 1993). By combining the virtues of attractor dynamics with the probabilistic semantics of feedforward networks, we feel that a more useful and interesting model emerges.

Appendix: Details of Mean Field Theory _____

In this appendix we derive the mean field approximation for large, layered networks whose probabilistic semantics are given by equations 2.1 and 2.2. Starting from the factorized distribution for $Q(H|V)$, equation 3.1, our goal is to minimize the KL divergence in equation 3.3, with respect to the parameters $\{\mu_i\}$. Note that this is equivalent to maximizing the lower bound on $\ln P(V)$, given in equation 3.15.

The first term on the right-hand side of equation 3.3 is simply minus the entropy of the factorial distribution, $Q(H|V)$, or:

$$\sum_H Q(H|V) \ln Q(H|V) = \sum_i \left[\mu_i \ln \mu_i + (1 - \mu_i) \ln(1 - \mu_i) \right]. \quad \text{(A.1)}$$

Here, for notational convenience, we have introduced parameters μ_i for all the units in the network, hidden *and* visible. For the visible units, we use these parameters simply as placeholders for the evidence. Thus, the visible units are clamped to either zero or one, and they do not contribute to the entropy in equation A.1.

Evaluating the second term on the right-hand side of equation 3.3 is not as straightforward as the entropy. In particular, for each unit, let

$$z_i = \sum_j W_{ij} S_j \quad \text{(A.2)}$$

denote its weighted sum of parents, and let $\sigma_i = \sigma(z_i)$ denote its squashed top-down signal. From equations 2.1 and 2.2, we can write the joint distribution in these networks as

$$\ln P(S) = \sum_i [S_i \ln \sigma_i + (1 - S_i) \ln(1 - \sigma_i)] \quad \text{(A.3)}$$

$$= \sum_i \left(S_i z_i - \ln \left[1 + e^{z_i} \right] \right). \quad \text{(A.4)}$$

Note that to evaluate the second term in equation 3.3, we must average the right-hand side of equation A.4 over the factorial distribution, $Q(H|V)$. The logarithm term in equation A.4, however, makes it impossible to compute this average in closed form.

Clearly, another approximation is needed to compute the expected value of $\ln[1 + e^{z_i}]$, averaged over the distribution, $Q(H|V)$. We can make progress by studying the sum of inputs, z_i, as a random variable in its own right. Under the distribution $Q(H|V)$, the right-hand side of equation A.2 is a weighted sum of independent random variables with means μ_j and variances $\mu_j(1 - \mu_j)$. The number of terms in this sum is equal to the number of hidden units in the preceding layer. In large networks, we expect the statistics of this sum—or, more precisely, the distribution $Q(z_i|V)$—to be governed by a central limit theorem. In other words, to a very good approximation, $Q(z_i|V)$ assumes a gaussian distribution with mean and variance:

$$\langle z_i \rangle = \sum_j W_{ij} \mu_j, \quad \text{(A.5)}$$

$$\langle \delta z_i^2 \rangle = \sum_j W_{ij}^2 \mu_j(1 - \mu_j), \quad \text{(A.6)}$$

where $\langle \cdot \rangle$ is used to denote the expected value. The gaussianity of $Q(z_i|V)$ emerges in the thermodynamic limit of large, layered networks where each unit receives an infinite number of inputs from the hidden units in the preceding layer. In particular, suppose that unit i has N_i parents and that the weights W_{ij} are bounded by $\sqrt{N_i}|W_{ij}| < c$ for some constant c. Then in the limit $N_i \rightarrow \infty$, the third- and higher-order cumulants of $\sum_j W_{ij}S_j$ vanish for any distribution under which S_j are independently distributed binary variables. The assumption that $\sqrt{N_i}W_{ij} < c$ implies that the weights are uniformly small and evenly distributed throughout the network; it is a natural assumption to make for robust, fault-tolerant networks whose computing abilities do not degrade catastrophically with random "lesions" in the weight matrix. Although only an approximation for finite networks, in what follows we make the simplifying assumption that $Q(z_i|V)$ is a gaussian distribution. This assumption—specifically tailored to large, layered networks whose evidence arrives in the bottom layer—leads to the simple mean field equations and attractor dynamics in section 3.[3]

The asymptotic form of $Q(z_i|V)$ and the logarithm term in equation 4.4 motivate us to consider the following lemma. Let z denote a gaussian random variable with mean $\langle z \rangle$ and variance $\langle \delta z^2 \rangle$, and consider the expected value, $\langle \ln[1 + e^z] \rangle$. Then, for any real number ξ, we have the upper bound (Seung, 1995):

$$\langle \ln[1 + e^z] \rangle = \langle \ln[e^{\xi z}e^{-\xi z}(1 + e^z)] \rangle, \tag{A.7}$$

$$= \xi \langle z \rangle + \langle \ln[e^{-\xi z} + e^{(1-\xi)z}] \rangle, \tag{A.8}$$

$$\leq \xi \langle z \rangle + \ln \langle e^{-\xi z} + e^{(1-\xi)z} \rangle, \tag{A.9}$$

where the last line follows from Jensen's inequality. Since z is gaussian, it is straightforward to perform the averages on the right-hand side. This gives us an upper bound on $\langle \ln[1 + e^z] \rangle$ expressed in terms of the mean and variance:

$$\langle \ln[1 + e^z] \rangle \leq \frac{1}{2}\xi^2 \langle \delta z^2 \rangle + \ln \left[1 + e^{\langle z \rangle + (1-2\xi)\langle \delta z^2 \rangle/2} \right]. \tag{A.10}$$

The right-hand side of equation A.10 is a convex function of ξ whose minimum occurs in the interval $\xi \in [0, 1]$.

We can use this lemma to compute an approximate value for $\langle \ln[1 + e^{z_i}] \rangle$, where the average is performed with respect to the distribution, $Q(H|V)$. This is done by introducing an extra parameter, ξ_i, for each unit in the network, then substituting ξ_i and the statistics of z_i into equation A.10. Note

---

[3] One can also proceed without making this assumption, as in Saul et al. (1996), to derive approximations for nonlayered networks. The resulting mean field equations, however, do not appear to lend themselves to a simple attractor dynamics.

that the terms $\ln[1 + e^{z_i}]$ appear in equation A.4 with an overall minus sign; thus, to the extent that $Q(z_i|V)$ is well approximated by a gaussian distribution, the upper bound in equation A.10 translates into a lower bound on $\langle \ln P(S) \rangle$. In particular, from equation A.4, we have:

$$\langle \ln P(S) \rangle \approx \sum_{ij} W_{ij}\mu_i\mu_j - \frac{1}{2}\sum_{ij} W_{ij}^2\xi_i^2\mu_j(1-\mu_j)$$

$$- \sum_i \ln\left\{ 1 + e^{\sum_j\left[W_{ij}\mu_j + \frac{1}{2}(1-2\xi_i)W_{ij}^2\mu_j(1-\mu_j)\right]} \right\}. \tag{A.11}$$

The right-hand side of equation A.11 becomes a lower bound on $\langle \ln P(S) \rangle$ in the thermodynamic limit where $Q(z_i|V)$ is described by a gaussian distribution.

The objective function for the mean field approximation is the difference between equations A.1 and A.11; these expressions correspond to the first two terms of equation 3.3. The difference of these two equations is in fact the Lyapunov function, L, from equation 3.10. This can be shown by appealing to the definition of h_i in equation 3.7 and by noting that

$$\int \sigma(h)\,dh = \ln[1 + e^h], \tag{A.12}$$

$$\int \sigma^{-1}(\mu)\,d\mu = \mu \ln \mu + (1 - \mu)\ln(1 - \mu), \tag{A.13}$$

where $\sigma^{-1}(\mu) = \ln[\frac{\mu}{1-\mu}]$ is the inverse sigmoid function. Thus we have derived the Lyapunov function by evaluating the KL divergence in equation 3.2. It follows that the Lyapunov function measures the discrepancy between the distributions $Q(H|V)$ and $P(H|V)$ in terms of the mean field parameters, $\{\mu_i, \xi_i\}$. Optimal values for these parameters are found by minimizing L; in particular, computing the gradients $\partial L/\partial \mu_i$ and $\partial L/\partial \xi_i$ and equating them to zero leads to the mean field equations, equations 3.4 and 3.5.

Acknowledgments

We are grateful to H. Seung for many useful discussions about attractor dynamics and Lyapunov functions. We also thank Hinton et al. (1995) for sharing their preprocessing software for images of handwritten digits.

References

Ackley, D. H., Hinton, G. E., & Sejnowski, T. J. (1985). A learning algorithm for Boltzmann machines. *Cognitive Science, 9*, 147–169.

Amit, D. J. (1989). *Modeling brain function*. Cambridge: Cambridge University Press.

Binder, J., Koller, D., Russell, S. J., & Kanazawa, K. (1997). Adaptive probabilistic networks with hidden variables. *Machine Learning, 29,* 213–244.

Buntine, W. (1994). Operations for learning with graphical models. *Journal of Artificial Intelligence Research, 2,* 159–225.

Cohen, M. A., & Grossberg, S. (1983). Absolute stability of global pattern formation and parallel memory storage by competitive neural networks. *IEEE Transactions on Systems, Man, and Cybernetics, 13,* 815–826.

Cooper, G. (1990). Computational complexity of probabilistic inference using Bayesian belief networks. *Artificial Intelligence, 42,* 393–405.

Dayan, P., Hinton, G. E., Neal, R. M., & Zemel, R. (1995). The Helmholtz machine. *Neural Computation, 7,* 889–904.

Galland, C. C. (1993). The limitations of deterministic Boltzmann machine learning. *Network: Computations in Neural Systems, 4,* 355–379.

Geman, S., & Geman, D. (1984). Stochastic relaxation, Gibbs distributions, and the Bayesian restoration of images. *IEEE Transactions on Pattern Analysis and Machine Intelligence, 6,* 721–741.

Hinton, G. E., Dayan, P., Frey, B. J., & Neal, R. M. (1995). The wake-sleep algorithm for unsupervised neural networks. *Science, 268,* 1158–1161.

Hinton, G. E., & Ghahramani, Z. (1997). Generative models for discovering sparse distributed representations. *Philosophical Transactions Royal Society B, 352,* 1177–1190.

Hopfield, J. J. (1982). Neural networks and physical systems with emergent collective computational abilities. *Proceedings of the National Academy of Sciences, USA, 79,* 2554–2558.

Hopfield, J. J. (1984). Neurons with graded responses have collective computational properties like those of two-state neurons. *Proceedings of the National Academy of Sciences, USA, 81,* 3088–3092.

Hopfield, J. J., & Tank, D. W. (1986). Computing with neural circuits: A model. *Science, 233,* 625–633.

Hoskins, D., Hwang, J., & Vagners, J. (1992). Iterative inversion of neural networks and its application to adaptive control. *IEEE Transactions on Neural Networks, 3,* 292–301.

Jordan, M. I., & Rumelhart, D. E. (1992). Forward models: Supervised learning with a distal teacher. *Cognitive Science, 16,* 307–354.

Koch, C., Marroquin, J., & Yuille, A. (1986). Analog "neuronal" networks in early vision. *Proceedings of the National Academy of Sciences, USA, 83,* 4263–4267.

Lauritzen, S. L. (1996). *Graphical models*. Oxford: Oxford University Press.

Lewicki, M. S., & Sejnowski, T. J. (1996). Bayesian unsupervised learning of higher order structure. In M. Mozer, M. Jordan, & T. Petsche (Eds.), *Advances in neural information processing systems, 9.* Cambridge, MA: MIT Press.

Metropolis, N., Rosenbluth, A. W., Rosenbluth, M. N., Teller, A. H., & Teller, E. (1953). Equation of state calculations for fast computing machines. *Journal of Chemical Physics, 21,* 1087–1092.

Neal, R. M. (1992). Connectionist learning of belief networks. *Artificial Intelligence, 56,* 71–113.

Parisi, G. (1988). *Statistical field theory*. Redwood City, CA: Addison-Wesley.

Pearl, J. (1988). *Probabilistic reasoning in intelligent systems*. San Mateo, CA: Morgan Kaufmann.

Peterson, C., & Anderson, J. R. (1987). A mean field theory learning algorithm for neural networks. *Complex Systems, 1*, 995–1019.

Saul, L. K., Jaakkola, T. S., & Jordan, M. I. (1996). Mean field theory for sigmoid belief networks. *Journal of Artificial Intelligence Research, 4*, 61–76.

Seung, H. S. (1995). Annealed theories of learning. In J.-H. Oh, C. Kwon, & S. Cho (Eds.), *Neural networks: The statistical mechanics perspective: Proceedings of the CTP-PRSRI Joint Workshop on Theoretical Physics*. Singapore: World Scientific.

Seung, H. S., Richardson, T. J., Lagarias, J. C., & Hopfield, J. J. (1998). Minimax and Hamiltonian dynamics of excitatory-inhibitory networks. In M. Jordan, M. Kearns, & S. Solla (Eds.), *Advances in neural information processing systems, 10*. Cambridge, MA: MIT Press.

6

Efficient Learning in Boltzmann Machines Using Linear Response Theory

H. J. Kappen
RWCP SNN Laboratory, Department of Biophysics, University of Nijmegen, NL 6525 EZ Nijmegen, The Netherlands

F. B. Rodríguez
Instituto de Ingeniería del Conocimiento y Departamento de Ingeniería Informática, Universidad Autónoma de Madrid, 28049 Madrid, Spain

The learning process in Boltzmann machines is computationally very expensive. The computational complexity of the exact algorithm is exponential in the number of neurons. We present a new approximate learning algorithm for Boltzmann machines, based on mean-field theory and the linear response theorem. The computational complexity of the algorithm is cubic in the number of neurons.

In the absence of hidden units, we show how the weights can be directly computed from the fixed-point equation of the learning rules. Thus, in this case we do not need to use a gradient descent procedure for the learning process. We show that the solutions of this method are close to the optimal solutions and give a significant improvement when correlations play a significant role. Finally, we apply the method to a pattern completion task and show good performance for networks up to 100 neurons.

1 Introduction

Boltzmann machines (Ackley, Hinton, & Sejnowski, 1985) are networks of binary neurons with a stochastic neuron dynamics, known as Glauber dynamics. Assuming symmetric connections between neurons, the probability distribution over neuron states $\vec{s}$ will become stationary and will be given by the Boltzmann-Gibbs distribution $P(\vec{s})$. The Boltzmann distribution is a known function of the weights and thresholds of the network. However, exact computation of $P(\vec{s})$ or any statistics involving $P(\vec{s})$, such as mean firing rates or correlations, requires exponential time in the number of neurons. This is due to the fact that $P(\vec{s})$ contains a normalization term Z, which involves a sum over all states in the network, of which there are exponentially many. This problem is particularly important for Boltzmann machine learning because the Boltzmann machine learning rule requires the computation of correlations between neurons. Thus, learning in Boltzmann machines requires exponential time.

For specific architectures, learning can be dramatically accelerated. For instance Saul and Jordan (1994) discuss how learning times become linear in the number of neurons for treelike architectures. Kappen (1995) shows how strong inhibition between hidden neurons reduces the computation time to polynomial in the number of neurons.

A well-known approximate method to compute correlations is the Monte Carlo method (Itzykson & Drouffe, 1989), which is a stochastic sampling of the state-space. Glauber dynamics is an example of such a method. The terms in the sum over states are proportional to a "Boltzmann factor" $\exp(-E)$. Monte Carlo methods can be more effective than the summation of all terms because the sampling is biased toward states with lower E. These terms will give the dominant contribution to the sum over states. This is the approach chosen for learning in the original Boltzmann machine (Ackley et al., 1985). Practical use requires that the Markov process converge sufficiently fast—in polynomial time—to the equilibrium distribution. This property is known as rapid mixing and probably does not hold in general for Glauber dynamics (Sinclair, 1993). Useful results can be obtained with Glauber dynamics when the network is not too large and has small weights.

In Peterson and Anderson (1987), an acceleration method for learning in Boltzmann machines is proposed. They suggest replacing the correlations in the Boltzmann machine learning rule by the naive mean-field approximation: $\langle s_i s_j \rangle = m_i m_j$, where m_i is the mean-field activity of neuron i. The mean fields are given by the solution of a set of n coupled mean-field equations, with n the number of neurons. The solution can be efficiently obtained by fixed-point iteration. The method was further elaborated in Hinton (1989). In this article, we will show that the naive mean-field approximation of the learning rules does not converge in general and explain why.

Another way to speed up learning is to observe that the Kullback-Leibler divergence is bounded from above by an effective free energy expression using Jensen's inequality. Such an approach can be applied to architectures whose probability distribution does not contain a sum over all states for normalization, such as the Helmholz machine (Dayan, Hinton, Neal, & Zemel, 1995) and the sigmoid belief network (Saul, Jaakkola, & Jordan, 1996). The application of such an approach to Boltzmann machines is not as simple because it requires in addition an upper bound on Z, which is computationally more complex (Jaakkola & Jordan, 1996).

We will argue that in the correct treatment of mean-field theory for Boltzmann machines, the correlations can be computed using the linear response theorem (Parisi, 1988). In the context of neural networks, this approach was first introduced by Ginzburg and Sompolinsky (1994) for the computation of time-delayed correlations and later by Kappen (1997) for the computation of stimulus-dependent correlations. We will show that this approximation can be used successfully to approximate the gradients in the Boltzmann machine.

In section 2, we introduce learning in Boltzmann machines and show why the naive mean-field approximation of the gradients does not work. In section 3, we derive the mean-field approximation for the correlations based on the linear response theory. We argue that an effective self-coupling term can be included to obtain better results. In the absence of hidden units, the fixed-point equations for the learning rules can be solved directly in terms of the weights and thresholds of the network. In section 4, we show results of simulations. We compare our methods with the exact computation of the optimal weights and with a factorized probability model that assumes absence of correlations. We use the Kullback-Leibler divergence as a criterion for comparison on small networks. For large networks, this criterion can no longer be computed, because it requires exponential time. We propose an approximate criterion for comparison on large networks and show that it correlates well with the Kullback-Leibler divergence for small problems. Subsequently we show good performance of our method for increasing problem size.

2 Boltzmann Machine Learning

2.1 General Dynamics of Boltzmann Machines. The Boltzmann machine is defined as follows. The possible configurations of the network can be characterized by a vector $\vec{s} = (s_1, .., s_i, .., s_n)$, where s_i is the state of the neuron i and n the total number of the neurons. Each neuron can be in two states ($s_i = \pm 1$), and its dynamics is governed by the following stochastic rule. At each time step, a neuron is selected at random. Its new value is determined as:

$$s_i = \begin{cases} +1 & \text{with probability } g(h_i) \\ -1 & \text{with probability } 1 - g(h_i), \end{cases} \tag{2.1}$$

with $g(h_i)$ and h_i (local field) defined by

$$g(h_i) = \frac{1}{1 + \exp\{-2\beta h_i)\}}, \quad h_i = \sum_{j \neq i} w_{ij} s_j + \theta_i. \tag{2.2}$$

The magnitude w_{ij} (weight) refers to the connection strength between the neuron i and neuron j, and θ_i is the threshold for neuron i. The weights are chosen symmetric, $w_{ij} = w_{ji}$. The parameter β controls the noise in the neuron dynamics. β is often interpreted as $\beta = 1/T$, where T acts like the temperature of a physical system. Since β is just a scaling of the weights and the thresholds, and the latter are optimized through learning, we can set $\beta = 1$ without loss of generality.

Let us define the energy of the system for a certain configuration $\vec{s}$ as

$$-E(\vec{s}) = \sum_{i<j} w_{ij} s_i s_j + \sum_i s_i \theta_i. \tag{2.3}$$

After long times, the probability of finding the network in a state $\vec{s}$ becomes independent of time (thermal equilibrium) and is given by the Boltzmann distribution

$$p(\vec{s}) = \frac{1}{Z}\exp\{-E(\vec{s})\}. \tag{2.4}$$

$Z = \sum_{\vec{s}}\exp\{-E(\vec{s})\}$ is the partition function that normalizes the probability distribution.

2.2 Slow Learning in Boltzmann Machines. A learning rule for Boltzmann machines was introduced by Ackley et al. (1985). Let us partition the neurons in a set of n_v visible units and n_h hidden units ($n_v + n_h = n$). Let α and β label the 2^{n_v} visible and 2^{n_h} hidden states of the network, respectively. Thus, every state $\vec{s}$ is uniquely described by a tuple $\alpha\beta$. Learning consists of adjusting the weights and thresholds in such a way that the Boltzmann distribution on the visible units $p_\alpha = \sum_\beta p_{\alpha\beta}$ approximates a target distribution q_α as closely as possible.

A suitable measure for the difference between the distributions p_α and q_α is the Kullback divergence (Kullback, 1959),

$$K = \sum_\alpha q_\alpha \log \frac{q_\alpha}{p_\alpha}. \tag{2.5}$$

It is easy to show that $K \geq 0$ for all distributions p_α and $K = 0$ iff $p_\alpha = q_\alpha$ for all α.

Therefore, learning consists of minimizing K using gradient descent, and the learning rules are given by Ackley et al. (1985) and Hertz, Krogh, and Palmer (1991):

$$\Delta\theta_i = \eta\left(\langle s_i\rangle_c - \langle s_i\rangle\right), \quad \Delta w_{ij} = \eta\left(\langle s_i s_j\rangle_c - \langle s_i s_j\rangle\right) i \neq j. \tag{2.6}$$

The parameter η is the learning rate. The brackets $\langle\cdot\rangle$ and $\langle\cdot\rangle_c$ denote the "free" and "clamped" expectation values, respectively. The "free" expectation values are defined as usual:

$$\langle s_i\rangle = \sum_{\alpha\beta} s_i^{\alpha\beta} p_{\alpha\beta}$$
$$\langle s_i s_j\rangle = \sum_{\vec{s}} s_i^{\alpha\beta} s_j^{\alpha\beta} p_{\alpha\beta}. \tag{2.7}$$

The "clamped" expectation values are obtained by clamping the visible units in a state α and taking the expectation value with respect to q_α:

$$\langle s_i\rangle_c = \sum_{\alpha\beta} s_i^{\alpha\beta} q_\alpha p_{\beta|\alpha}$$
$$\langle s_i s_j\rangle_c = \sum_{\alpha\beta} s_i^{\alpha\beta} s_j^{\alpha\beta} q_\alpha p_{\beta|\alpha}. \tag{2.8}$$

$s_i^{\alpha\beta}$ is the value of neuron i when the network is in state $\alpha\beta$. $p_{\beta|\alpha}$ is the conditional probability to observe hidden state β given that the visible state is α. Note that in equations 2.6 through 2.8, i and j run over both visible and hidden units.

Thus, the Boltzmann machine learning rules contain clamped and free expectation values of the Boltzmann distribution. The computation of the free expectation values is intractible, because the sums in equations 2.7 consist of 2^n terms. If q_α is given in the form of a training set of p patterns, the computation of the clamped expectation values (see equations 2.8) contains $p2^{n_h}$ terms. This is intractible as well, but usually less expensive than the free expectation values. As a result, the Boltzmann machine learning algorithm cannot be applied to practical problems.

2.3 The Naive Mean-Field Approximation.
Peterson and Anderson (1987) proposed an approximation to calculate the expectation values based on mean-field theory. In their approach, the free and clamped expectation values in equation 2.6 are approximated by their mean-field values,

$$\langle s_i \rangle \approx m_i, \quad \langle s_i s_j \rangle \approx m_i m_j, \quad i \neq j, \tag{2.9}$$

where m_i is the solution to the set of coupled mean-field equations,

$$m_i = \tanh\left(\sum_{j \neq i} w_{ij} m_j + \theta_i\right). \tag{2.10}$$

We will refer to this method as the naive mean-field approximation. In each step of the gradient descent procedure, one must solve the mean-field equations given by equation 2.10. This can be done quite easily using fixed-point iteration. In section 3, we will give more details about mean-field theory.

Peterson and Anderson found that this method was 10 to 30 times faster than the Monte Carlo method. However, there are many data sets for which the naive mean-field approximation does not work. Here, we show the consequences of their approach in the case that there are no hidden units.

Consider a network with only two visible neurons and no hidden neurons. We want to learn the probability distribution given by two patterns $(1, 1)$ and $(-1, -1)$ with equal probability. Thus, $\langle s_1 \rangle_c = \langle s_2 \rangle_c = 0$ and $\langle s_1 s_2 \rangle_c = 1$.

On this particular problem, the gradient descent procedure combined with the naive mean-field computation does not converge. The reason is simple. If we assume that the learning process converges to a fixed point ($\Delta w_{ij} = 0$ and $\Delta\theta_i = 0$), then we obtain from equations 2.6 and 2.9,

$$\langle s_i \rangle_c = m_i, \quad \langle s_i s_j \rangle_c = m_i m_j \quad i \neq j.$$

126   H. J. Kappen and F. B. Rodríguez

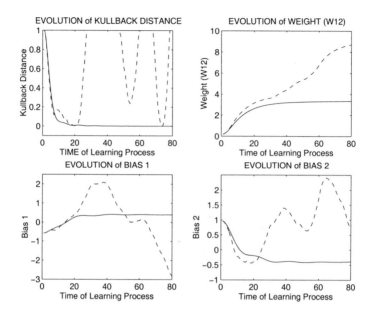

Figure 1: Gradient descent learning. The network consists of two visible neurons and no hidden neurons. The target distribution q is given by two patterns, $(1, 1)$ and $(-1, -1)$, with equal probability. The solid line shows the evolution of the Kullback divergence and the different network parameters when the exact gradient descent method is used. The dotted line shows the evolution of the different network parameters when the naive mean-field approximation gradient descent procedure is used. Learning rate $\eta = 0.1$, momentum $\alpha = 0.9$.

Thus, the fixed-point equations of the learning process combined with the naive mean-field approximation imply that the data set has no nontrivial correlations. In our example, this condition is clearly violated since $0 = \langle s_1 \rangle_c \langle s_2 \rangle_c \neq \langle s_1 s_2 \rangle_c = 1$.

Thus, we expect that if we use the naive mean-field approximation for the computation of the gradients, the resulting learning process will not converge. This is illustrated in Figure 1. We compare the exact gradient descent method, where the correlations are calculated using equations 2.7 and gradient descent using the naive mean-field approximation. Although the mean-field method sometimes reaches close to optimal solutions, the gradients in equations 2.6 are not zero at these points, and therefore the solution does not remain there.

From this example, we conclude that the naive mean-field approximation leads to a converging gradient descent algorithm *only* when the data are such that

$$\langle s_i s_j \rangle_c = \langle s_i \rangle_c \langle s_j \rangle_c \quad i \neq j. \tag{2.11}$$

For i and j visible units, this is simply a property of the data. It is equivalent to the statement that the target probability distribution q_α is factorized in all its variables: $q(\vec{s}) = \Pi_i q_i(s_i)$. The quality of the naive mean-field approximation will depend on to what extent equation 2.11 is violated. This conclusion holds regardless of whether the network has hidden units.

3 The Mean-Field Method and the Linear Response Correction _____

In this section we introduce an improved method to compute correlations within the mean-field framework. We will consider the mean-field approximation and its formulation in the first subsection. Then we will derive our main result based on the linear response theory. In the special case that the network has no hidden units, the optimal weights and thresholds can be computed directly from the fixed-point equations; that is, no gradient procedure needs to be applied.

3.1 Mean-Field Formulation. The basic idea of mean-field theory is to replace the quadratic term in the energy, $w_{ij} s_i s_j$ in equation 2.3 by a term linear in s_i. Such a linearized form allows for efficient computation of the sum over all states, such as equations 2.7 and 2.8 and the partition function Z. We define the mean-field energy

$$-E_{mf}(\vec{s}) = \sum_i s_i \{W_i + \theta_i\}, \tag{3.1}$$

where we introduce n mean fields W_i. The mean fields approximate the lateral interaction between neurons. The values of W_i must be chosen such that this approximation is as good as possible. How to do this will be shown below.

We define the mean-field probability distribution as

$$p_{mf}(\vec{s}) = \frac{\exp\{-E_{mf}(\vec{s})\}}{Z_{mf}}, \tag{3.2}$$

with

$$Z_{mf} = \sum_{\vec{s}} \exp\{-E_{mf}(\vec{s})\} = \prod_i 2 \cosh(\theta_i + W_i) \tag{3.3}$$

the mean-field partition function.

The expectations values for s_i and s_is_j in the mean-field approximation are given by:

$$\langle s_i \rangle_{mf} \equiv \sum_{\vec{s}} s_i p_{mf}(\vec{s}) = \tanh(W_i + \theta_i) \equiv m_i, \tag{3.4}$$

$$\langle s_is_j \rangle_{mf} \equiv \sum_{\vec{s}} s_is_j p_{mf}(\vec{s}) = m_i m_j \; i \neq j, \tag{3.5}$$

where we have introduced the parameters m_i, which are still to be fixed because of their dependence on W_i.

The real partition function Z (see equation 2.4) can be computed in the mean-field approximation (Itzykson & Drouffe, 1989):

$$Z = \sum_{\vec{s}} \exp(-E) = \sum_{\vec{s}} \exp(-E_{mf} + E_{mf} - E)$$

$$= Z_{mf} \langle \exp(E_{mf} - E) \rangle_{mf} \approx Z_{mf} \exp(\langle E_{mf} - E \rangle_{mf}) = Z'. \tag{3.6}$$

The mean-field approximation is in the last step and is related to the convexity of the exponential function $\langle \exp f \rangle \geq \exp\langle f \rangle$ (Itzykson & Drouffe, 1989). Note that $\langle \cdot \rangle_{mf}$ denotes expectation with respect to the mean-field distribution in equation 3.2 and not with respect to the Boltzmann distribution in equation 2.4. Therefore, the free energy in the mean-field approximation can be easily computed and is given by

$$-F = \log Z' = \sum_i \log(2\cosh(\theta_i + W_i)) - \sum_i W_i m_i + \sum_{i<j} w_{ij} m_i m_j. \tag{3.7}$$

We can calculate the mean fields W_i by minimizing the free energy:

$$\frac{\partial F}{\partial W_i} = (1 - m_i^2)\left(W_i - \sum_{j\neq i} w_{ij} m_j\right) = 0. \tag{3.8}$$

It can be shown, that the solutions $m_i^2 = 1$ maximize F. The required minima are therefore given by $W_i = \sum_{j\neq i} w_{ij} m_j$, which, combined with equation equation 3.4, give the mean-field equations in equation 2.10. These equations can be solved for m_i in terms of w_{ij} and θ_i using fixed-point iteration. The mean fields W_i can then be directly computed using equation 3.8.

3.2 Derivation of Linear Response Correction. We can go beyond the naive mean-field prediction $\langle s_is_j \rangle_{mf} = m_i m_j$ of equation 3.5 in the following way. First, observe that the mean firing rates and correlations are

$$\langle s_i \rangle = \frac{1}{Z}\frac{dZ}{d\theta_j} \approx \frac{1}{Z'}\frac{dZ'}{d\theta_j}, \quad \langle s_is_j \rangle \approx \frac{1}{Z'}\frac{d^2Z'}{d\theta_i d\theta_j}. \tag{3.9}$$

We will compute these quantities using the approximation in equation 3.6. While computing $dZ/d\theta_j$, using equation 3.7, we must be aware that the mean fields W_i depend on θ_i through equation 2.10 and equation 3.8:

$$\langle s_i \rangle \approx \frac{d}{d\theta_i} \log Z' = \left(\frac{\partial}{\partial \theta_i} + \sum_j \frac{\partial W_j}{\partial \theta_i} \frac{\partial}{\partial W_j} \right) \log Z' = m_i \qquad (3.10)$$

$$\langle s_i s_j \rangle \approx \frac{1}{Z'} \frac{d}{d\theta_j} (Z' m_i) = m_i m_j + A_{ij}, \qquad (3.11)$$

with $A_{ij} = dm_i/d\theta_j$. The last step in equation 3.10 follows when we use the mean-field equations in equation 3.8. Thus, there are no linear response corrections to the mean firing rate. Equation 3.11 is known as the linear response theorem (Parisi, 1988). The inverse of the matrix A can be directly obtained by differentiating equation 2.10 with respect to θ_i. The result is:

$$(A^{-1})_{ij} = \frac{\delta_{ij}}{1 - m_i^2} - w_{ij}. \qquad (3.12)$$

When the network is divided into visible and hidden units, the above approximation can be directly applied to computation of the free expectation values in equations 2.7.

When the visible units are clamped, the above derivation can be repeated to compute the expectation values for the hidden units. The only difference is that the thresholds θ_i for the hidden units receive an extra contribution from the clamped visible neurons. Let us assume that the visible units are clamped in state α. The mean firing rates of the hidden units are denoted by $\langle s_i \rangle^\alpha = m_i^\alpha, i \in H$ where m_i^α satisfy the mean-field equations

$$m_i^\alpha = \tanh \left(\sum_{j \in H} w_{ij} m_j^\alpha + \sum_{j \in V} w_{ij} s_j^\alpha + \theta_i \right), i \in H. \qquad (3.13)$$

V and H denote the subsets of visible and hidden units, respectively. Note that m_i^α depends on the clamped state α. The correlations $\langle s_i s_j \rangle^\alpha$ are given as follows:

$$i, j \in H : \langle s_i s_j \rangle^\alpha = m_i^\alpha m_j^\alpha + A_{ij}^\alpha \qquad (3.14)$$

$$i \in V, j \in H : \langle s_i s_j \rangle^\alpha = s_i^\alpha m_j^\alpha \qquad (3.15)$$

$$i, j \in V : \langle s_i s_j \rangle^\alpha = s_i^\alpha s_j^\alpha \qquad (3.16)$$

$$(A^{\alpha,-1})_{ij} = \frac{\delta_{ij}}{1 - (m_i^\alpha)^2} - w_{ij}. \qquad (3.17)$$

Finally, the clamped expectation values are given by taking the expectation value over q_α: $\langle s_i \rangle_c = \sum_\alpha \langle s_i \rangle^\alpha q_\alpha$ and $\langle s_i s_j \rangle_c = \sum_\alpha \langle s_i s_j \rangle^\alpha q_\alpha$.

Thus, our approximation consists of replacing the clamped and free expectation values in equations 2.6 by their linear response approximations. Equations 2.10 and 3.10 through 3.12 and equations 3.13 through 3.17 define the linear response approximations in the free phase and the clamped phase, respectively. The complexity of the method is dominated by the computations in the free phase. The computation of the linear response correlations involves the inversion of the matrix A, which requires $\mathcal{O}(n^3)$ operations. The computation of the mean firing rates through fixed-point iteration of equation 2.10 requires $\mathcal{O}(n^2)$ or $\mathcal{O}(n^2 \log n)$ operations, depending on whether fixed precision in the components of m_i or in the vector norm $\sum_i m_i^2$ is required. Thus, the full mean-field approximation, including the linear response correction, computes the gradients in $\mathcal{O}(n^3)$ operations.

3.3 TAP Correction to the Mean-Field Equations.

It is well known that the standard mean-field description (see equation 3.7) is inadequate for the description of frustrated systems. In general, terms involving higher powers of the coupling matrix w_{ij} must be included. For example, for the Sherrington-Kirkpatrick (SK) model, the appropriate mean-field free energy becomes (Thouless, Anderson, & Palmer [TAP], 1977)

$$-F = \sum_i \log(2 \cosh(\theta_i + W_i)) - \sum_i W_i m_i + \frac{1}{2} \sum_{i,j} w_{ij} m_i m_j$$
$$+ \frac{1}{4} \sum_{i,j} w_{ij}^2 (1 - m_i^2)(1 - m_j^2), \qquad (3.18)$$

and the corresponding mean-field equations become the TAP equations:

$$m_i = \tanh \left(\sum_{j \neq i} w_{ij} m_j + \theta_i - m_i \sum_{j \neq i} w_{ij}^2 (1 - m_j^2) \right). \qquad (3.19)$$

The additional term is called the Onsager reaction term (Onsager, 1936). It describes how the mean firing of neuron i affects the polarization of the surrounding spins and thus affects the local field of spin i. The effect of this additional term, but in the absence of the linear response correction, was studied by Galland (1993). In general, there is an infinite sum of terms, each involving a higher power of the couplings w_{ij} (Fischer & Hertz, 1991). It is interesting to note that all higher-order terms in the fixed-point equation are proportional to m_i and thus represent corrections to the self-coupling term. In the case of the SK model, it can be shown that all terms beyond the Onsager term are negligible (Plefka, 1982). (For unfrustrated systems, like the Ising model, the Onsager term itself is negligible.)

One can obtain the linear response corrections for TAP and higher-order mean-field corrections in a similar way, as described (by variation around the TAP equations). These extensions will be explored in a future publication. In this article, we restrict ourselves to the linear response corrections to the lowest-order mean-field equations and ignore higher-order corrections. However, we will consider the effect of an *effective* self-coupling term $w_{ii}m_i$. The mean-field equations (see equation 2.10) become

$$m_i = \tanh\left(\sum_j w_{ij}m_j + \theta_i\right), \tag{3.20}$$

where the sum now includes the diagonal term. The derivation of the linear response correction is unaltered, except that w_{ij} now has nonzero diagonal terms (e.g., in equation 3.12). We propose to fix the value of w_{ii} through learning. We will demonstrate that the inclusion of the self-coupling term is (1) beneficial to obtain a closed-form solution for the learning problem in the absence of hidden units and (2) gives significantly better results than without the self-coupling term.

3.4 No Hidden Units. For the special case of a network without hidden units and with the effective self-coupling, we can make significant simplifications. In this case, the gradients in equations 2.6 can be set equal to zero and can be solved directly in terms of the weights and thresholds; no gradient-based learning is required. First note that $\langle s_i \rangle_c$ and $\langle s_i s_j \rangle_c$ can be computed exactly from the data for all i and j. Let us define $C_{ij} = \langle s_i s_j \rangle_c - \langle s_i \rangle_c \langle s_j \rangle_c$.

The fixed-point equation for $\Delta\theta_i$ gives

$$\Delta\theta_i = 0 \Leftrightarrow m_i = \langle s_i \rangle_c. \tag{3.21}$$

The fixed-point equation for Δw_{ij}, using equation 3.21, gives

$$\Delta w_{ij} = 0 \Leftrightarrow A_{ij} = C_{ij}\, i \neq j. \tag{3.22}$$

Because we have introduced n self-coupling parameters, we must specify n additional constraints. An obvious choice is to ensure that $\langle s_i^2 \rangle = 1$ is also true in the linear response approximation: $1 = \langle s_i^2 \rangle_{lr} = m_i^2 + A_{ii} \Leftrightarrow A_{ii} = C_{ii}$. Then equation 3.22 is equivalent to $(A^{-1})_{ij} = (C^{-1})_{ij}$ if C is invertible. Using equation 3.12, we obtain

$$w_{ij} = \frac{\delta_{ij}}{1 - m_i^2} - (C^{-1})_{ij}. \tag{3.23}$$

In this way we have solved m_i and w_{ij} directly from the fixed-point equations. The thresholds θ_i can now be computed from equation 2.10:

$$\theta_i = \tanh^{-1}(m_i) - \sum_j w_{ij}m_j. \tag{3.24}$$

Note that this method does not require fixed-point iterations to obtain mean firing rates m_i in terms of w_{ij} and θ_i. Instead, the "inverse" computation of θ_i given m_i and w_{ij} is required in equation 3.24. Note also that the thresholds depend on the diagonal weights. The solution of the example task of two neurons discussed in section 2.3 is computed in the appendix.

Although the choice of constraint is particularly convenient, keep in mind that in principle other choices could be made, leading to other solutions. The justification for our choice is that it gives a closed-form solution of high quality, as we will show.

4 Results

In this section we will compare the accuracy of the linear response correction with and without self-coupling with the exact method and with a factorized model that ignores correlations. We restrict ourselves to networks without hidden units. Of course, there are many probability estimation problems, for which the Boltzmann machine without hidden units is a poor model. Our main concern is whether the linear response approximation will give a solution sufficiently close to the optimal solution, not whether the optimal solution is good or bad.

The correct way to compare our method to the exact method is by means of the Kullback divergence. However, this comparison can be done only for small networks. The reason is that the computation of the Kullback divergence requires the computation of the Boltzmann distribution, (see equation 2.4), which requires exponential time due to the partition function Z. In addition, the exact learning method requires exponential time. The comparison by Kullback divergence on small problems is the subject of section 4.1.

For networks with a large number of units, we will demonstrate the quality of the linear response method by means of a pattern completion task; the network must be able to generate the rest of a pattern when part of the pattern is shown. The comparison of pattern completion on larger problems is the subject of section 4.2.

4.1 Comparison Using Kullback Divergence. In order to show the performance of the linear response correction, we have compared it with the results obtained with a factorized model and with the exact method.

For the exact method (ex) we have used conjugate gradient. The mean firing rates and correlations are computed using equations 2.7. For the linear response method without self-coupling term (lr0) we have solved the fixed-point equations 3.22 for $i \neq j$ using least squares and the Levenberg-Marquardt method. The matrix A is given by equation 3.12 with $w_{ii} = 0$. For the linear response method with self-coupling (lr) we obtain the weights and thresholds from equations 3.23 and 3.24. This method can be applied when $\det(C) > 0$. When $\det(C)=0$, we have solved the fixed-point equations 3.22

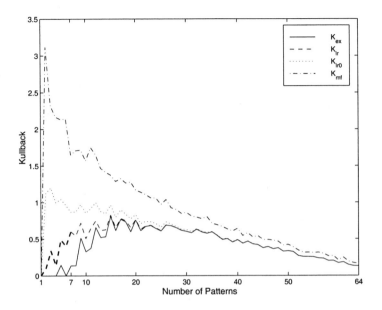

Figure 2: Average Kullback divergence over five random training sets as a function of the number of patterns in the training set. The network consists of six neurons.

for all i, j using least squares and the Levenberg-Marquardt method. The matrix A is given by equation 3.12 with w_{ii} free parameters.

In the case of the factorized model, we assume

$$p_{mf}(\vec{s}) = \prod_i \frac{1}{2}(1 + s_i m_i). \tag{4.1}$$

The mean firing rates are given by $m_i = \langle s_i \rangle_c$. The four methods are compared by computing the Kullback divergence, using equation 2.5.

In Figure 2, we present the results for a network of six neurons. The number of patterns in the training set is varied from $p = 1$ until $p = 64$. For each p, five data sets were randomly generated. Each of the p patterns in the data set is assigned a random probability such that the total probability on the p patterns sums to 1.

The lr method used least-squares minimization for $2 \leq p \leq 6$. For the methods lr0 and lr, we observed for $2 \leq p \leq 6$ in approximately 10% of the cases that the fixed-point equations could not be solved. This can happen because the equations are approximations to the true gradients and therefore do not need to have a fixed-point solution. These cases were deleted from the computation of the average Kullbacks in Figure 2.

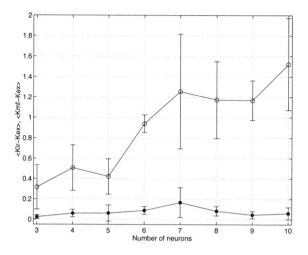

Figure 3: Kullback divergence relative to exact method, for mean-field approximation (open circles) and linear response method with self-coupling (closed circles). The number of patterns $p = 2n$. Results are averaged over four data sets. The error bars indicate the variance over the data sets.

We see that the exact method approaches the target distribution ($K = 0$) for very small number of patterns and for $p \to 2^n$. For $p = 1$, the correlations in the target distribution are absent, and all methods yield Kullback zero. For $p \to 2^n$ the factorized model approaches the exact model. This is because the target distribution becomes more or less constant over all patterns, and correlations are absent in the constant distribution. The most difficult learning tasks are for low and intermediate values of p. The difference between K_{mf} and K_{ex} shows that correlations play a significant role. The linear response solutions with and without the self-coupling term give a significant improvement. Linear response with a self-coupling term gives the best approximation. In the remaining numerical studies, we will consider only the linear response method with self-coupling.

We compare the performance of the various methods on networks with 3 to 10 neurons in Figure 3. For each problem size, training data were randomly generated with $p = 2n$. Each neuron value $s_i^\mu = \pm 1, i = 1, \ldots, n, \mu = 1, \ldots, p$ is generated randomly and independently with equal probability. For each data set, we compute $K_{lr} - K_{ex}$ and $K_{mf} - K_{ex}$. In the figure, we show these values averaged over all data sets, as well as their variances. From the difference between K_{ex} and K_{mf}, we see that correlations play an increasingly important role. The linear response approximation is often quite close to the exact result. The quality of the approximation does not deteriorate with increasing problem size.

4.2 Comparison on Pattern Completion. In this subsection, we demonstrate the quality of the linear response method for larger networks. As we mentioned above, this cannot be done by comparison of the Kullback divergence. Therefore, we propose to compare the different methods on n pattern completion tasks.

We first train the networks as before, as if the problem were a joint probability estimation problem—with no distinction between input and output. Subsequently, we measure the quality of the different solutions by computing

$$Q = -\frac{1}{np} \sum_{i\mu} \log(p(s_i^\mu | \tilde{s}_i^\mu)), \quad \tilde{s}_i^\mu = (s_1^\mu, \ldots, s_{i-1}^\mu, s_{i+1}^\mu, \ldots, s_n^\mu) \qquad (4.2)$$

The quantity $p(s_i^\mu | \tilde{s}_i^\mu)$ is the conditional probability of finding neuron i in the state s_i^μ, given that the rest of the state is $\tilde{s}_i^\mu$. We can do this for the exact method (for small networks) for the linear response method and for the factorized model. Note that the computation of Q is fast because it does not require the computation of the partition function.

In order to use Q to assess the quality of the various methods, we must establish that low Q implies low Kullback divergence K, and vice versa. This is shown in Figure 4. The left graph shows for the linear response solutions and for the factorized model solutions separately that there is a more or less linear relation between the quality in terms of K and in terms of Q. In the right graph, we show for the same data sets the difference in pattern completion quality, $Q_{mf} - Q_{lr}$, versus the difference in Kullback divergence, $K_{mf} - K_{lr}$. From this we see that if one method has a lower Q than another method, we can expect that its Kullback divergence is lower as well.

Thus, one can use the more or less linear relation between Q and K to test the performance of the linear response method for problems with a large number of neurons. In Figure 5, we show the pattern completion quality for the different methods as a function of the network size. The exact method was computed only up to 10 neurons because of the time required. (Depending on the stop criterion, the exact method requires approximately 10 to 30 minutes on a network of 10 neurons on a SPARC 5.) We can see that the linear response method is very close to the exact method. The much higher value of the factorized model indicates the obvious fact that correlations play an important role in this task. Note that the mean-field method approaches $q = \log 2$ for large n, which is due to the fact that the mean-field method assigns $p(s_i^\mu) \approx \frac{1}{2}$ ($m_i \approx 0$) for all i and μ.

5 Discussion

We have proposed a new, efficient method for learning in Boltzmann machines. The method is generally applicable to networks with or without

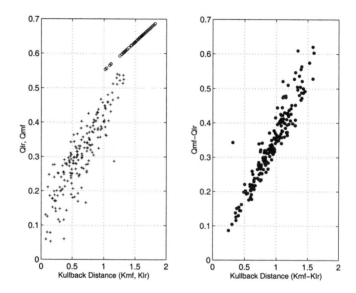

Figure 4: Variation of the pattern completion quality Q with respect to the Kullback divergence K, for 200 data sets on six neurons. Each data set consists of 10 patterns. In the left graph, the plus signs represent the linear response method and the open circles represent the factorized model. In the right graph we plot the difference between the two pattern completion qualities $(Q_{mf} - Q_{lr})$ versus the difference of the Kullback divergence $(K_{mf} - K_{lr})$ for the same data sets.

hidden units. It makes use of the linear response theorem for the computation of the correlations within the mean-field framework.

In our numerical experiments, we restricted ourselves to networks without hidden units. We believe that this is sufficient to show the advantage of the method, since the free expectation values are the most time-consuming part of the computation.

We have observed numerically that the inclusion of self-coupling is important for good results. This is probably also true in the presence of hidden units. In that case, a gradient-based procedure is required, and no closed-form solution exists. The presence of self-coupling was motivated from the TAP equations. A full treatment of the linear response correction in this case is the subject of a future publication.

In the presence of hidden units, both the exact method and the linear response method require a gradient descent algorithm. The advantage of our method is that the gradients can be computed in $\mathcal{O}(n^3)$ instead of in $\mathcal{O}(2^n)$, time. The required number of iterations may be somewhat more for the linear response method, because the gradients are computed only approximately.

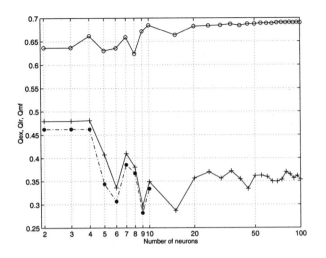

Figure 5: Prediction quality for 27 different random problems with different number of neurons. In every problem, the number of patterns $p = 2n$. The plus signs represent the linear response correction (Q_{lr}). The open circles represent the factorized model (Q_{mf}). The closed circles represent the exact method (Q_{ex}).

This brings us to an interesting point, which is the convergence of the gradient descent algorithm in the linear response approximation. Convergence requires the existence of a Lyapunov function. The Kullback divergence is clearly a Lyapunov function for the exact method, but we were not able to find a Lyapunov function for the linear response approximation. In fact, we would like to construct a cost function such that its gradients are equal to the gradients of K in the linear response approximation. Whether such a function exists is unknown to our knowledge.

In addition to probability estimation, Boltzmann machines have been proposed for combinatoric optimization (Hopfield & Tank, 1985; Durbin & Willshaw, 1987; Yuille & Kosowsky, 1994). For optimization the naive mean-field framework can be successfully applied to combinatoric optimization problems (Yuille, Geiger, & Bülthoff, 1991; Kosowsky & Yuille, 1994). This method is known as deterministic annealing. Clearly the situation is different here, since one is mainly concerned with the quality of the solution at the end of the annealing schedule—when $T \to 0$. Correlations vanish in this limit in unfrustrated systems but can be quite complex in spin glasses (see, for instance, Young, 1983, for numerical results). Whether the linear response correction can improve deterministic annealing is an open question.

The naive mean-field approach arises as a special case of the variational techniques that have been recently proposed. Whether the linear response correction can be applied in this context as well should be investigated further.

Appendix

In this appendix we illustrate the consequences of the linear response method for the simple case of two neurons, considered numerically in section 2.3.

The general probability distribution in two neurons is parameterized by three numbers. Consider the symmetric case where $\langle s_1 \rangle = \langle s_2 \rangle$. Then only two parameters are needed, which we choose such that

$$p(+, +) = \frac{1}{2}(1 + m) - a$$
$$p(+, -) = p(-, +) = a$$
$$p(-, -) = \frac{1}{2}(1 - m) - a.$$

We must require that $0 < a < \frac{1}{2}$ and $2a - 1 < m < 1 - 2a$ to ensure that all probabilities are positive. In this parameterization $\langle s_1 s_2 \rangle = 1 - 4a$ and $\langle s_1 \rangle = \langle s_2 \rangle = m$. The special case of section 2.3 is obtained for $m = a = 0$. The matrix C as defined in section 3.4 is given as

$$C = \begin{pmatrix} 1 - m^2 & 1 - 4a - m^2 \\ 1 - 4a - m^2 & 1 - m^2 \end{pmatrix}.$$

Equation 3.23 gives directly

$$w = \frac{1}{8a} \frac{1 - m^2 - 4a}{1 - m^2 - 2a} \begin{pmatrix} -1 + \frac{4a}{1-m^2} & 1 \\ 1 & -1 + \frac{4a}{1-m^2} \end{pmatrix},$$

and the thresholds are computed using equation 3.24. Note that the diagonal weights play an important role in the computation of the thresholds.

One can also compute the optimal weights and thresholds using the exact method. Setting $\Delta w_{ij} = 0$ and $\Delta \theta_i = 0$ in equation 2.6, we obtain

$$w_{12} = \log \left(\frac{(1 - 2a)^2 - m^2}{4a^2} \right).$$
$$\theta_i = \frac{1}{2} \tanh^{-1} \left(\frac{m}{1 - 2a} \right).$$

The differences are illustrated for $m = 0.1$ and $m = 0.5$ for all allowed values of a in Figure 6.

Note that the linear response approximation is very good when the optimal weights are small. For larger weights, the difference between the two methods increases.

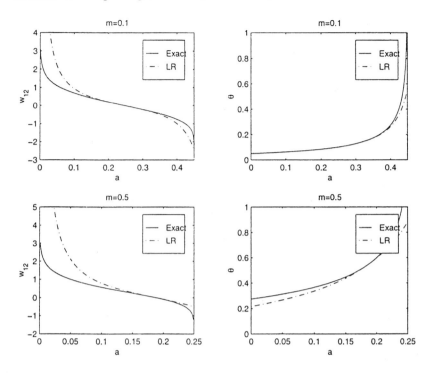

Figure 6: Examples of lateral connection and threshold(s) obtained by exact method and linear response method (LR) for a network of two neurons with $m = 0.1$ and $m = 0.5$.

Acknowledgments

We thank the anonymous referees for valuable suggestions for improvement on earlier versions of this article.

References

Ackley, D., Hinton, G., & Sejnowski, T. (1985). A learning algorithm for Boltzmann machines. *Cognitive Science, 9,* 147–169.

Dayan, P., Hinton, G., Neal, R., & Zemel, R. (1995). The Helmholtz machine. *Neural Computation, 7,* 889–904.

Durbin, R., & Willshaw, D. (1987). An analogue approach to the travelling salesman problem using an elastic net method. *Nature, 326,* 689–691.

Fischer, K., & Hertz, J. (1991). *Spin glasses.* Cambridge: Cambridge University Press.

Galland, C. (1993). The limitations of deterministic Boltzmann machine learning. *Network, 4*, 355–380.

Ginzburg, I., & Sompolinsky, H. (1994). Theory of correlations in stochastic neural networks. *Physical Review E, 50*, 3171–3191.

Hertz, J., Krogh, A., & Palmer, R. (1991). *Introduction to the theory of neural computation.* Redwood City, CA: Addison-Wesley.

Hinton, G. (1989). Deterministic Boltzmann learning performs steepest descent in weight-space. *Neural Computation, 1*, 143–150.

Hopfield, J., & Tank, D. (1985). Neural computation of decision in optimization problems. *Biological Cybernetics, 52*, 141–152.

Itzykson, C., & Drouffe, J.-M. (1989). *Statistical field theory.* Cambridge: Cambridge University Press.

Jaakkola, T., & Jordan, M. (1996). *Recursive algorithms for approximating probabilities in graphical models.* (MIT Computational Cognitive Science Tech. Rep. No. 9604). Cambridge, MA: MIT.

Kappen, H. (1995). Deterministic learning rules for Boltzmann machines. *Neural Networks, 8*, 537–548.

Kappen, H. (1997). Stimulus dependent correlations in stochastic networks. *Physical Review E, 55*, 5849–5858.

Kosowsky, J., & Yuille, A. (1994). The invisible hand algorithm: Solving the assignment problem with statistical physics. *Neural Networks, 3*, 477–490.

Kullback, S. (1959). *Information theory and statistics.* New York: Wiley.

Onsager, L. (1936). Electric moments of molecules in liquids. *Journal of the American Chemical Society, 58*, 1486–1493.

Parisi, G. (1988). *Statistical field theory.* Reading, MA: Addison-Wesley.

Peterson, C., & Anderson, J. (1987). A mean field theory learning algorithm for neural networks. *Complex Systems, 1*, 995–1019.

Plefka, T. (1982). Convergence condition of the TAP equation for the infinite-range Ising spin glass model. *Journal of Physics A, 24*, 2173.

Saul, L., Jaakkola, T., & Jordan, M. (1996). Mean field theory for sigmoid belief networks. *Journal of Artificial Intelligence Research, 4*, 61–76.

Saul, L., & Jordan, M. (1994). Learning in Boltzmann trees. *Neural Computation, 6*, 1174–1184.

Sinclair, A. (1993). *Algorithms for random generation and counting: A Markov chain approach.* Basel: Birkhäuser.

Thouless, D., Anderson, P., & Palmer, R. (1977). Solution of "solvable model of a spin glass." *Philosophical Magazine, 35*, 593–601.

Young, A. (1983). Direct determination of the probability distribution for the spin-glass order parameter. *Physical Review Letters, 51*, 1206–1209.

Yuille, A., Geiger, D., & Bülthoff, H. (1991). Stereo integration, mean field theory and psychophysics. *Network, 2*, 423–442.

Yuille, A., & Kosowsky, J. (1994). Statistical physics algorithms that converge. *Neural Computation, 6*, 341–356.

7

Asymmetric Parallel Boltzmann Machines are Belief Networks

Radford M. Neal
Department of Computer Science, University of Toronto,
10 King's College Road, Toronto, Canada M5S 1A4

A recent paper in this journal (Apolloni and de Falco 1991) presents a learning algorithm for "asymmetric parallel Boltzmann machines." The networks described there can be viewed as particular forms of the "belief networks" (also known as "Bayesian networks") that are discussed in Pearl (1988). I have investigated connectionist learning rules for two types of belief network (Neal 1990, 1992), finding a learning rule for networks with sigmoidal units that is mathematically equivalent to that of Apolloni and de Falco. However, my computational implementation of this rule is different.

The networks of Apolloni and de Falco consist, when unfolded in time, of some number of layers of 0/1-valued units, each with weighted connections from the units of the preceding layer. Given some probability distribution for units in the first layer, a probability distribution for the subsequent layers is defined by letting the conditional probability that unit i in layer ℓ takes the value 1, given the values in the preceding layers, be $\sigma(\sum_j w_{ij}^\ell s_j^{\ell-1})$, where $s_j^{\ell-1}$ is the value of unit j in layer $\ell - 1$, w_{ij}^ℓ is the weight from that unit to unit i, and $\sigma(x) = 1/(1 + e^{-x})$. The learning problem is to adjust the network weights so as to make the distribution so defined for the last, "output," layer match that observed in the environment. There is also a version that learns a conditional distribution for an "output" given an "input."

A "belief network" also defines a probability distribution over units, expressed as the product of the conditional probabilities for each unit given the values of units that precede it in some ordering. Many types of belief networks are possible, differing in how these conditional probabilities are expressed. The networks of Apolloni and de Falco are belief networks in which the units have values of 0 and 1 and conditional probabilities are defined in terms of a weighted sum from preceding units, using the sigmoid function. Note that when viewed as belief networks, the layer structure is seen to be inessential. It is necessary only that the units be ordered in some way such that the connections all go forward; output units can be situated anywhere. Mixture models and hidden

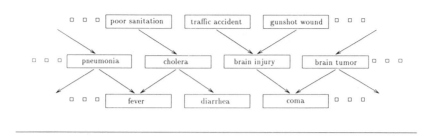

Figure 1: A fragment of a belief network for medical diagnosis.

Markov models can also be regarded as belief networks. In these cases, the networks have a tree structure that permits particularly efficient computation.

A fragment of a hypothetical belief network that might be used for medical diagnosis is shown in Figure 1. The arrows into a unit indicate which other units are relevant in specifying its conditional probability distribution. If these probabilities are specified in terms of a weighted sum of inputs, each arrow will have a weight associated with it. In manually constructed belief networks such as this, it is typical for the arrows to also correspond to the direction in which causal influences are thought to operate, but this is not necessary if the objective is simply to represent probabilities.

Weights for such a network can be learned as follows. For each training case, a sample is taken from the distribution over all units conditional on the output units having their observed values. For each state thus sampled, the weights are updated by amounts

$$\Delta w_{ij}^{\ell} \propto \left[s_i^{\ell} - \sigma \left(\sum_k w_{ik}^{\ell} s_k^{\ell-1} \right) \right] s_j^{\ell-1}$$

Apolloni and de Falco sample states compatible with the known outputs by simply generating states from the unconditional distribution and discarding those that fail to match the output. If the number of outputs is at all large, this procedure is extremely slow.

The stochastic simulation procedure now known as "Gibbs sampling" is generally preferable (Pearl 1988, section 4.4.3). In this method, of which the standard Boltzmann machine simulation procedure is a particular case, one clamps the values of observed units to their known values, sets the unclamped units to arbitrary initial values, and then repeatedly chooses a new value for each unclamped unit from its conditional distribution given the current values of all other units. This results in a stationary distribution equal to the conditional distribution given the observational data. I have successfully used this procedure to learn sigmoidal belief networks, as well as belief networks of the "noisy-OR" type

(Neal 1990, 1992). The method is similar to Boltzmann machine learning, but without the "negative phase." Lack of a negative phase allows learning to proceed significantly faster than in a Boltzmann machine.

I believe that connectionist forms of belief networks are a promising way to attack unsupervised learning problems, at which backpropagation does not excel. They may also be useful in integrating empirical knowledge with knowledge derived from human experts, representation of which was the original motivation for work on belief networks.

References

Apolloni, B., and de Falco, D. 1991. Learning by asymmetric parallel Boltzmann machines. *Neural Comp.* **3**, 402–408.

Neal, R. M. 1990. *Learning stochastic feedforward networks.* Tech. Rep. CRG-TR-90-7, University of Toronto, Department of Computer Science, Connectionist Research Group.

Neal, R. M. 1992. Connectionist learning of belief networks. *Artificial Intelligence* **56**, 71–113.

Pearl, J. 1988. *Probabilistic Reasoning in Intelligent System: Networks of Plausible Inference.* Morgan Kaufmann, San Mateo, CA.

8

Variational Learning in Nonlinear Gaussian Belief Networks

Brendan J. Frey
Beckman Institute, University of Illinois at Urbana-Champaign, Urbana, IL 61801, U.S.A.

Geoffrey E. Hinton
Gatsby Computational Neuroscience Unit, University College London, London, England WC1N 3AR, U.K.

We view perceptual tasks such as vision and speech recognition as inference problems where the goal is to estimate the posterior distribution over latent variables (e.g., depth in stereo vision) given the sensory input. The recent flurry of research in independent component analysis exemplifies the importance of inferring the continuous-valued latent variables of input data. The latent variables found by this method are linearly related to the input, but perception requires nonlinear inferences such as classification and depth estimation. In this article, we present a unifying framework for stochastic neural networks with nonlinear latent variables. Nonlinear units are obtained by passing the outputs of linear gaussian units through various nonlinearities. We present a general variational method that maximizes a lower bound on the likelihood of a training set and give results on two visual feature extraction problems. We also show how the variational method can be used for pattern classification and compare the performance of these nonlinear networks with other methods on the problem of handwritten digit recognition.

1 Introduction

There have been many proposals for unsupervised, multilayer neural networks that contain a stochastic generative model and learn by adjusting their parameters to maximize the likelihood of generating the observed data. Two of the most tractable models of this kind are factor analysis (Everitt, 1984) and independent component analysis (Comon, Jutten, & Herault, 1991; Bell & Sejnowski, 1995; Amari, Cichocki, & Yang, 1996; MacKay, 1997).

1.1 Linear Generative Models. In factor analysis there is one hidden layer that contains fewer units than the visible layer. In the generative model, the hidden units are driven by zero-mean, unit-variance, independent gaussian noise. The hidden units provide top-down input to the linear visible units via the generative weights and each visible unit has its own level of added gaussian noise. Given the generative weights and the noise levels of the visible units, it is tractable to compute the posterior distribution of the hidden activities induced by an observed vector of visible activities. This posterior distribution is a full covariance gaussian whose mean depends on the visible activities. Once this distribution has been computed, it is straightforward to adjust the generative weights to maximize the likelihood of the observed data using either a gradient method or the expectation-maximization (EM) algorithm (Rubin & Thayer, 1982). Unfortunately, factor analysis ignores all the statistical structure in the data that is not contained in the covariance matrix and its hidden representations are linearly related to the data, so it is unable to extract many of the hidden causes of the data that are important in tasks such as vision and speech recognition.

In independent component analysis the generative model is still linear, but the independent noise levels for the hidden units are nongaussian. This makes it difficult to compute the full posterior distribution across the hidden units given a visible vector. However, by using the same number of hidden and visible units and by setting the noise levels of the visible units to zero, it is possible to collapse the posterior distribution across the hidden units to a point that is found by multiplying the visible activities by the inverse of the matrix of hidden-to-visible generative weights. To maximize the likelihood of the data, the weights are adjusted to make the posterior points have high log probability under the noise models of the hidden units, while keeping the determinant of the generative weight matrix small so that probability density in the space of hidden activities gets concentrated when it is mapped into the visible space. Unfortunately, independent component analysis extracts components that are a linear function of the data and it assumes the data are noise-free, so it too is unable to extract hidden causes that are nonlinearly related to observed, noisy data. Recently, attempts have been made to enhance the representational capabilities of independent component analysis by adding noise to the visible units (Olshausen & Field, 1996; Lewicki & Sejnowski, 1998).

1.2 Very Nonlinear Generative Models. An appealing approach to understanding how the cortex constructs models of sensory data is to assume that it uses maximum likelihood to learn a hierarchical generative model. For tasks such as vision and speech recognition, the cortex probably requires distributed representations that are a nonlinear function of the data and allow noise at every level of the hierarchy. Attempts at developing learning algorithms capable of constructing such generative models have been less successful in practice than the simpler linear models. This is because it is hard to compute (or even to represent) the posterior probability distribution across the hidden representations when given a visible vector and a set of weights and noise variances.

The unsupervised version of the Boltzmann machine (Hinton & Sejnowski, 1986) is a multilayer generative model that learns distributed representations that are a nonlinear function of the data. It uses symmetrically connected stochastic binary units and has a relatively simple learning rule that follows the gradient of the log-likelihood of the data under the generative model. Unfortunately, to get this gradient, it is necessary to perform Gibbs sampling in the hidden activities until they reach thermal equilibrium with a data vector clamped on the visible units. This is very time-consuming, and the problem is made even worse by the need to compute derivatives of the partition function, which requires the network to reach thermal equilibrium with the visible units unclamped. The sampling noise and the difficulty in reaching equilibrium in networks with large weights make the learning algorithm painfully slow.

When binary stochastic units are connected in a directed acyclic graph, we get a "binary sigmoidal belief network" (Pearl, 1988; Neal, 1992). (Here, "acyclic" means that there are not any closed paths when following edge directions. There may be closed paths when the edge directions are ignored.) The net input to each unit is given by a weighted sum of the activities of the unit's parents. Learning is easier in this network than in a Boltzmann machine because there is no need to compute the derivative of a partition function and the gradient of the log-likelihood does not involve a difference in sampled statistics. Most important, it is no longer necessary for the Gibbs sampling to converge to thermal equilibrium before the weights are adjusted. Using the analysis of EM provided by Neal and Hinton (1993), it can be shown that on average, the learning algorithm improves a bound on the log probability of the data even when the Gibbs sampling is too brief to get close to equilibrium (Hinton, Sallans, & Ghahramani, 1998).

There have been several attempts to avoid Gibbs sampling altogether when fitting a sigmoidal belief network to data. (See Frey, 1998, for a review of these methods.) They all rely on the idea that learning can still improve a bound on the log-likelihood of the data even when the posterior distribution over hidden states is computed incorrectly. The stochastic Helmholtz machine (Hinton, Dayan, Frey, & Neal, 1995) uses a separate, stochastic recognition network to compute a quick and dirty approximation to a sample from the posterior distribution over the hidden units when given a visible vector. There is a very simple rule for learning both the generative weights and the recognition weights, but the approximation produced by the recognition network is often poor, and the method of learning the recognition weights is not guaranteed to improve it. The deterministic Helmholtz machine (Dayan, Hinton, Neal, & Zemel, 1995) makes even more restrictive assumptions than the stochastic version about the probability distribution that is used to approximate the full posterior distribution over the binary hidden states when given a data vector. It assumes that the approximating distribution can be written as a product of separate probabilities for each hidden unit. It also assumes that the approximating product distribution can be computed by a deterministic recognition network in a single bottom-up pass. This latter assumption is relaxed in variational approaches

(Saul, Jaakkola, & Jordan, 1996; Jaakkola, Saul, & Jordan, 1996), which eliminate the separate recognition model and use the generative weights and
numerical optimization to find the set of probabilities that minimizes the
asymmetric divergence from the true posterior distribution.

1.3 Continuous Sigmoidal Belief Networks. For real-valued data that
come from real physical processes, binary units are often an inappropriate
model because they fail to capture the approximately linear structure of the
data over small ranges. For example, very small changes in the position,
orientation, or scale of an object lead to linear changes in the pixel intensities. One way to endow the linear gaussian networks described above with
representations that are nonlinear functions of the data is to apply a smooth
sigmoidal squashing function to the output of each gaussian before passing
the activity down the network. The nonlinear squashing function allows
each unit to take on a variety of behaviors, ranging from nearly gaussian to
nearly binary. Frey (1997a, b) showed that a Markov chain Monte Carlo and
a variational method could be used to train small networks of these units.
However, the smoothness of the squashing function prevents units from
placing probability mass on a single point, and so these units are unable
to produce activities exactly equal to zero. The ability of a network to set
activities exactly equal to zero is important for sparse representations where
many units do not participate in explaining an input pattern.

1.4 Piecewise Linear Belief Networks. In an attempt to produce sparse
distributed representations of real-valued data, Hinton and Ghahramani
(1997) investigated generative models composed of multiple layers of rectified linear units. In the generative model, each unit receives top-down input
that is a linear function of the rectified states in the layer above and it adds
gaussian noise to get its own real-valued unrectified state,

$$x_i = w_{i0} + \sum_{j \in A_i} w_{ij} f(x_j) + \text{noise}, \quad \text{where} \quad f(x_j) = \begin{cases} 0 & \text{if } x_j < 0, \\ x_j & \text{if } x_j \geq 0, \end{cases} \quad (1.1)$$

and A_i is the set of indices for the parents of unit i. The output that a unit
sends to the layer below is equal to its unrectified state if it is positive but
is equal to 0 if it is negative.

Networks of these units can set the activities of some units exactly equal
to zero so that they do not participate in explaining the current input pattern.
Hinton and Ghahramani (1997) showed that Gibbs sampling was feasible in
such networks and that multilayer networks of rectified linear units could
learn to extract sparse hidden representations that were nonlinearly related
to images.

1.5 Nonlinear Gaussian Belief Networks. Linear generative models,
binary sigmoidal belief networks, continuous sigmoidal belief networks,

and piecewise linear belief networks can all be viewed as networks of gaussian units that apply various nonlinearities to their gaussian states. The probability density function over the pre-nonlinearity variables $\mathbf{x} = (x_1, \ldots, x_N)$ in such a nonlinear gaussian belief network (NLGBN) is

$$p(\mathbf{x}) = \prod_{i=1}^{N} p(x_i | \{x_j\}_{j \in A_i}) = \prod_{i=1}^{N} \frac{1}{\psi_i} \phi \left(\frac{x_i - \sum_{j \in A_i} w_{ij} f_j(x_j)}{\psi_i} \right), \tag{1.2}$$

where A_i is the set of indices for the parents of unit i and $\phi(\cdot)$ is the standard normal density function:

$$\phi(y) = \frac{1}{\sqrt{2\pi}} e^{-y^2/2}. \tag{1.3}$$

ψ_i^2 is the variance of the gaussian noise for unit i and $f_j(\cdot)$ is the nonlinear function for unit j. For example, some units may use a step function (making them binary sigmoidal units with a cumulative gaussian activation function), whereas other units may use the rectification function (making them real-valued units that encourage sparse representat ons). We define $f_0(x_0) = 1$ so that w_{i0} represents a constant bias for unit i i. equation 1.2.

In this article, we generalize the variational method developed by Jaakkola et al. (1996) for networks of binary units and show that it can be successfully applied to performing approximate inference and learning in nonlinear gaussian belief networks. The variational method can still be applied when different types of nonlinearity are used in the same network, such as networks of the kind described in Hinton, Sallans, & Ghahramani (1998), where binary and linear units come in pairs and the output of each linear unit is gated by its associated binary unit.

2 Variational Expectation Maximization

A surprisingly simple variational technique can be used for inference and learning in NLGBNs. In this method, once some variables have been observed, we postulate a simple parametric variational distribution $q(\cdot)$ over the remaining unobserved variables. (The variational distribution $q(\cdot)$ is separate from the generative distribution $p(\cdot)$.) A numerical optimization method (e.g., conjugate gradients) is then used to adjust the variational parameters to bring $q(\cdot)$ as close to the true posterior as possible. We use a function that not only measures closeness in the Kullback-Leibler sense, but also bounds from below the log-likelihood of the input pattern. This choice of function leads to an efficient generalized EM learning algorithm.

2.1 A Function That Bounds the Log-Probability. Let V be the set of indices of the observed variables for the current input pattern and let H be the set of indices of the unobserved variables for the current input pattern,

so that $V \cup H = \{1, \ldots, N\}$. The variational bound (Neal & Hinton, 1993) is

$$F = \langle \log p(\mathbf{x}) \rangle - \langle \log q(\{x_i\}_{i \in H}) \rangle \leq \log p(\{x_i\}_{i \in V}), \tag{2.1}$$

where $\langle \cdot \rangle$ indicates an expectation over the unobserved variables with respect to $q(\cdot)$. It is easily shown that for unconstrained $q(\cdot)$, F is maximized by setting $q(\{x_i\}_{i \in H}) = p(\{x_i\}_{i \in H} | \{x_i\}_{i \in V})$, in which case the bound in equation 2.1 is tight. This gives exact probabilistic inference, whereas using a constrained form for $q(\cdot)$ gives approximate probabilistic inference.

The variational distribution we consider here is a product of gaussians:

$$q(\{x_i\}_{i \in H}) = \prod_{i \in H} q(x_i) = \prod_{i \in H} \frac{1}{\sigma_i} \phi \left(\frac{x_i - \mu_i}{\sigma_i} \right), \tag{2.2}$$

where μ_i and σ_i, $i \in H$ are the variational parameters. By adjusting these parameters, we can obtain an axis-aligned gaussian approximation to the true posterior distribution over the prenonlinearity hidden variables.

For this variational distribution, it turns out that F can be expressed in terms of the mean and variance of the postnonlinearity activities. Let $M_i(\mu, \sigma)$ be the mean output of unit i when the input is gaussian noise with mean μ and variance σ^2:

$$M_i(\mu, \sigma) = \int_x \frac{1}{\sigma} \phi \left(\frac{x - \mu}{\sigma} \right) f_i(x) dx. \tag{2.3}$$

Let $V_i(\mu, \sigma)$ be the variance at the output of unit i when the input is gaussian noise with mean μ and variance σ^2:

$$V_i(\mu, \sigma) = \int_x \frac{1}{\sigma} \phi \left(\frac{x - \mu}{\sigma} \right) \{ f_i(x) - M_i(\mu, \sigma) \}^2 dx. \tag{2.4}$$

We assume that these can be easily computed, closely approximated, or in the case of $V_i(\cdot, \cdot)$, bounded from above (the latter will give a new lower bound on F). (See appendix C for these functions in the case of linear units, binary units, rectified units, and sigmoidal units.)

The variational bound, equation 2.1, simplifies to[1]

$$F = -\sum_{i=1}^{N} \frac{1}{2\psi_i^2} \left\{ \left[\mu_i - \sum_{j \in A_i} w_{ij} M_j(\mu_j, \sigma_j) \right]^2 + \sum_{j \in A_i} w_{ij}^2 V_j(\mu_j, \sigma_j) \right\}$$

$$+ \sum_{i \in H} \frac{1}{2} \left(1 + \log 2\pi \sigma_i^2 - \frac{\sigma_i^2}{\psi_i^2} \right) - \sum_{i=1}^{N} \frac{1}{2} \log 2\pi \psi_i^2. \tag{2.5}$$

---

[1] To see how $\langle \log p(\mathbf{x}) \rangle$ simplifies, add and subtract both μ_i and $\sum_{j \in A_i} w_{ij} M_j(\mu_j, \sigma_j)$ in the numerator of the argument of $\phi(\cdot)$ in equation 1.2, so that $\langle \log p(\mathbf{x}) \rangle = -\sum_i \log(2\pi \psi_i^2)/2 - \sum_i \langle ([x_i - \mu_i] + [\mu_i - \sum_{j \in A_i} w_{ij} M_j(\mu_j, \sigma_j)] + \sum_{j \in A_i} w_{ij} [M_j(\mu_j, \sigma_j) - f_j(x_j)])^2 \rangle / 2\psi_i^2$. The cross-terms produced by the square vanish under the expectation.

To make this formula concise, we have introduced dummy variational parameters for the observed variables: if x_i is observed to have the value x_i^*, we *fix* $\mu_i = x_i^*$ and $\sigma_i = 0$.

For unit i in equation 2.5, the term in curly braces measures the mean squared error under $q(\cdot)$ between μ_i and the input to unit i as given by its parents: $\langle[\mu_i - \sum_{j\in A_i} w_{ij}f_j(x_j)]^2\rangle$. It is down-weighted by the model noise variance ψ_i^2, since for larger noise variances, a particular mean squared prediction error is less important.

2.2 Probabilistic Inference. Variational inference consists of first fixing $\mu_i = x_i^*$ and $\sigma_i = 0, i \in V$ in equation 2.5 and then maximizing F with respect to μ_i and $\log\sigma_i^2, i \in H$. (The optimization for the variances is performed in the log-domain, since $\log\sigma_i^2$ is allowed to go negative.) We use the conjugate gradient method to perform this optimization, although other techniques can be used (e.g., steepest descent or possibly a covariant method; Amari, 1985). The derivatives of F with respect to μ_i and $\log\sigma_i^2, i \in H$ are given in appendix A. After optimization, the means and variances of the variational distribution represent the inference statistics.

2.3 Learning. We bound the log-probability of an entire training set by $\mathcal{F}$, which is equal to the sum of the bounds for the individual training patterns. The variational EM algorithm based on $\mathcal{F}$ consists of iterating the following two steps:

- *E-step*: Perform variational inference by maximizing $\mathcal{F}$ with respect to the sets of variational parameters corresponding to the different input patterns.

- *M-step*: Maximize $\mathcal{F}$ with respect to the model parameters ($w_{..}$'s and $\psi_.$'s).

Notice that by maintaining sufficient statistics while scanning through the training set in the E-step, it is not necessary to store the sets of variational parameters. These sufficient statistics are described in appendix B. However, to speed up the current E-step, we initialize the set of variational parameters to the set found at the end of the last E-step for the same pattern.

It turns out that the M-step can be performed very efficiently (see appendix B for details). Since the values of the model variances do not affect the values of the weights that maximize F in equation 2.5, we first maximize F with respect to the weights. As pointed out by Jaakkola et al. (1996) for their binary gaussian belief networks, F is quadratic in the weights, so we can use singular value decomposition to solve for the weights exactly. Next, the optimal model variances are computed directly.

2.4 Software. A set of UNIX programs that implement variational learning in NLGBNs is available at http://www.cs.utoronto.ca/~frey. The software includes linear units, binary units, rectified units, and sigmoidal units. New types of unit can be added easily by providing the nonlinear function and its derivatives.

3 Visual Feature Extraction

Approximate maximum likelihood estimation in latent variable models can be used to learn latent structure that is perceptually significant (Hinton et al., 1995). In this section, we consider two unsupervised feature extraction tasks and for each task we compare the representations learned by the variational method applied to two types of NLGBN and the representations learned by Gibbs sampling applied to a piecewise linear NLGBN. If the hidden units all use a piecewise linear activation function, then Gibbs sampling can be efficiently used for learning, as described in Hinton and Ghahramani (1997). One of the NLGBNs used for variational learning contains only binary hidden units of the type described in Jaakkola et al. (1996). In this section we see how the variational technique compares to another learning method for continuous hidden units, as well as how the generalization of the variational method from binary to continuous units compares to variational learning in binary networks.

3.1 The Continuous Bars Problem.
An important problem in vision is modeling surface edges in a way that is consistent with physical constraints. The goal of the much simpler bars problem (Dayan & Zemel, 1995) is to learn without supervision to detect bars of two orthogonal orientations and to model the constraint that each image consists of bars of the same orientation. In Hinton and Ghahramani (1997), a continuous form of this problem was presented. Each training image is formed by first choosing between vertical and horizontal orientation with equal probability. Then each bar of that orientation is turned on with a probability of 0.3 with an intensity that is drawn uniformly from [0, 5]. Eight examples from a training set of 1000 6×6 images of this sort are shown in Figure 1a, where the area of each tiny white square indicates the pixel intensity. A noisy version of these data in which unit variance gaussian noise is added to each pixel is shown in Figure 1e (a black square indicates a negative pixel value).

For each of the two data sets, we used 100 iterations of variational EM to train a three-layer NLGBN with 1 binary top-layer unit, 16 rectified middle-layer units, and 36 linear visible bottom-layer units. (Using more units in the hidden layers had little effect on the features extracted during learning.) The resulting weights projecting from each of the 16 middle-layer units to the 6×6 image are shown in Figures 1b and 1f. Surprisingly, clearer bar features were extracted from the noisy data. The weights (not shown) from the top-layer binary unit to the middle-layer units tend to make the top-layer unit active for one orientation and inactive for the other. The weights look similar if a rectified unit is used at the top, but a binary unit properly represents

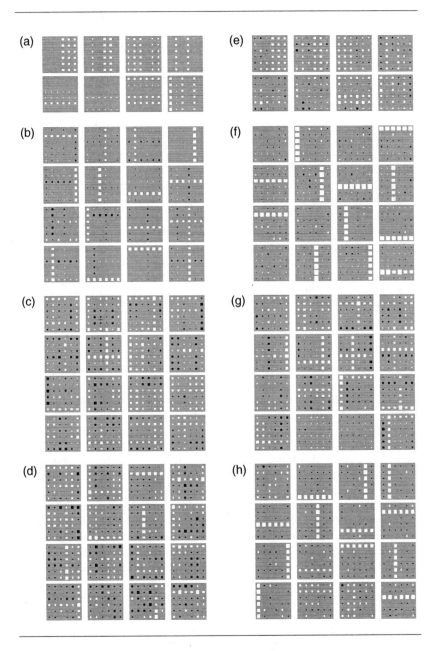

Figure 1: Learning in NLGBNs using the variational method and Gibbs sampling, for noise-free (a–d) and noisy (e–h) bar patterns. (a, e) Training examples. (b, f) Weights learned by the variational method with rectified units. (c, g) Weights learned by the variational method with binary units. (d, h) Weights learned by Gibbs sampling with rectified units.

the discrete choice between horizontal and vertical. Figures 1c and 1g show the weights learned by variational EM in a network where all of the hidden units are binary. The individual bars are not properly extracted for either the noise-free or noisy training data. The log-probability bounds for the trained binary-rectified-linear NLGBNs are 27.4 nats and −60.3 nats, whereas the bounds for the trained binary-binary-linear NLGBNs are −48.3 nats and −65.6 nats, significantly lower.

We also trained a three-layer NLGBN with rectified hidden units using Gibbs sampling. For this method, a learning rate must be chosen, and we used 0.1. Sixteen sweeps of Gibbs sampling were performed for each pattern presentation before the parameters were adjusted online. The weights obtained after 10 passes through each data set are shown in Figures 1d and 1h. The features for the noise-free data are not as clear as the ones extracted using the variational method. The features for the noisy data can be cleaned up if some weight decay is used (Hinton & Ghahramani, 1997). We did not estimate the log-probability of the data in this case, since Gibbs sampling does not readily provide a straightforward way to obtain such estimates. In our experiments, variational EM and the Gibbs sampling method took roughly the same time. However, an online version of variational EM may be faster.

3.2 The Continuous Stereo Disparity Problem. Another vision problem where the latent variables are nonlinearly related to the input is the estimation of depth from a stereo pair of sensory images. In the simplified version of this problem presented in Becker and Hinton (1992), the goal is to learn that the visual input consists of randomly positioned dots on a one-dimensional surface placed at one of two depths.

In our experiments, four blurred dots (gaussian functions) were randomly positioned uniformly on the continuous interval [0, 12] and the brightness of each dot (magnitude of the gaussian) was drawn uniformly from [0, 5]. Next, a left or a right shift was applied with equal probability to obtain a second activity pattern. Finally, two sensory images containing 12 real values each were obtained by dividing each interval into 12 pixels and assigning to each pixel the net activity within the pixel. Twelve examples from a training set of 1000 pairs of images obtained in this manner are shown in Figure 2a, where the images are positioned so that the relative shift is evident. A noisy version of these data in which unit variance gaussian noise is added to each sensor is shown in Figure 2e.

The stereo disparity problem is much more difficult than the bars problem, since there is more overlap between the underlying features. To see this, imagine a "multieyed" disparity problem in which there are as many sensory images as there are one-dimensional sensors. We expect the depth inference to be easier in this case, since there is more evidence for each of the two possible directions of shift. Imagine stacking the sensory images on top of each other, so that each resulting square image will contain blurred

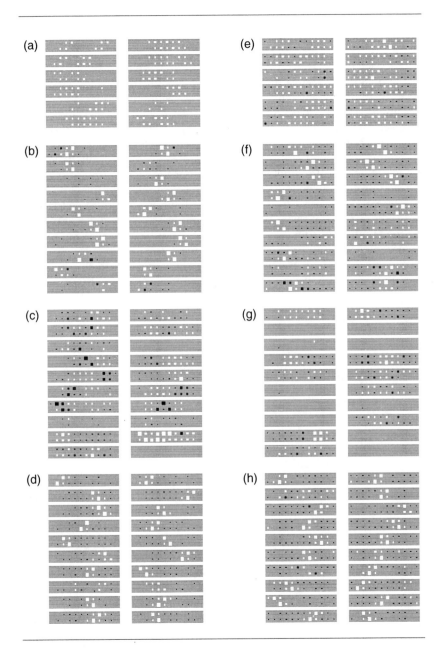

Figure 2: Learning in NLGBNs using the variational method and Gibbs sampling, for noise-free (a–d) and noisy (e–h) stereo disparity patterns. (a, e) Training examples. (b, f) Weights learned by the variational method with rectified units. (c, g) Weights learned by the variational method with binary units. (d, h) Weights learned by Gibbs sampling with rectified units.

diagonal bars that are oriented either up and to the right or up and to the left. Extracting disparity from these data is roughly equivalent to extracting bar orientation in the data from the previous section.

For each of the noisy and noise-free data sets, we used 100 iterations of variational EM to train a three-layer NLGBN with 1 binary top-layer unit, 20 rectified middle-layer units, and 24 linear visible bottom-layer units. The resulting weights projecting from each of the 20 middle-layer units to the two sets of 12 pixels are shown in Figures 2b and 2f. In both cases, the algorithm has extracted features that are spatially local and represent each of the two possible depths. Figures 2c and 2g show the weights learned by variational EM in a network where all of the hidden units are binary. The log-probability bounds for the trained binary-rectified-linear NLGBNs are 1.0 nats and -43.7 nats, whereas the bounds for the trained binary-binary-linear NLGBNs are -37.8 nats and -46.1 nats. The Gibbs sampling method with rectified hidden units and using the same learning parameters as described in the previous section produced the weight patterns shown in Figures 2d and 2h. For the noisy data, the features extracted by Gibbs sampling appear to be slightly cleaner than those extracted by variational EM.

4 Handwriting Recognition

Variational inference and learning in NLGBNs can be used to do real-valued pattern classification by training one NLGBN on each class of data. If C_i is the event that a pattern comes from class $i \in \{0, 1, \ldots\}$, then the posterior class probabilities are given by Bayes' rule

$$P(C_i | \{x_k\}_{k \in V}) = \frac{p(\{x_k\}_{k \in V} | C_i) P(C_i)}{\sum_j p(\{x_k\}_{k \in V} | C_j) P(C_j)}, \tag{4.1}$$

where $P(C_j)$ is the prior probability that a pattern comes from class j. The likelihood $p(\{x_k\}_{k \in V} | C_j)$ for class j is approximated by the value of the variational bound obtained from a generalized E-step.

In this section, we report the performances of several completely automated learning procedures on the problem of recognizing gray-level 8×8 images of handwritten digits from the CEDAR CDROM 1 database of zip codes (Hull, 1994). The DELVE evaluation platform (Rasmussen et al., 1996) was used to obtain fair comparisons, including levels of statistical significance.

For each of three different sizes of training set, we empirically estimated the performances of k-nearest neighbors, with the neighborhood for each class of data determined using leave-one-out cross validation; mixture of diagonal (axis-aligned) gaussians, with the number of gaussians for each class determined using a validation set; factor analysis, with the number of factors for each class determined using a validation set; and one- and two-hidden layer NLGBNs using rectified hidden units and linear visible units, with the number of hidden units determined using a validation set. For each of the latter four methods, the training set was first split according to class, and then one-third of the data was set aside for validation. Models with different complexities (number of gaussians or number of hidden units) were trained on the remaining two-thirds of the data using EM or generalized EM until convergence. The model that gave the highest validation set log-probability (or log-probability bound) was further trained to convergence on all of the data for the corresponding class. To prevent degenerate overfitting of a pixel that happens to have the same value in all of the training cases, the variances for the visible units were not allowed to fall below 0.01 in the latter four methods. For each method, equation 4.1 was used to classify each test pattern.

To obtain robust estimates of the relative performances of these methods on the problem of handwritten digit recognition, we trained and tested each method multiple times using disjoint training set–test set pairs. The original data set of 11,000 8×8 images was partitioned into a set of 8000 images used for training and a set of 3000 images used for testing. For training set sizes of 1000 and 2000 patterns, four disjoint training set–test set pairs were extracted from the two partitions (each test set had 750 images). For the training set size of 4000 patterns, two disjoint training set–test set pairs were extracted (each test set had 1500 images).

The results are shown in Figure 3, where each horizontal bar gives an estimate of the expected error rate for a particular method using a particular training set size. The methods are ordered from left to right for each training set size as follows: k-nearest neighbors, mixture of gaussians, factor analysis, one-hidden layer NLGBN, and two-hidden layer NLGBN. Each vertical bar gives an estimate of the error (one standard deviation) in the corresponding estimate of the expected error rate. Integers in the boxes lying beneath the x-axis are p-values (in percent) for a paired t-test that compares the performances of the corresponding methods. Select a method from the list in the lower left-hand corner of the figure, and scan from left to right. Whenever you see a number, that means another method has performed better than the method you selected, with the given statistical significance. A low p-value indicates the difference in the misclassification rates is significant. More precisely, the p-value is an estimate of the probability of obtaining a difference in performance that is equal to or greater than the observed difference, given that the true difference is zero (the null hypothesis).

On the largest training set size, the two-hidden layer NLGBN performs better than k-nearest neighbors ($p = 5\%$), mixture of gaussians ($p = 9\%$), factor analysis ($p = 5\%$), and the one-hidden layer NLGBN ($p = 16\%$). The performance of the NLGBN with one hidden layer is fairly indistinguishable from the performance of factor analysis ($p = 25\%$). However, on average the NLGBN used only half as many hidden units as were used by factor analysis, indicating that the NLGBN provides a more compact

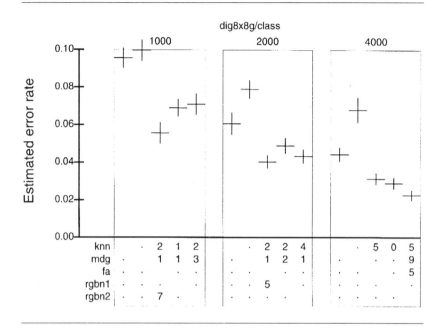

Figure 3: Estimated error rates on gray-level handwritten digit recognition using different sizes of training set (1000, 2000, and 4000 images) for the following methods: k-nearest neighbor, mixture of diagonal (axis-aligned) gaussians, factor analysis, and rectified gaussian belief networks with one and two hidden layers. For each size of training set, the error rates for the different methods are given in the above order. The numbers in the boxes are p-values (in percent) for a paired t-test on the null hypothesis that the corresponding two methods have identical performance. A dot indicates the p-value was above 9%.

representation of the input. It is also interesting that this more compact representation emerged despite the fact that the posterior distribution over the hidden units in the NLGBN was approximated by an axis-aligned gaussian distribution, whereas in factor analysis, the exact full-covariance posterior distribution over the hidden units is used.

5 Conclusions

Results on visual feature extraction show that the variational technique can extract perceptually significant continuous nonlinear latent structure. In contrast with networks with continuous hidden variables, networks with binary hidden variables do not extract spatially local features from the data. Similarly, linear methods like factor analysis and independent component analysis fail to extract spatially local features (Zoubin Ghahramani, personal communication). Results also show that the variational method presented in this article is a viable alternative to Gibbs sampling in stochastic neural networks with rectified hidden variables.

Advantages of the variational method over Gibbs sampling include the absence of a learning rate and the ability to compute the log-probability bound very efficiently. The latter is particularly useful for pattern classifiers that train one network on each class of data and then classify a novel pattern by picking the network that gives the highest estimate of the log-probability (Frey, 1998). Results show that for handwritten digit recognition, there is a regime of training set size in which NLGBNs perform better than k-nearest neighbors, mixture of gaussians, and the linear factor analysis method.

The variational method may be made more powerful by making each distribution $q(x_i)$ in equation 2.1 a mixture of gaussians, by making the entire distribution $q(\cdot)$ a mixture of product form distributions (Jaakkola & Jordan, 1998), or by grouping together small numbers of hidden variables over which full-covariance gaussians are fit during variational inference.

We considered three types of continuous nonlinear unit in this article: binary, rectified, and sigmoidal. The variational method can be easily extended to other types of units (such as "twinned" units; Hinton et al., 1998) as long as the output mean function $M(\mu, \sigma)$ and the output variance function $V(\mu, \sigma)$ can be computed. To perform a gradient-based E-step, the gradients of these functions with respect to their arguments are also needed.

Although we have not focused our attention on implementations of the variational algorithm that are suited to biology, we believe that with some modifications, they can be made so. The inference algorithm uses the log-probability bound derivatives given in equation A.3, and these are computed from simple differences passed locally in the network. A partial M-step can be used for online learning, in which case the derivative of the bound for just the current input pattern is followed. This derivative can be followed by applying a delta-type rule based on locally computed differences.

Appendix A: The E-Step

Here we show how to compute F and its derivatives with respect to the variational parameters. For the current set of variational parameters (including the ones fixed by the current input pattern), we first compute for each unit the current values of the mean output $m_i \leftarrow M_i(\mu_i, \sigma_i)$, the output variance $v_i \leftarrow V_i(\mu_i, \sigma_i)$, and the mean net input:

$$n_i \leftarrow \sum_{j \in A_i} w_{ij} m_j. \tag{A.1}$$

Then the bound on the log-probability of the input pattern is computed from

$$F \leftarrow -\sum_{i=1}^{N} \frac{1}{2\psi_i^2} \left[(\mu_i - n_i)^2 + \sum_{j \in A_i} w_{ij}^2 v_j \right]$$

$$+ \sum_{i \in H} \frac{1}{2} \left(1 + \log 2\pi \sigma_i^2 - \frac{\sigma_i^2}{\psi_i^2} \right) - \sum_{i=1}^{N} \frac{1}{2} \log 2\pi \psi_i^2. \tag{A.2}$$

To perform a gradient-based optimization in the E-step, the derivatives of the bound with respect to μ_j and $\log \sigma_j^2$ for $j \in H$ are computed as follows:

$$\frac{\partial F}{\partial \mu_j} \leftarrow \frac{n_j - \mu_j}{\psi_j^2} - \frac{\partial M_j(\mu_j, \sigma_j)}{\partial \mu_j} \sum_{i \in C_j} \frac{w_{ij}(n_i - \mu_i)}{\psi_i^2}$$

$$- \frac{\partial V_j(\mu_j, \sigma_j)}{\partial \mu_j} \sum_{i \in C_j} \frac{w_{ij}^2}{2\psi_i^2},$$

$$\frac{\partial F}{\partial \log \sigma_j^2} \leftarrow - \frac{\partial V_j(\mu_j, \sigma_j)}{\partial \log \sigma_j^2} \sum_{i \in C_j} \frac{w_{ij}^2}{2\psi_i^2} - \frac{\partial M_j(\mu_j, \sigma_j)}{\partial \log \sigma_j^2} \sum_{i \in C_j} \frac{w_{ij}(n_i - \mu_i)}{\psi_i^2}$$

$$- \frac{\sigma_j^2}{2\psi_j^2} + \frac{1}{2}, \tag{A.3}$$

where C_j is the set of indices for the children of unit j. Appendix C gives expressions for the derivatives of the nonlinear functions for binary units, rectified units, and sigmoidal units.

An E-step produces one set of variational parameters $\mu_i^{(t)}, \sigma_i^{(t)}, i = 1, \ldots,$ N and the corresponding $m_i^{(t)}, v_i^{(t)},$ and $n_i^{(t)}, i = 1, \ldots, N$ for each training pattern, $t = 1, \ldots, T$. These are used to initialize the next E-step.

Appendix B: The M-Step

In the log-probability bound in equation 2.5, the model variances do not influence the optimal weights. So in the M-step, we first maximize the total bound with respect to the weights. Since the bound is quadratic in the weights, we use singular value decomposition to solve for them exactly. In fact, the weights associated with the input to each variable are decoupled from the other weights in the network. That is, the value of w_{ij} does not affect the optimal value of w_{kl} if $i \neq k$. Consequently, solving for the optimal weights is a matter of solving N linear systems, where system $i, i = 1, \ldots, N,$ has dimensionality equal to the number of parents for unit i and once solved gives the weights on the incoming connections to unit i.

Consider the input means $\mu_i^{(t)}$, output means $m_i^{(t)}$, input variances $\sigma_i^{(t)}$, output variances $v_i^{(t)}$, and mean net inputs $n_i^{(t)}$, $i = 1, \ldots, N$, which are computed for training pattern t in the E-step. It is not necessary to store all of these sets for all T training patterns. However, they are used to compute the following sufficient statistics:

$$a_{jk} \leftarrow \frac{1}{T}\sum_t m_j^{(t)}m_k^{(t)}, \quad b_j \leftarrow \frac{1}{T}\sum_t v_j^{(t)}, \quad c_{ij} \leftarrow \frac{1}{T}\sum_t \mu_i^{(t)}m_j^{(t)},$$

$$d_j \leftarrow \frac{1}{T}\sum_t (n_j^{(t)} - \mu_j^{(t)})^2, \quad e_j \leftarrow \frac{1}{T}\sum_t \sigma_j^{(t)2}, \tag{B.1}$$

for $j = 0, \ldots, N$, $k = 0, \ldots, N$, and $i \in c_j$. These can be accumulated while scanning through the training set during the E-step.

Once the sufficient statistics have been computed, we first solve for the weights. The system of equations for the weights associated with the input to unit i is

$$\sum_{k \in A_i} a_{jk}w_{ik} + b_j w_{ij} = c_{ij}, \quad j \in A_i, \tag{B.2}$$

where i is fixed in this set of equations. We use singular value decomposition to solve for each set of weights. In fact, the system of equations for unit i has dimensionality equal to the number of parents for unit i (including its bias). Finally, the model variances are computed from

$$\psi_j^2 \leftarrow d_j + e_j + \sum_{k \in A_j} w_{jk}^2 b_k. \tag{B.3}$$

Appendix C: $M(\mu, \sigma)$, $V(\mu, \sigma)$ and Their Derivatives for Interesting Nonlinear Functions

In this appendix, we give the output means and variances for some useful types of units: linear units, binary units, rectified units, and sigmoidal units.

C.1 Linear Units. Although this article is about how to deal with nonlinear units, it is often useful to include some units (e.g., visible units) that are linear:

$$f(x) = x. \tag{C.1}$$

For this unit, the output mean and variance are

$$M(\mu, \sigma) = \mu, \quad V(\mu, \sigma) = \sigma^2. \tag{C.2}$$

The derivatives are

$$\frac{\partial M(\mu, \sigma)}{\partial \mu} = 1, \qquad \frac{\partial M(\mu, \sigma)}{\partial \log \sigma^2} = 0,$$

$$\frac{\partial V(\mu, \sigma)}{\partial \mu} = 0, \qquad \frac{\partial V(\mu, \sigma)}{\partial \log \sigma^2} = \sigma^2. \tag{C.3}$$

C.2 Binary Units. To obtain a stochastic binary unit, take

$$f(x) = \begin{cases} 0 & \text{if } x < 0, \\ 1 & \text{if } x \geq 0. \end{cases} \tag{C.4}$$

For this unit, the output mean and variance are

$$M(\mu, \sigma) = \Phi\left(\frac{\mu}{\sigma}\right), \qquad V(\mu, \sigma) = \Phi\left(\frac{\mu}{\sigma}\right)\left[1 - \Phi\left(\frac{\mu}{\sigma}\right)\right], \tag{C.5}$$

where $\Phi(\cdot)$ is the cumulative gaussian function:

$$\Phi(y) = \int_{\alpha=-\infty}^{y} \phi(\alpha)d\alpha. \tag{C.6}$$

The derivatives are

$$\frac{\partial M(\mu, \sigma)}{\partial \mu} = \frac{1}{\sigma}\phi\left(\frac{\mu}{\sigma}\right), \qquad \frac{\partial M(\mu, \sigma)}{\partial \log \sigma^2} = -\frac{\mu}{2\sigma}\phi\left(\frac{\mu}{\sigma}\right),$$

$$\frac{\partial V(\mu, \sigma)}{\partial \mu} = \frac{1}{\sigma}\phi\left(\frac{\mu}{\sigma}\right)\left[1 - 2\Phi\left(\frac{\mu}{\sigma}\right)\right],$$

$$\frac{\partial V(\mu, \sigma)}{\partial \log \sigma^2} = -\frac{\mu}{2\sigma}\phi\left(\frac{\mu}{\sigma}\right)\left[1 - 2\Phi\left(\frac{\mu}{\sigma}\right)\right]. \tag{C.7}$$

C.3 Rectified Units. A rectified unit is linear if its input exceeds 0 and outputs 0 otherwise:

$$f(x) = \begin{cases} 0 & \text{if } x < 0, \\ x & \text{if } x \geq 0. \end{cases} \tag{C.8}$$

For this unit, the output mean and variance are

$$M(\mu, \sigma) = \mu\Phi\left(\frac{\mu}{\sigma}\right) + \sigma\phi\left(\frac{\mu}{\sigma}\right),$$

$$V(\mu, \sigma) = (\mu^2 + \sigma^2)\Phi\left(\frac{\mu}{\sigma}\right) + \mu\sigma\phi\left(\frac{\mu}{\sigma}\right) - M(\mu, \sigma)^2. \tag{C.9}$$

The derivatives are

$$\frac{\partial M(\mu,\sigma)}{\partial \mu} = \Phi\left(\frac{\mu}{\sigma}\right), \qquad \frac{\partial M(\mu,\sigma)}{\partial \log \sigma^2} = \frac{\sigma}{2}\phi\left(\frac{\mu}{\sigma}\right),$$

$$\frac{\partial V(\mu,\sigma)}{\partial \mu} = 2\mu\Phi\left(\frac{\mu}{\sigma}\right) + 2\sigma\phi\left(\frac{\mu}{\sigma}\right) - 2M(\mu,\sigma)\Phi\left(\frac{\mu}{\sigma}\right),$$

$$\frac{\partial V(\mu,\sigma)}{\partial \log \sigma^2} = \sigma^2\Phi\left(\frac{\mu}{\sigma}\right) - \sigma M(\mu,\sigma)\Phi\left(\frac{\mu}{\sigma}\right). \tag{C.10}$$

C.4 Sigmoidal Units. The cumulative gaussian squashing function,

$$f(x) = \Phi(x), \tag{C.11}$$

leads to closed-form expressions for the output mean and its derivatives. We have not found a closed-form expression for the output variance, but it can be approximately bounded by a new function $V'(\mu,\sigma)$, giving a new lower bound on F. The output mean and variance bound are

$$M(\mu,\sigma) = \Phi\left(\frac{\mu}{\sqrt{1+\sigma^2}}\right),$$

$$V(\mu,\sigma) \leq V'(\mu,\sigma) = \Phi\left(\frac{\mu}{\sqrt{1+\sigma^2}}\right)\left[1 - \Phi\left(\frac{\mu}{\sqrt{1+\sigma^2}}\right)\right]$$

$$\times \frac{\sigma^2}{\sigma^2 + \pi/2}. \tag{C.12}$$

The derivatives are

$$\frac{\partial M(\mu,\sigma)}{\partial \mu} = \frac{1}{\sqrt{1+\sigma^2}}\phi\left(\frac{\mu}{\sqrt{1+\sigma^2}}\right),$$

$$\frac{\partial M(\mu,\sigma)}{\partial \log \sigma^2} = -\frac{\mu\sigma^2}{2(1+\sigma^2)^{3/2}}\phi\left(\frac{\mu}{\sqrt{1+\sigma^2}}\right),$$

$$\frac{\partial V'(\mu,\sigma)}{\partial \mu} = \frac{\sigma^2}{(\sigma^2+\pi/2)\sqrt{1+\sigma^2}}\phi\left(\frac{\mu}{\sqrt{1+\sigma^2}}\right)\left[1 - 2\Phi\left(\frac{\mu}{\sqrt{1+\sigma^2}}\right)\right],$$

$$\frac{\partial V'(\mu,\sigma)}{\partial \log \sigma^2} = \frac{\sigma^2}{\sigma^2+\pi/2}\left\{\frac{\pi/2}{\sigma^2+\pi/2}\Phi\left(\frac{\mu}{\sqrt{1+\sigma^2}}\right)\left[1 - \Phi\left(\frac{\mu}{\sqrt{1+\sigma^2}}\right)\right]\right.$$

$$\left. - \frac{\mu\sigma^2}{2(1+\sigma^2)^{3/2}}\phi\left(\frac{\mu}{\sqrt{1+\sigma^2}}\right)\left[1 - 2\Phi\left(\frac{\mu}{\sqrt{1+\sigma^2}}\right)\right]\right\}. \tag{C.13}$$

Acknowledgments

We thank Peter Dayan, Zoubin Ghahramani, and Tommi Jaakkola for helpful discussions. We also appreciate the useful feedback provided by Michael

Jordan, an anonymous reviewer, and Karla Miller. The Gibbs sampling experiments were performed using software developed by Zoubin Ghahramani (see http://www.cs.utoronto.ca/~zoubin). This research was funded by grants from the Arnold and Mabel Beckman Foundation, the Natural Science and Engineering Research Council of Canada, and the Information Technology Research Center of Ontario.

References

Amari, S.-I. (1985). *Differential-geometrical methods in statistics.* New York: Springer-Verlag.

Amari, S.-I., Cichocki, A., & Yang, H. (1996). A new learning algorithm for blind signal separation. In D. S. Touretzky, M. C. Mozer, & M. E. Hasselmo (Eds.), *Advances in neural information processing systems, 8.* Cambridge, MA: MIT Press.

Becker, S., & Hinton, G. E. (1992). A self-organizing neural network that discovers surfaces in random-dot stereograms. *Nature, 355,* 161–163.

Bell, A. J., & Sejnowski, T. J. (1995). An information maximization approach to blind separation and blind deconvolution. *Neural Computation, 7,* 1129–1159.

Comon, P., Jutten, C., & Herault, J. (1991). Blind separation of sources. *Signal Processing, 24,* 11–20.

Dayan, P., Hinton, G. E., Neal, R. M., & Zemel, R. S. (1995). The Helmholtz machine. *Neural Computation, 7,* 889–904.

Dayan, P., & Zemel, R. S. (1995). Competition and multiple cause models. *Neural Computation, 7,* 565–579.

Everitt, B. S. (1984). *An introduction to latent variable models.* New York: Chapman and Hall.

Frey, B. J. (1997a). Continuous sigmoidal belief networks trained using slice sampling. In M. C. Mozer, M. I. Jordan, & T. Petsche (Eds.), *Advances in neural information processing systems, 9.* Cambridge, MA: MIT Press. Available online at: http://www.cs.utoronto.ca/~frey.

Frey, B. J. (1997b). Variational inference for continuous sigmoidal Bayesian networks. In *Sixth International Workshop on Artificial Intelligence and Statistics.*

Frey, B. J. (1998). *Graphical models for machine learning and digital communication.* Cambridge, MA: MIT Press. Available online at: http://mitpress.mit.edu/book-home.tcl?isbn=026206202X.

Hinton, G. E., Dayan, P., Frey, B. J., & Neal, R. M. (1995). The wake-sleep algorithm for unsupervised neural networks. *Science, 268,* 1158–1161.

Hinton, G. E., & Ghahramani, Z. (1997). Generative models for discovering sparse distributed representations. *Philosophical Transactions of the Royal Society of London B, 352,* 1177–1190.

Hinton, G. E., Sallans, B., & Ghahramani, Z. (1998). A hierarchical community of experts. In M. I. Jordan (Ed.), *Learning and inference in graphical models.* Norwell, MA: Kluwer.

Hinton, G. E., & Sejnowski, T. J. (1986). Learning and relearning in Boltzmann machines. In D. E. Rumelhart & J. L. McClelland (Eds.), *Parallel distributed processing: Explorations in the microstructure of cognition* (vol. 1, pp. 282–317). Cambridge, MA: MIT Press.

Hull, J. J. (1994). A database for handwritten text recognition research. *IEEE Transactions on Pattern Analysis and Machine Intelligence, 16*, 550–554.

Jaakkola, T. S., & Jordan, M. I. (1998). Approximating posteriors via mixture models. In M. I. Jordan (Ed.), *Learning and inference in graphical models*. Norwell MA: Kluwer.

Jaakkola, T., Saul, L. K., & Jordan, M. I. (1996). Fast learning by bounding likelihoods in sigmoid type belief networks. In D. S. Touretzky, M. C. Mozer, & M. E. Hasselmo (Eds.), *Advances in neural information processing systems, 8*. Cambridge, MA: MIT Press.

Lewicki, M. S., & Sejnowski, T. J. (1998). Learning nonlinear overcomplete representations for efficient coding. In M. I. Jordan, M. I. Kearns, & S. A. Solla (Eds.), *Advances in neural information processing systems, 10*. Cambridge, MA: MIT Press.

MacKay, D. J. C. (1997). *Maximum likelihood and covariant algorithms for independent component analysis*. Unpublished manuscript. Available online at: http://wol.ra.phy.cam.ac.uk/mackay.

Neal, R. M. (1992). Connectionist learning of belief networks. *Artificial Intelligence, 56*, 71–113.

Neal, R. M., & Hinton, G. E. (1993). *A new view of the EM algorithm that justifies incremental and other variants*. Unpublished manuscript. Available via FTP at: ftp://ftp.cs.utoronto.ca/pub/radford/em.ps.Z.

Olshausen, B. A., & Field, D. J. (1996). Emergence of simple-cell receptive-field properties by learning a sparse code for natural images. *Nature, 381*, 607–609.

Pearl, J. (1988). *Probabilistic reasoning in intelligent systems*. San Mateo, CA: Morgan Kaufmann.

Rasmussen, C. E., Neal, R. M., Hinton, G. E., van Camp, D., Revow, M., Ghahramani, Z., Kustra, R., & Tibshirani, R. (1996). *The DELVE manual*. Toronto: University of Toronto. Available online at: http://www.cs.utoronto.ca/~delve.

Rubin, D., & Thayer, D. (1982). EM algorithms for ML factor analysis. *Psychometrika, 47*, 69–76.

Saul, L. K., Jaakkola, T., & Jordan, M. I. (1996). Mean field theory for sigmoid belief networks. *Journal of Artificial Intelligence Research, 4*, 61–76.

9

Mixtures of Probabilistic Principal Component Analyzers

Michael E. Tipping
Christopher M. Bishop
Microsoft Research, St. George House, Cambridge CB2 3NH, U.K.

Principal component analysis (PCA) is one of the most popular techniques for processing, compressing, and visualizing data, although its effectiveness is limited by its global linearity. While nonlinear variants of PCA have been proposed, an alternative paradigm is to capture data complexity by a combination of local linear PCA projections. However, conventional PCA does not correspond to a probability density, and so there is no unique way to combine PCA models. Therefore, previous attempts to formulate mixture models for PCA have been ad hoc to some extent. In this article, PCA is formulated within a maximum likelihood framework, based on a specific form of gaussian latent variable model. This leads to a well-defined mixture model for probabilistic principal component analyzers, whose parameters can be determined using an expectation-maximization algorithm. We discuss the advantages of this model in the context of clustering, density modeling, and local dimensionality reduction, and we demonstrate its application to image compression and handwritten digit recognition.

1 Introduction

Principal component analysis (PCA) (Jolliffe, 1986) has proved to be an exceedingly popular technique for dimensionality reduction and is discussed at length in most texts on multivariate analysis. Its many application areas include data compression, image analysis, visualization, pattern recognition, regression, and time-series prediction.

The most common definition of PCA, due to Hotelling (1933), is that for a set of observed d-dimensional data vectors $\{t_n\}$, $n \in \{1 \ldots N\}$, the q principal axes w_j, $j \in \{1, \ldots, q\}$, are those orthonormal axes onto which the retained variance under projection is maximal. It can be shown that the vectors w_j are given by the q dominant eigenvectors (those with the largest associated eigenvalues) of the sample covariance matrix $S = \sum_n (t_n - \bar{t})(t_n - \bar{t})^T / N$ such that $Sw_j = \lambda_j w_j$ and where $\bar{t}$ is the sample mean. The vector $x_n = W^T(t_n - \bar{t})$, where $W = (w_1, w_2, \ldots, w_q)$, is thus a q-dimensional reduced representation of the observed vector t_n.

A complementary property of PCA, and that most closely related to the original discussions of Pearson (1901), is that the projection onto the principal subspace minimizes the squared reconstruction error $\sum \|\mathbf{t}_n - \hat{\mathbf{t}}_n\|^2$. The optimal linear reconstruction of $\mathbf{t}_n$ is given by $\hat{\mathbf{t}}_n = \mathbf{W}\mathbf{x}_n + \bar{\mathbf{t}}$, where $\mathbf{x}_n = \mathbf{W}^T(\mathbf{t}_n - \bar{\mathbf{t}})$, and the orthogonal columns of $\mathbf{W}$ span the space of the leading q eigenvectors of $\mathbf{S}$. In this context, the principal component projection is often known as the Karhunen-Loève transform.

One limiting disadvantage of these definitions of PCA is the absence of an associated probability density or generative model. Deriving PCA from the perspective of density estimation would offer a number of important advantages, including the following:

- The corresponding likelihood would permit comparison with other density-estimation techniques and facilitate statistical testing.

- Bayesian inference methods could be applied (e.g., for model comparison) by combining the likelihood with a prior.

- In classification, PCA could be used to model class-conditional densities, thereby allowing the posterior probabilities of class membership to be computed. This contrasts with the alternative application of PCA for classification of Oja (1983) and Hinton, Dayan, and Revow (1997).

- The value of the probability density function could be used as a measure of the "degree of novelty" of a new data point, an alternative approach to that of Japkowicz, Myers, and Gluck (1995) and Petsche et al. (1996) in autoencoder-based PCA.

- The probability model would offer a methodology for obtaining a principal component projection when data values are missing.

- The single PCA model could be extended to a mixture of such models.

This final advantage is particularly significant. Because PCA defines only a *linear* projection of the data, the scope of its application is necessarily somewhat limited. This has naturally motivated various developments of *nonlinear* PCA in an effort to retain a greater proportion of the variance using fewer components. Examples include principal curves (Hastie & Stuetzle, 1989; Tibshirani, 1992), multilayer autoassociative neural networks (Kramer, 1991), the kernel-function approach of Webb (1996), and the generative topographic mapping (GTM) of Bishop, Svensén, and Williams (1998). An alternative paradigm to such global nonlinear approaches is to model nonlinear structure with a collection, or mixture, of local linear submodels. This philosophy is an attractive one, motivating, for example, the mixture-of-experts technique for regression (Jordan & Jacobs, 1994).

A number of implementations of "mixtures of PCA" have been proposed in the literature, each defining a different algorithm or a variation. The variety of proposed approaches is a consequence of ambiguity in the formulation of the overall model. Current methods for local PCA generally necessitate a two-stage procedure: a partitioning of the data space followed by estimation of the principal subspace within each partition. Standard Euclidean distance-based clustering may be performed in the partitioning phase, but more appropriately, the reconstruction error may be used as the criterion for cluster assignments. This conveys the advantage that a common cost measure is used in both stages. However, even recently proposed models that adopt this cost measure still define different algorithms (Hinton et al., 1997; Kambhatla & Leen, 1997), while a variety of alternative approaches for combining local PCA models have also been proposed (Broomhead, Indik, Newell, & Rand, 1991; Bregler & Omohundro, 1995; Hinton, Revow, & Dayan, 1995; Dony & Haykin, 1995). None of these algorithms defines a probability density.

One difficulty in implementation is that when using "hard" clustering in the partitioning phase (Kambhatla & Leen, 1997), the overall cost function is inevitably nondifferentiable. Hinton et al. (1997) finesse this problem by considering the partition assignments as missing data in an expectation-maximization (EM) framework, and thereby propose a "soft" algorithm where instead of any given data point being assigned exclusively to one principal component analyzer, the responsibility for its generation is shared among all of the analyzers. The authors concede that the absence of a probability model for PCA is a limitation to their approach and propose that the responsibility of the jth analyzer for reconstructing data point t_n be given by $r_{nj} = \exp{(-E_j^2/2\sigma^2)}/\{\sum_{j'} \exp{(-E_{j'}^2/2\sigma^2)}\}$, where E_j is the corresponding reconstruction cost. This allows the model to be determined by the maximization of a pseudo-likelihood function, and an explicit two-stage algorithm is unnecessary. Unfortunately, this also requires the introduction of a variance parameter σ^2 whose value is somewhat arbitrary, and again, no probability density is defined.

Our key result is to derive a probabilistic model for PCA. From this a mixture of local PCA models follows as a natural extension in which all of the model parameters may be estimated through the maximization of a single likelihood function. Not only does this lead to a clearly defined and unique algorithm, but it also conveys the advantage of a probability density function for the final model, with all the associated benefits as outlined above.

In section 2, we describe the concept of latent variable models. We then introduce probabilistic principal component analysis (PPCA) in section 3, showing how the principal subspace of a set of data vectors can be obtained within a maximum likelihood framework. Next, we extend this result to mixture models in section 4, and outline an efficient EM algorithm for estimating all of the model parameters in a mixture of probabilistic principal component analyzers. The partitioning of the data and the estimation of local principal axes are automatically linked. Furthermore, the algorithm implicitly incorporates a soft clustering similar to that implemented by Hinton et al. (1997), in which the parameter σ^2 appears naturally within the model.

Indeed, σ^2 has a simple interpretation and is determined by the same EM procedure used to update the other model parameters.

The proposed PPCA mixture model has a wide applicability, and we discuss its advantages from two distinct perspectives. First, in section 5, we consider PPCA for dimensionality reduction and data compression in local linear modeling. We demonstrate the operation of the algorithm on a simple toy problem and compare its performance with that of an explicit reconstruction-based nonprobabilistic modeling method on both synthetic and real-world data sets.

A second perspective is that of general gaussian mixtures. The PPCA mixture model offers a way to control the number of parameters when estimating covariance structures in high dimensions, while not overconstraining the model flexibility. We demonstrate this property in section 6 and apply the approach to the classification of images of handwritten digits.

Proofs of key results and algorithmic details are provided in the appendixes.

2 Latent Variable Models and PCA

2.1 Latent Variable Models. A latent variable model seeks to relate a d-dimensional observed data vector $\mathbf{t}$ to a corresponding q-dimensional vector of latent variables $\mathbf{x}$:

$$\mathbf{t} = \mathbf{y}(\mathbf{x}; \mathbf{w}) + \boldsymbol{\epsilon}, \tag{2.1}$$

where $\mathbf{y}(\cdot; \cdot)$ is a function of the latent variables $\mathbf{x}$ with parameters $\mathbf{w}$, and $\boldsymbol{\epsilon}$ is an $\mathbf{x}$-independent noise process. Generally, $q < d$ such that the latent variables offer a more parsimonious description of the data. By defining a prior distribution over $\mathbf{x}$, together with the distribution of $\boldsymbol{\epsilon}$, equation 2.1 induces a corresponding distribution in the data space, and the model parameters may then be determined by maximum likelihood techniques. Such a model may also be termed generative, as data vectors $\mathbf{t}$ may be generated by sampling from the $\mathbf{x}$ and $\boldsymbol{\epsilon}$ distributions and applying equation 2.1.

2.2 Factor Analysis. Perhaps the most common example of a latent variable model is that of statistical factor analysis (Bartholomew, 1987), in which the mapping $\mathbf{y}(\mathbf{x}; \mathbf{w})$ is a linear function of $\mathbf{x}$:

$$\mathbf{t} = \mathbf{W}\mathbf{x} + \boldsymbol{\mu} + \boldsymbol{\epsilon}. \tag{2.2}$$

Conventionally, the latent variables are defined to be independent and gaussian with unit variance, so $\mathbf{x} \sim \mathcal{N}(\mathbf{0}, \mathbf{I})$. The noise model is also gaussian such that $\boldsymbol{\epsilon} \sim \mathcal{N}(\mathbf{0}, \boldsymbol{\Psi})$, with $\boldsymbol{\Psi}$ diagonal, and the $(d \times q)$ parameter matrix $\mathbf{W}$ contains the factor loadings. The parameter $\boldsymbol{\mu}$ permits the data model to have nonzero mean. Given this formulation, the observation vectors are also normally distributed $t \sim \mathcal{N}(\mu, C)$, where the model covariance is $C = \Psi + WW^T$. (As a result of this parameterization, C is invariant under postmultiplication of W by an orthogonal matrix, equivalent to a rotation of the x coordinate system.) The key motivation for this model is that because of the diagonality of Ψ, the observed variables t are conditionally independent given the latent variables, or factors, x. The intention is that the dependencies between the data variables t are explained by a smaller number of latent variables x, while ϵ represents variance unique to each observation variable. This is in contrast to conventional PCA, which effectively treats both variance and covariance identically. There is no closed-form analytic solution for W and Ψ, so their values must be determined by iterative procedures.

2.3 Links from Factor Analysis to PCA. In factor analysis, the subspace defined by the columns of W will generally not correspond to the principal subspace of the data. Nevertheless, certain links between the two methods have been noted. For instance, it has been observed that the factor loadings and the principal axes are quite similar in situations where the estimates of the elements of Ψ turn out to be approximately equal (e.g., Rao, 1955). Indeed, this is an implied result of the fact that if $\Psi = \sigma^2 I$ and an isotropic, rather than diagonal, noise model is assumed, then PCA emerges if the $d - q$ smallest eigenvalues of the sample covariance matrix S are exactly equal. This homoscedastic residuals model is considered by Basilevsky (1994, p. 361), for the case where the model covariance is identical to its data sample counterpart. Given this restriction, the factor loadings W and noise variance σ^2 are identifiable (assuming correct choice of q) and can be determined analytically through eigendecomposition of S, without resort to iteration (Anderson, 1963).

This established link with PCA requires that the $d - q$ minor eigenvalues of the sample covariance matrix be equal (or, more trivially, be negligible) and thus implies that the covariance model must be exact. Not only is this assumption rarely justified in practice, but when exploiting PCA for dimensionality reduction, we do not require an exact characterization of the covariance structure in the minor subspace, as this information is effectively discarded. In truth, what is of real interest in the homoscedastic residuals model is the form of the maximum likelihood solution when the model covariance is not identical to its data sample counterpart.

Importantly, we show in the following section that PCA still emerges in the case of an approximate model. In fact, this link between factor analysis and PCA had been partially explored in the early factor analysis literature by Lawley (1953) and Anderson and Rubin (1956). Those authors showed that the maximum likelihood solution in the approximate case was related to the eigenvectors of the sample covariance matrix, but did not show that these were the *principal* eigenvectors but instead made this additional assumption. In the next section (and in appendix A) we extend this earlier work to give a full characterization of the properties of the model we term probabilistic PCA. Specifically, with $\epsilon \sim \mathcal{N}\left(0, \sigma^2 I\right)$, the columns of the maximum likelihood estimator W_{ML} are shown to span the principal subspace of the data even when $C \neq S$.

3 Probabilistic PCA

3.1 The Probability Model.
For the case of isotropic noise $\epsilon \sim \mathcal{N}\left(0, \sigma^2 I\right)$, equation 2.2 implies a probability distribution over t-space for a given x of the form

$$p(t|x) = (2\pi\sigma^2)^{-d/2} \exp\left\{-\frac{1}{2\sigma^2}\|t - Wx - \mu\|^2\right\}. \tag{3.1}$$

With a gaussian prior over the latent variables defined by

$$p(x) = (2\pi)^{-q/2} \exp\left\{-\frac{1}{2}x^T x\right\}, \tag{3.2}$$

we obtain the marginal distribution of t in the form

$$p(t) = \int p(t|x)p(x)dx, \tag{3.3}$$

$$= (2\pi)^{-d/2}|C|^{-1/2} \exp\left\{-\frac{1}{2}(t - \mu)^T C^{-1}(t - \mu)\right\}, \tag{3.4}$$

where the model covariance is

$$C = \sigma^2 I + WW^T. \tag{3.5}$$

Using Bayes' rule, the posterior distribution of the latent variables x given the observed t may be calculated:

$$p(x|t) = (2\pi)^{-q/2}|\sigma^{-2}M|^{1/2}$$

$$\times \exp\left[-\frac{1}{2}\left\{x - M^{-1}W^T(t - \mu)\right\}^T (\sigma^{-2}M)\right.$$

$$\left.\left\{x - M^{-1}W^T(t - \mu)\right\}\right], \tag{3.6}$$

where the posterior covariance matrix is given by

$$\sigma^2 M^{-1} = \sigma^2(\sigma^2 I + W^T W)^{-1}. \tag{3.7}$$

Note that M is $q \times q$ while C is $d \times d$.

The log-likelihood of observing the data under this model is

$$\mathcal{L} = \sum_{n=1}^{N} \ln \{p(\mathbf{t}_n)\},$$

$$= -\frac{N}{2} \left\{ d \ln(2\pi) + \ln |\mathbf{C}| + \mathrm{tr}\left(\mathbf{C}^{-1}\mathbf{S}\right)\right\}, \qquad (3.8)$$

where

$$\mathbf{S} = \frac{1}{N} \sum_{n=1}^{N} (\mathbf{t}_n - \boldsymbol{\mu})(\mathbf{t}_n - \boldsymbol{\mu})^{\mathrm{T}}, \qquad (3.9)$$

is the sample covariance matrix of the observed $\{\mathbf{t}_n\}$.

3.2 Properties of the Maximum Likelihood Estimators. The maximum likelihood estimate of the parameter $\boldsymbol{\mu}$ is given by the mean of the data:

$$\boldsymbol{\mu}_{\mathrm{ML}} = \frac{1}{N} \sum_{n=1}^{N} \mathbf{t}_n. \qquad (3.10)$$

We now consider the maximum likelihood estimators for the parameters $\mathbf{W}$ and σ^2.

3.2.1 The Weight Matrix $\mathbf{W}$.   The log-likelihood (see equation 3.8) is maximized when the columns of $\mathbf{W}$ span the principal subspace of the data. To show this we consider the derivative of equation 3.8 with respect to $\mathbf{W}$:

$$\frac{\partial \mathcal{L}}{\partial \mathbf{W}} = N(\mathbf{C}^{-1}\mathbf{S}\mathbf{C}^{-1}\mathbf{W} - \mathbf{C}^{-1}\mathbf{W}). \qquad (3.11)$$

In appendix A it is shown that with $\mathbf{C}$ given by equation 3.5, the only nonzero stationary points of equation 3.11 occur for

$$\mathbf{W} = \mathbf{U}_q (\boldsymbol{\Lambda}_q - \sigma^2 \mathbf{I})^{1/2} \mathbf{R}, \qquad (3.12)$$

where the q column vectors in the $d \times q$ matrix $\mathbf{U}_q$ are eigenvectors of $\mathbf{S}$, with corresponding eigenvalues in the $q \times q$ diagonal matrix $\boldsymbol{\Lambda}_q$, and $\mathbf{R}$ is an arbitrary $q \times q$ orthogonal rotation matrix. Furthermore, it is also shown that the stationary point corresponding to the global maximum of the likelihood occurs when $\mathbf{U}_q$ comprises the principal eigenvectors of $\mathbf{S}$, and thus $\boldsymbol{\Lambda}_q$ contains the corresponding eigenvalues $\lambda_1, \ldots, \lambda_q$, where the eigenvalues of $\mathbf{S}$ are indexed in order of decreasing magnitude. All other combinations of eigenvectors represent saddle points of the likelihood surface. Thus, from equation 3.12, the latent variable model defined by equation 2.2 effects a mapping from the latent space into the principal subspace of the observed data.

3.2.2 The Noise Variance σ^2. It may also be shown that for $\mathbf{W} = \mathbf{W}_{\mathrm{ML}}$, the maximum likelihood estimator for σ^2 is given by

$$\sigma_{\mathrm{ML}}^2 = \frac{1}{d-q} \sum_{j=q+1}^{d} \lambda_j, \tag{3.13}$$

where $\lambda_{q+1}, \ldots, \lambda_d$ are the smallest eigenvalues of $\mathbf{S}$, and so σ_{ML}^2 has a clear interpretation as the average variance "lost" per discarded dimension.

3.3 Dimensionality Reduction and Optimal Reconstruction. To implement probabilistic PCA, we would generally first compute the usual eigendecomposition of $\mathbf{S}$ (we consider an alternative, iterative approach shortly), after which σ_{ML}^2 is found from equation 3.13 followed by $\mathbf{W}_{\mathrm{ML}}$ from equation 3.12. This is then sufficient to define the associated density model for PCA, allowing the advantages listed in section 1 to be exploited.

In conventional PCA, the reduced-dimensionality transformation of a data point $\mathbf{t}_n$ is given by $\mathbf{x}_n = \mathbf{U}_q^{\mathrm{T}}(\mathbf{t}_n - \boldsymbol{\mu})$ and its reconstruction by $\hat{\mathbf{t}}_n = \mathbf{U}_q \mathbf{x}_n + \boldsymbol{\mu}$. This may be similarly achieved within the PPCA formulation. However, we note that in the probabilistic framework, the generative model defined by equation 2.2 represents a mapping from the lower-dimensional latent space to the data space. So in PPCA, the probabilistic analog of the dimensionality reduction process of conventional PCA would be to invert the conditional distribution $p(\mathbf{t}|\mathbf{x})$ using Bayes' rule, in equation 3.6, to give $p(\mathbf{x}|\mathbf{t})$. In this case, each data point $\mathbf{t}_n$ is represented in the latent space not by a single vector, but by the gaussian posterior distribution defined by equation 3.6. As an alternative to the standard PCA projection, then, a convenient summary of this distribution and representation of $\mathbf{t}_n$ would be the posterior mean $\langle \mathbf{x}_n \rangle = \mathbf{M}^{-1} \mathbf{W}_{\mathrm{ML}}^{\mathrm{T}} (\mathbf{t}_n - \boldsymbol{\mu})$, a quantity that also arises naturally in (and is computed in) the EM implementation of PPCA considered in section 3.4. Note also from equation 3.6 that the covariance of the posterior distribution is given by $\sigma^2 \mathbf{M}^{-1}$ and is therefore constant for all data points.

However, perhaps counterintuitively given equation 2.2, $\mathbf{W}_{\mathrm{ML}}\langle \mathbf{x}_n \rangle + \boldsymbol{\mu}$ is *not* the optimal linear reconstruction of $\mathbf{t}_n$. This may be seen from the fact that for $\sigma^2 > 0$, $\mathbf{W}_{\mathrm{ML}}\langle \mathbf{x}_n \rangle + \boldsymbol{\mu}$ is not an orthogonal projection of $\mathbf{t}_n$, as a consequence of the gaussian prior over $\mathbf{x}$ causing the posterior mean projection to become skewed toward the origin. If we consider the limit as $\sigma^2 \to 0$, the projection $\mathbf{W}_{\mathrm{ML}}\langle \mathbf{x}_n \rangle = \mathbf{W}_{\mathrm{ML}}(\mathbf{W}_{\mathrm{ML}}^{\mathrm{T}} \mathbf{W}_{\mathrm{ML}})^{-1} \mathbf{W}_{\mathrm{ML}}^{\mathrm{T}} (\mathbf{t}_n - \boldsymbol{\mu})$ does become orthogonal and is equivalent to conventional PCA, but then the density model is singular and thus undefined.

Taking this limit is not necessary, however, since the optimal least-squares linear reconstruction of the data from the posterior mean vectors $\langle \mathbf{x}_n \rangle$ may be obtained from (see appendix B)

$$\hat{t}_n = W_{ML} \left(W_{ML}^T W_{ML} \right)^{-1} M \langle x_n \rangle + \mu, \tag{3.14}$$

with identical reconstruction error to conventional PCA.

For reasons of probabilistic elegance, therefore, we might choose to exploit the posterior mean vectors $\langle x_n \rangle$ as the reduced-dimensionality representation of the data, although there is no material benefit in so doing. Indeed, we note that in addition to the conventional PCA representation $U_q^T(t_n - \mu)$, the vectors $\hat{x}_n = W_{ML}^T(t_n - \mu)$ could equally be used without loss of information and reconstructed using

$$\hat{t}_n = W_{ML} \left(W_{ML}^T W_{ML} \right)^{-1} \hat{x}_n + \mu.$$

3.4 An EM Algorithm for PPCA. By a simple extension of the EM formulation for parameter estimation in the standard linear factor analysis model (Rubin & Thayer 1982), we can obtain a principal component projection by maximizing the likelihood function (see equation 3.8). We are not suggesting that such an approach necessarily be adopted for probabilistic PCA; normally the principal axes would be estimated in the conventional manner, via eigendecomposition of S, and subsequently incorporated in the probability model using equations 3.12 and 3.13 to realize the advantages outlined in the introduction. However, as discussed in appendix A.5, there may be an advantage in the EM approach for large d since the presented algorithm, although iterative, requires neither computation of the $d \times d$ covariance matrix, which is $O(Nd^2)$, nor its explicit eigendecomposition, which is $O(d^3)$. We derive the EM algorithm and consider its properties from the computational perspective in appendix A.5.

3.5 Factor Analysis Revisited. The probabilistic PCA algorithm was obtained by introducing a constraint into the noise matrix of the factor analysis latent variable model. This apparently minor modification leads to significant differences in the behavior of the two methods. In particular, we now show that the covariance properties of the PPCA model are identical to those of conventional PCA and are quite different from those of standard factor analysis.

Consider a nonsingular linear transformation of the data variables, so that $t \rightarrow At$. Using equation 3.10, we see that under such a transformation, the maximum likelihood solution for the mean will be transformed as $\mu_{ML} \rightarrow A\mu_{ML}$. From equation 3.9, it then follows that the covariance matrix will transform as $S \rightarrow ASA^T$.

The log-likelihood for the latent variable model, from equation 3.8, is given by

$$\mathcal{L}(\mathbf{W}, \boldsymbol{\Psi}) = -\frac{N}{2} \left\{ d \ln(2\pi) + \ln |\mathbf{W}\mathbf{W}^T + \boldsymbol{\Psi}| \right.$$

$$\left. + \text{tr} \left[(\mathbf{W}\mathbf{W}^T + \boldsymbol{\Psi})^{-1} \mathbf{S} \right] \right\}, \qquad (3.15)$$

where $\boldsymbol{\Psi}$ is a general noise covariance matrix. Thus, using equation 3.15, we see that under the transformation $\mathbf{t} \to \mathbf{At}$, the log-likelihood will transform as

$$\mathcal{L}(\mathbf{W}, \boldsymbol{\Psi}) \to \mathcal{L}(\mathbf{A}^{-1}\mathbf{W}, \mathbf{A}^{-1}\boldsymbol{\Psi}\mathbf{A}^{-T}) - N \ln |\mathbf{A}|, \qquad (3.16)$$

where $\mathbf{A}^{-T} \equiv (\mathbf{A}^{-1})^T$. Thus, if $\mathbf{W}_{\text{ML}}$ and $\boldsymbol{\Psi}_{\text{ML}}$ are maximum likelihood solutions for the original data, then $\mathbf{A}\mathbf{W}_{\text{ML}}$ and $\mathbf{A}\boldsymbol{\Psi}_{\text{ML}}\mathbf{A}^T$ will be maximum likelihood solutions for the transformed data set.

In general, the form of the solution will not be preserved under such a transformation. However, we can consider two special cases. First, suppose $\boldsymbol{\Psi}$ is a diagonal matrix, corresponding to the case of factor analysis. Then $\boldsymbol{\Psi}$ will remain diagonal provided $\mathbf{A}$ is also a diagonal matrix. This says that factor analysis is covariant under component-wise rescaling of the data variables: the scale factors simply become absorbed into rescaling of the noise variances, and the rows of $\mathbf{W}$ are rescaled by the same factors. Second, consider the case $\boldsymbol{\Psi} = \sigma^2 \mathbf{I}$, corresponding to PPCA. Then the transformed noise covariance $\sigma^2 \mathbf{A}\mathbf{A}^T$ will be proportional to the unit matrix only if $\mathbf{A}^T = \mathbf{A}^{-1}$— in other words, if $\mathbf{A}$ is an orthogonal matrix. Transformation of the data vectors by multiplication with an orthogonal matrix corresponds to a rotation of the coordinate system. This same covariance property is shared by standard nonprobabilistic PCA since a rotation of the coordinates induces a corresponding rotation of the principal axes. Thus we see that factor analysis is covariant under componentwise rescaling, while PPCA and PCA are covariant under rotations, as illustrated in Figure 1.

4 Mixtures of Probabilistic Principal Component Analyzers _____

The association of a probability model with PCA offers the tempting prospect of being able to model complex data structures with a combination of local PCA models through the mechanism of a mixture of probabilistic principal component analysers (Tipping & Bishop, 1997). This formulation would permit all of the model parameters to be determined from maximum likelihood, where both the appropriate partitioning of the data and the determination of the respective principal axes occur automatically as the likelihood is maximized. The log-likelihood of observing the data set for such a mixture

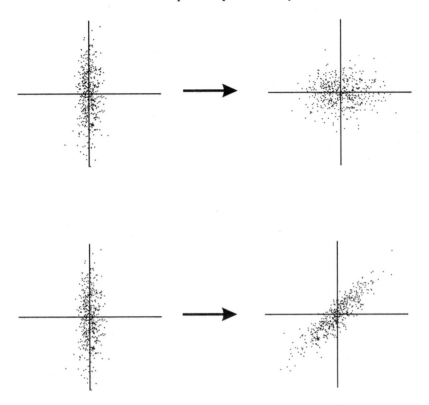

Figure 1: Factor analysis is covariant under a componentwise rescaling of the data variables (top plots), while PCA and probabilistic PCA are covariant under rotations of the data space coordinates (bottom plots).

model is:

$$\mathcal{L} = \sum_{n=1}^{N} \ln \left\{ p(\mathbf{t}_n) \right\}, \tag{4.1}$$

$$= \sum_{n=1}^{N} \ln \left\{ \sum_{i=1}^{M} \pi_i p(\mathbf{t}_n | i) \right\}, \tag{4.2}$$

where $p(\mathbf{t}|i)$ is a single PPCA model and π_i is the corresponding mixing proportion, with $\pi_i \geq 0$ and $\sum \pi_i = 1$. Note that a separate mean vector $\boldsymbol{\mu}_i$ is now associated with each of the M mixture components, along with the parameters $\mathbf{W}_i$ and σ_i^2. A related model has recently been exploited for data visualization (Bishop & Tipping, 1998), and a similar approach, based on the standard factor analysis diagonal ($\mathbf{\Psi}$) noise model, has been employed for handwritten digit recognition (Hinton et al. 1997), although it does not implement PCA.

The corresponding generative model for the mixture case now requires the random choice of a mixture component according to the proportions π_i, followed by sampling from the $\mathbf{x}$ and $\boldsymbol{\epsilon}$ distributions and applying equation 2.2 as in the single model case, taking care to use the appropriate parameters $\boldsymbol{\mu}_i$, $\mathbf{W}_i$, and σ_i^2. Furthermore, for a given data point $\mathbf{t}$, there is now a posterior distribution associated with each latent space, the mean of which for space i is given by $(\sigma_i^2 \mathbf{I} + \mathbf{W}_i^T \mathbf{W}_i)^{-1} \mathbf{W}_i^T (\mathbf{t} - \boldsymbol{\mu}_i)$.

We can develop an iterative EM algorithm for optimization of all of the model parameters π_i, $\boldsymbol{\mu}_i$, $\mathbf{W}_i$, and σ_i^2. If $R_{ni} = p(i|\mathbf{t}_n)$ is the posterior responsibility of mixture i for generating data point $\mathbf{t}_n$, given by

$$R_{ni} = \frac{p(\mathbf{t}_n|i)\pi_i}{p(\mathbf{t}_n)}, \tag{4.3}$$

then in appendix C it is shown that we obtain the following parameter updates:

$$\widetilde{\pi}_i = \frac{1}{N} \sum_{n=1}^{N} R_{ni}, \tag{4.4}$$

$$\widetilde{\boldsymbol{\mu}}_i = \frac{\sum_{n=1}^{N} R_{ni} \mathbf{t}_n}{\sum_{n=1}^{N} R_{ni}}. \tag{4.5}$$

Thus the updates for $\widetilde{\pi}_i$ and $\widetilde{\boldsymbol{\mu}}_i$ correspond exactly to those of a standard gaussian mixture formulation (e.g., see Bishop, 1995). Furthermore, in appendix C, it is also shown that the combination of the E- and M-steps leads to the intuitive result that the axes $\mathbf{W}_i$ and the noise variance σ_i^2 are determined from the local responsibility–weighted covariance matrix:

$$\mathbf{S}_i = \frac{1}{\widetilde{\pi}_i N} \sum_{n=1}^{N} R_{ni} (\mathbf{t}_n - \widetilde{\boldsymbol{\mu}}_i)(\mathbf{t}_n - \widetilde{\boldsymbol{\mu}}_i)^T, \tag{4.6}$$

by standard eigendecomposition in exactly the same manner as for a single PPCA model. However, as noted in section 3.4 (and also in appendix A.5), for larger values of data dimensionality d, computational advantages can be obtained if $\mathbf{W}_i$ and σ_i^2 are updated iteratively according to an EM schedule. This is discussed for the mixture model in appendix C.

Iteration of equations 4.3, 4.4, and 4.5 in sequence followed by computation of $\mathbf{W}_i$ and σ_i^2, from either equation 4.6 using equations 2.12 and 2.13 or using the iterative updates in appendix C, is guaranteed to find a local maximum of the log-likelihood in equation 4.2. At convergence of the algorithm each weight matrix $\mathbf{W}_i$ spans the principal subspace of its respective $\mathbf{S}_i$.

In the next section we consider applications of this PPCA mixture model, beginning with data compression and reconstruction tasks. We then consider general density modeling in section 6.

5 Local Linear Dimensionality Reduction

In this section we begin by giving an illustration of the application of the PPCA mixture algorithm to a synthetic data set. More realistic examples are then considered, with an emphasis on cases in which a principal component approach is motivated by the objective of deriving a reduced-dimensionality representation of the data, which can be reconstructed with minimum error. We will therefore contrast the clustering mechanism in the PPCA mixture model with that of a hard clustering approach based explicitly on reconstruction error as used in a typical algorithm.

5.1 Illustration for Synthetic Data. For a demonstration of the mixture of PPCA algorithm, we generated a synthetic data set comprising 500 data points sampled uniformly over the surface of a hemisphere, with additive gaussian noise. Figure 2a shows this data.

A mixture of 12 probabilistic principal component analyzers was then fitted to the data using the EM algorithm outlined in the previous section, with latent space dimensionality $q = 2$. Because of the probabilistic formalism, a generative model of the data is defined, and we emphasize this by plotting a second set of 500 data points, obtained by sampling from the fitted generative model. These data points are shown in Figure 2b. Histograms of the distances of all the data points from the hemisphere are also given to indicate more clearly the accuracy of the model in capturing the structure of the underlying generator.

5.2 Clustering Mechanisms. Generating a local PCA model of the form illustrated above is often prompted by the ultimate goal of accurate data reconstruction. Indeed, this has motivated Kambhatla and Leen (1997) and Hinton et al. (1997) to use squared reconstruction error as the clustering criterion in the partitioning phase. Dony and Haykin (1995) adopt a similar approach to image compression, although their model has no set of independent mean parameters μ_i. Using the reconstruction criterion, a data point is assigned to the component that reconstructs it with lowest error, and the principal axes are then reestimated within each cluster. For the mixture of PPCA model, however, data points are assigned to mixture components (in a soft fashion) according to the responsibility R_{ni} of the mixture component for its generation. Since $R_{ni} = p(\mathbf{t}_n|i)\pi_i/p(\mathbf{t}_n)$ and $p(\mathbf{t}_n)$ is constant for all components, $R_{ni} \propto p(\mathbf{t}_n|i)$, and we may gain further insight into the clustering by considering the probability density associated with component i at

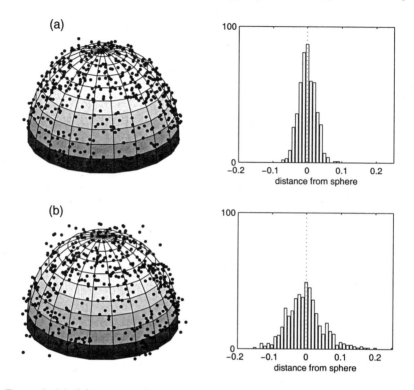

Figure 2: Modeling noisy data on a hemisphere. (a) On the left, the synthetic data; on the right, a histogram of the Euclidean distances of each data point to the sphere. (b) Data generated from the fitted PPCA mixture model with the synthetic data on the left and the histogram on the right.

data point $\mathbf{t}_n$:

$$p(\mathbf{t}_n|i) = (2\pi)^{-d/2}|\mathbf{C}_i|^{-1/2} \exp\left\{-E_{ni}^2/2\right\},\tag{5.1}$$

where

$$E_{ni}^2 = (\mathbf{t}_n - \boldsymbol{\mu}_i)^{\mathrm{T}}\mathbf{C}_i^{-1}(\mathbf{t}_n - \boldsymbol{\mu}_i),\tag{5.2}$$

$$\mathbf{C}_i = \sigma_i^2\mathbf{I} + \mathbf{W}_i\mathbf{W}_i^{\mathrm{T}}.\tag{5.3}$$

It is helpful to express the matrix $\mathbf{W}_i$ in terms of its singular value decomposition (and although we are considering an individual mixture component i, the i subscript will be omitted for notational clarity):

$$\mathbf{W} = \mathbf{U}_q(\mathbf{K}_q - \sigma^2\mathbf{I})^{1/2}\mathbf{R},\tag{5.4}$$

where $\mathbf{U}_q$ is a $d \times q$ matrix of orthonormal column vectors and $\mathbf{R}$ is an arbitrary $q \times q$ orthogonal matrix. The singular values are parameterized, without loss of generality, in terms of $(\mathbf{K}_q - \sigma^2 \mathbf{I})^{1/2}$, where $\mathbf{K}_q = \mathrm{diag}(k_1, k_2, \ldots, k_q)$ is a $q \times q$ diagonal matrix. Then

$$E_n^2 = (\mathbf{t}_n - \boldsymbol{\mu})^{\mathrm{T}} \left\{ \sigma^2 \mathbf{I} + \mathbf{U}_q (\mathbf{K}_q - \sigma^2 \mathbf{I}) \mathbf{U}_q^{\mathrm{T}} \right\}^{-1} (\mathbf{t}_n - \boldsymbol{\mu}). \tag{5.5}$$

The data point $\mathbf{t}_n$ may also be expressed in terms of the basis of vectors $\mathbf{U} = (\mathbf{U}_q, \mathbf{U}_{d-q})$, where $\mathbf{U}_{d-q}$ comprises $(d-q)$ vectors perpendicular to $\mathbf{U}_q$, which complete an orthonormal set. In this basis, we define $\mathbf{z}_n = \mathbf{U}^{\mathrm{T}}(\mathbf{t}_n - \boldsymbol{\mu})$ and so $\mathbf{t}_n - \boldsymbol{\mu} = \mathbf{U}\mathbf{z}_n$, from which equation 5.5 may then be written as

$$E_n^2 = \mathbf{z}_n^{\mathrm{T}} \mathbf{U}^{\mathrm{T}} \left\{ \sigma^2 \mathbf{I} + \mathbf{U}_q (\mathbf{K}_q - \sigma^2 \mathbf{I}) \mathbf{U}_q^{\mathrm{T}} \right\}^{-1} \mathbf{U}\mathbf{z}_n, \tag{5.6}$$

$$= \mathbf{z}_n^{\mathrm{T}} \mathbf{D}^{-1} \mathbf{z}_n, \tag{5.7}$$

where $\mathbf{D} = \mathrm{diag}(k_1, k_2, \ldots, k_q, \sigma^2, \ldots, \sigma^2)$ is a $d \times d$ diagonal matrix. Thus:

$$E_n^2 = \mathbf{z}_{\mathrm{in}}^{\mathrm{T}} \mathbf{K}_q^{-1} \mathbf{z}_{\mathrm{in}} + \frac{\mathbf{z}_{\mathrm{out}}^{\mathrm{T}} \mathbf{z}_{\mathrm{out}}}{\sigma^2}, \tag{5.8}$$

$$= E_{\mathrm{in}}^2 + E_{\mathrm{rec}}^2 / \sigma^2, \tag{5.9}$$

where we have partitioned the elements of $\mathbf{z}$ into $\mathbf{z}_{\mathrm{in}}$, the projection of $\mathbf{t}_n - \boldsymbol{\mu}$ onto the subspace spanned by $\mathbf{W}$, and $\mathbf{z}_{\mathrm{out}}$, the projection onto the corresponding perpendicular subspace. Thus, E_{rec}^2 is the squared reconstruction error, and E_{in}^2 may be interpreted as an in-subspace error term. At the maximum likelihood solution, $\mathbf{U}_q$ is the matrix of eigenvectors of the local covariance matrix and $\mathbf{K}_q = \boldsymbol{\Lambda}_q$.

As $\sigma_i^2 \to 0$, $R_{ni} \propto \pi_i \exp\left(-E_{\mathrm{rec}}^2 / 2\right)$ and, for equal prior probabilities, cluster assignments are equivalent to a soft reconstruction-based clustering. However, for $\sigma_A^2, \sigma_B^2 > 0$, consider a data point that lies in the subspace of a relatively distant component A, which may be reconstructed with zero error yet lies closer to the mean of a second component B. The effect of the noise variance σ_B^2 in equation 5.9 is to moderate the contribution of E_{rec}^2 for component B. As a result, the data point may be assigned to the nearer component B even though the reconstruction error is considerably greater, given that it is sufficiently distant from the mean of A such that E_{in}^2 for A is large.

It should be expected, then, that mixture of PPCA clustering would result in more localized clusters, but with the final reconstruction error inferior to that of a clustering model based explicitly on a reconstruction criterion. Conversely, it should also be clear that clustering the data according to the proximity to the subspace alone will not necessarily result in localized partitions (as noted by Kambhatla, 1995, who also considers the relationship

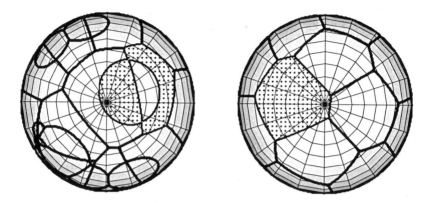

Figure 3: Comparison of the partitioning of the hemisphere effected by a
VQPCA-based model (left) and a PPCA mixture model (right). The illustrated
boundaries delineate regions of the hemisphere that are best reconstructed by a
particular local PCA model. One such region is shown shaded to emphasize that
clustering according to reconstruction error results in a nonlocalized partitioning. In the VQPCA case, the circular effects occur when principal component
planes intersect beneath the surface of the hemisphere.

of such an algorithm to a probabilistic model). That this is so is simply
illustrated in Figure 3, in which a collection of 12 conventional PCA models
have been fitted to the hemisphere data, according to the VQPCA (vector-
quantization PCA) algorithm of Kambhatla and Leen (1997), defined as
follows:

1. Select initial cluster centers μ_i at random from points in the data set,
   and assign all data points to the nearest (in terms of Euclidean distance) cluster center.

2. Set the $\mathbf{W}_i$ vectors to the first two principal axes of the covariance
   matrix of cluster i.

3. Assign data points to the cluster that best reconstructs them, setting
   each μ_i to the mean of those data points assigned to cluster i.

4. Repeat from step 2 until the cluster allocations are constant.

In Figure 3, data points have been sampled over the hemisphere, without noise, and allocated to the cluster that best reconstructs them. The left
plot shows the partitioning associated with the best (i.e., lowest reconstruction error) model obtained from 100 runs of the VQPCA algorithm. The right
plot shows a similar partitioning for the best (i.e., greatest likelihood) PPCA
mixture model using the same number of components, again from 100 runs.
Note that the boundaries illustrated in this latter plot were obtained using

Table 1: Data Sets Used for Comparison of Clustering Criteria.

Data Set	N	d	M	q	Description
Hemisphere	500	3	12	2	Synthetic data used above
Oil	500	12	12	2	Diagnostic measurements from oil pipeline flows
Digit_1	500	64	10	10	8 × 8 gray-scale images of handwritten digit 1
Digit_2	500	64	10	10	8 × 8 gray-scale images of handwritten digit 2
Image	500	64	8	4	8 × 8 gray-scale blocks from a photographic image
EEG	300	30	8	5	Delay vectors from an electroencephalogram time-series signal

assignments based on reconstruction error for the final model, in identical fashion to the VQPCA case, and not on probabilistic responsibility. We see that the partitions formed when clustering according to reconstruction error alone can be nonlocal, as exemplified by the shaded component. This phenomenon is rather contrary to the philosophy of local dimensionality reduction and is an indirect consequence of the fact that reconstruction-based local PCA does not model the data in a probabilistic sense.

However, we might expect that algorithms such as VQPCA should offer better performance in terms of the reconstruction error of the final solution, having been designed explicitly to optimize that measure. In order to test this, we compared the VQPCA algorithm with the PPCA mixture model on six data sets, detailed in Table 1.

Figure 4 summarizes the reconstruction error of the respective models, and in general, VQPCA performs better, as expected. However, we also note two interesting aspects of the results.

First, in the case of the oil data, the final reconstruction error of the PPCA model on both training and test sets is counterintuitively superior, despite the fact that the partitioning of the data space was based only partially on reconstruction error. This behavior is, we hypothesize, a result of the particular structure of that data set. The oil data are known to comprise a number of disjoint, but locally smooth, two-dimensional cluster structures (see Bishop & Tipping, 1998, for a visualization).

For the oil data set, we observed that many of the models found by the VQPCA algorithm exhibit partitions that are not only often nonconnected (similar to those shown for the hemisphere in Figure 3) but may also span more than one of the disjoint cluster structures. The evidence of Figure 4 suggests that these models represent poor local minima of the reconstruc-

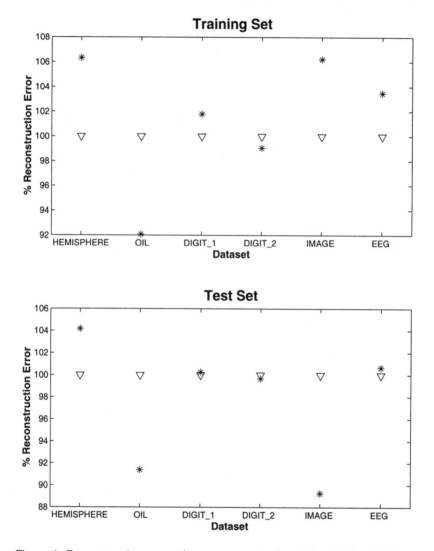

Figure 4: Reconstruction errors for reconstruction-based local PCA (VQPCA) and the PPCA mixture. Errors for the latter (∗) have been shown relative to the former (∇), and are averaged over 100 runs with random initial configurations.

tion error cost function. The PPCA mixture algorithm does not find such suboptimal solutions, which would have low likelihood due to the locality implied by the density model. The experiment indicates that by avoiding these poor solutions, the PPCA mixture model is able to find solutions with lower reconstruction error (on average) than VQPCA.

These observations apply only to the case of the oil data set. For the hemisphere, digit 1, image, and electroencephalogram (EEG) training sets, the data manifolds are less disjoint, and the explicit reconstruction-based algorithm, VQPCA, is superior. For the digit 2 case, the two algorithms appear approximately equivalent.

A second aspect of Figure 4 is the suggestion that the PPCA mixture model algorithm may be less sensitive to overfitting. As would be expected, compared with the training set, errors on the test set increase for both algorithms (although, because the errors have been normalized to allow comparisons between data sets, this is not shown in Figure 4). However, with the exception of the case of the digit 2 data set, for the PPCA mixture model this increase is proportionately smaller than for VQPCA. This effect is most dramatic for the image data set, where PPCA is much superior on the test set. For that data set, the test examples were derived from a separate portion of the image (see below), and as such, the test set statistics can be expected to differ more significantly from the respective training set than for the other examples.

A likely explanation is that because of the soft clustering of the PPCA mixture model, there is an inherent smoothing effect occurring when estimating the local sets of principal axes. Each set of axes is determined from its corresponding local responsibility–weighted covariance matrix, which in general will be influenced by many data points, not just the subset that would be associated with the cluster in a "hard" implementation. Because of this, the parameters in the W_i matrix in cluster i are also constrained by data points in neighboring clusters ($j \neq i$) to some extent. This notion is discussed in the context of regression by Jordan and Jacobs (1994) as motivation for their mixture-of-experts model, where the authors note how soft partitioning can reduce variance (in terms of the bias-variance decomposition). Although it is difficult to draw firm conclusions from this limited set of experiments, the evidence of Figure 4 does point to the presence of such an effect.

5.3 Application: Image Compression. As a practical example, we consider an application of the PPCA mixture model to block transform image coding. Figure 5 shows the original image. This 720×360 pixel image was segmented into 8×8 nonoverlapping blocks, giving a total data set of 4050 64-dimensional vectors. Half of these data, corresponding to the left half of the picture, were used as training data. The right half was reserved for testing; a magnified portion of the test image is also shown in Figure 5. A reconstruction of the entire image based on the first four principal components of a single PCA model determined from the block-transformed left half of the image is shown in Figure 6.

Figure 7 shows the reconstruction of the original image when modeled by a mixture of probabilistic principal component analyzers. The model parameters were estimated using only the left half of the image. In this example, 12

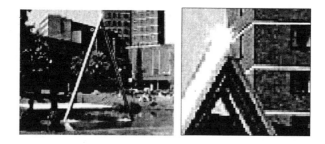

Figure 5: (Left) The original image. (Right) Detail.

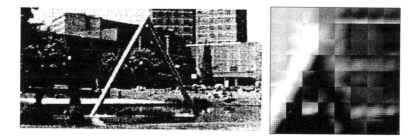

Figure 6: The PCA reconstructed image, at 0.5 bit per pixel. (Left) The original image. (Right) Detail.

components were used, of dimensionality 4; after the model likelihood had been maximized, the image coding was performed in a "hard" fashion, by allocating data to the component with the lowest reconstruction error. The resulting coded image was uniformly quantized, with bits allocated equally to each transform variable, before reconstruction, in order to give a final bit rate of 0.5 bits per pixel (and thus compression of 16 to 1) in both Figures 6 and 7. In the latter case, the cost of encoding the mixture component label was included. For the simple principal subspace reconstruction, the normalized test error was 7.1×10^{-2}; for the mixture model, it was 5.7×10^{-2}. The VQPCA algorithm gave a test error of 6.2×10^{-2}.

6 Density Modeling

A popular approach to semiparametric density estimation is the gaussian mixture model (Titterington, Smith, & Makov, 1985). However, such models suffer from the limitation that if each gaussian component is described by a full covariance matrix, then there are $d(d + 1)/2$ independent covariance parameters to be estimated for each mixture component. Clearly, as the dimensionality of the data space increases, the number of data points required to specify those parameters reliably will become prohibitive. An alternative

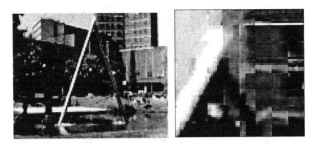

Figure 7: The mixture of PPCA reconstructed image, using the same bit rate as Figure 6. (Left) The original image. (Right) Detail.

approach is to reduce the number of parameters by placing a constraint on the form of the covariance matrix. (Another would be to introduce priors over the parameters of the full covariance matrix, as implemented by Ormoneit & Tresp, 1996.) Two common constraints are to restrict the covariance to be isotropic or to be diagonal. The isotropic model is highly constrained as it assigns only a single parameter to describe the entire covariance structure in the full d dimensions. The diagonal model is more flexible, with d parameters, but the principal axes of the elliptical gaussians must be aligned with the data axes, and thus each individual mixture component is unable to capture correlations among the variables.

A mixture of PPCA models, where the covariance of each gaussian is parameterized by the relation $\mathbf{C} = \sigma^2 \mathbf{I} + \mathbf{W}\mathbf{W}^T$, comprises $dq + 1 - q(q-1)/2$ free parameters.[1] (Note that the $q(q-1)/2$ term takes account of the number of parameters needed to specify the arbitrary rotation $\mathbf{R}$.) It thus permits the number of parameters to be controlled by the choice of q. When $q = 0$, the model is equivalent to an isotropic gaussian. With $q = d - 1$, the general covariance gaussian is recovered.

6.1 A Synthetic Example: Noisy Spiral Data. The utility of the PPCA mixture approach may be demonstrated with the following simple example. A 500-point data set was generated along a three-dimensional spiral configuration with added gaussian noise. The data were then modeled by both a mixture of PPCA models and a mixture of diagonal covariance gaussians, using eight mixture components. In the mixture of PPCA case, $q = 1$ for each component, and so there are four variance parameters per component compared with three for the diagonal model. The results are visualized in Figure 8, which illustrates both side and end projections of the data.

---

[1] An alternative would be a mixture of factor analyzers, implemented by Hinton et al. (1997), although that comprises more parameters.

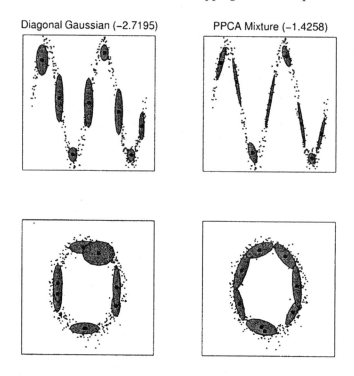

Figure 8: Comparison of an eight-component diagonal variance gaussian mixture model with a mixture of PPCA model. The upper two plots give a view perpendicular to the major axis of the spiral; the lower two plots show the end elevation. The covariance structure of each mixture component is shown by projection of a unit Mahalanobis distance ellipse, and the log-likelihood per data point is given in parentheses above the figures.

The orientation of the ellipses in the diagonal model can be seen not to coincide with the local data structure, which is a result of the axial alignment constraint. A further consequence of the diagonal parameterization is that the means are also implicitly constrained because they tend to lie where the tangent to the spiral is parallel to either axis of the end elevation. This qualitative superiority of the PPCA approach is underlined quantitatively by the log-likelihood per data point given in parentheses in the figure. Such a result would be expected given that the PPCA model has an extra parameter in each mixture component, but similar results are observed if the spiral is embedded in a space of much higher dimensionality where the extra parameter in PPCA is proportionately less relevant.

It should be intuitive that the axial alignment constraint of the diagonal model is, in general, particularly inappropriate when modeling a smooth

Table 2: Log-Likelihood per Data Point Measured on Training and Test Sets for Gaussian Mixture Models with Eight Components and a 100-Point Training Set.

	Isotropic	Diagonal	Full	PPCA
Training	−3.14	−2.74	−1.47	−1.65
Test	−3.68	−3.43	−3.09	−2.37

and continuous lower dimensional manifold in higher dimensions, regardless of the intrinsic dimensionality. Even with $q = 1$, the PPCA approach is able to track the spiral manifold successfully.

Finally, we demonstrate the importance of the use of an appropriate number of parameters by modeling a three-dimensional spiral data set of 100 data points (the number of data points was reduced to emphasize the overfitting) as above with isotropic, diagonal, and full covariance gaussian mixture models, along with a PPCA mixture model. For each model, the log-likelihood per data point for both the training data set and an unseen test set of 1000 data points is given in Table 2.

As would be expected in this case of limited data, the full covariance model exhibits the best likelihood on the training set, but test set performance is worse than for the PPCA mixture. For this simple example, there is only one intermediate PPCA parameterization with $q = 1$ ($q = 0$ and $q = 2$ are equivalent to the isotropic and full covariance cases respectively). In realistic applications, where the dimensionality d will be considerably larger, the PPCA model offers the choice of a range of q, and an appropriate value can be determined using standard techniques for model selection. Finally, note that these advantages are not limited to mixture models, but may equally be exploited for the case of a single gaussian distribution.

6.2 Application: Handwritten Digit Recognition. One potential application for high-dimensionality density models is handwritten digit recognition. Examples of gray-scale pixel images of a given digit will generally lie on a lower-dimensional smooth continuous manifold, the geometry of which is determined by properties of the digit such as rotation, scaling, and thickness of stroke. One approach to the classification of such digits (although not necessarily the best) is to build a model of each digit separately, and classify unseen digits according to the model to which they are most similar.

Hinton et al. (1997) gave an excellent discussion of the handwritten digit problem and applied a mixture of PCA approach, using soft reconstruction–based clustering, to the classification of scaled and smoothed 8 × 8 gray-scale images taken from the CEDAR U.S. Postal Service database (Hull, 1994). The models were constructed using an 11,000-digit subset of the *br*

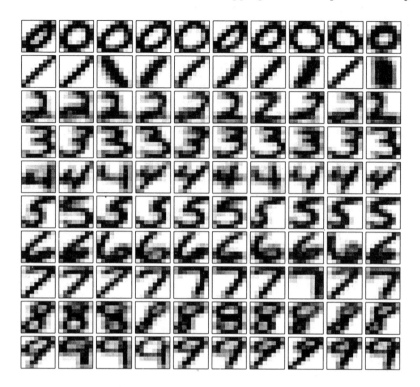

Figure 9: Mean vectors μ_i, illustrated as gray-scale digits, for each of the 10 digit models. The model for a given digit is a mixture of 10 PPCA models, one centered at each of the pixel vectors shown on the corresponding row. Note how different components can capture different styles of digit.

data set (which was further split into training and validation sets), and the *bs* test set was classified according to which model best reconstructed each digit (in the squared-error sense). We repeated the experiment with the same data using the PPCA mixture approach using the same choice of parameter values ($M = 10$ and $q = 10$). To help visualize the final model, the means of each component μ_i are illustrated in digit form in Figure 9.

The digits were again classified, using the same method of classification, and the best model on the validation set misclassified 4.64% of the digits in the test set. Hinton et al. (1997) reported an error of 4.91%, and we would expect the improvement to be a result partly of the localized clustering of the PPCA model, but also the use of individually estimated values of σ_i^2 for each component, rather than a single, arbitrarily chosen, global value.

One of the advantages of the PPCA methodology is that the definition of the density model permits the posterior probabilities of class membership to be computed for each digit and used for subsequent classification, rather than using reconstruction error as above. Classification according to the largest posterior probability for the $M = 10$ and $q = 10$ model resulted in an increase in error, and it was necessary to invest significant effort to optimize the parameters M and q for each model to provide comparable performance. Using this approach, our best classifier on the validation set misclassified 4.61% of the test set. An additional benefit of the use of posterior probabilities is that it is possible to reject a proportion of the test samples about which the classifier is most "unsure" and thus hopefully improve the classification performance. Using this approach to reject 5% of the test examples resulted in a misclassification rate of 2.50%. (The availability of posteriors can be advantageous in other applications, where they may be used in various forms of follow-on processing.)

7 Conclusions

Modeling complexity in data by a combination of simple linear models is an attractive paradigm offering both computational and algorithmic advantages along with increased ease of interpretability. In this article, we have exploited the definition of a probabilistic model for PCA in order to combine local PCA models within the framework of a probabilistic mixture in which all the parameters are determined from maximum likelihood using an EM algorithm. In addition to the clearly defined nature of the resulting algorithm, the primary advantage of this approach is the definition of an observation density model.

A possible disadvantage of the probabilistic approach to combining local PCA models is that by optimizing a likelihood function, the PPCA mixture model does not directly minimize squared reconstruction error. For applications where this is the salient criterion, algorithms that explicitly minimize reconstruction error should be expected to be superior. Experiments indeed showed this to be generally the case, but two important caveats must be considered before any firm conclusions can be drawn concerning the suitability of a given model. First, and rather surprisingly, for one of the data sets ('oil') considered in the article, the final PPCA mixture model was actually superior in the sense of squared reconstruction error, even on the training set. It was demonstrated that algorithms incorporating reconstruction-based clustering do not necessarily generate local clusters, and it was reasoned that for data sets comprising a number of disjoint data structures, this phenomenon may lead to poor local minima. Such minima are not found by the PPCA density model approach. A second consideration is that there was also evidence that the smoothing implied by the soft clustering inherent in the PPCA mixture model helps to reduce overfitting, particularly in the case of the image compression experiment where the statistics of the test data set differed from the training data much more so than for other examples. In that instance, the reconstruction test error for the PPCA model was, on average, more than 10% lower.

In terms of a gaussian mixture model, the mixture of probabilistic principal component analyzers enables data to be modeled in high dimensions with relatively few free parameters, while not imposing a generally inappropriate constraint on the covariance structure. The number of free parameters may be controlled through the choice of latent space dimension q, allowing an interpolation in model complexity from isotropic to full covariance structures. The efficacy of this parameterization was demonstrated by performance on a handwritten digit recognition task.

Appendix A: Maximum Likelihood PCA

A.1 The Stationary Points of the Log-Likelihood. The gradient of the log-likelihood (see equation 3.8) with respect to $\mathbf{W}$ may be obtained from standard matrix differentiation results (e.g., see Krzanowski & Marriott, 1994, p. 133):

$$\frac{\partial \mathcal{L}}{\partial \mathbf{W}} = N(\mathbf{C}^{-1}\mathbf{S}\mathbf{C}^{-1}\mathbf{W} - \mathbf{C}^{-1}\mathbf{W}). \tag{A.1}$$

At the stationary points

$$\mathbf{S}\mathbf{C}^{-1}\mathbf{W} = \mathbf{W}, \tag{A.2}$$

assuming that $\sigma^2 > 0$, and thus that $\mathbf{C}^{-1}$ exists. This is a necessary and sufficient condition for the density model to remain nonsingular, and we will restrict ourselves to such cases. It will be seen shortly that $\sigma^2 > 0$ if $q < \text{rank}(\mathbf{S})$, so this assumption implies no loss of practicality.

There are three possible classes of solutions to equation A.2:

1. $\mathbf{W} = \mathbf{0}$. This is shown later to be a minimum of the log-likelihood.

2. $\mathbf{C} = \mathbf{S}$, where the covariance model is exact, such as is discussed by Basilevsky (1994, pp. 361–363) and considered in section 2.3. In this unrealistic case of an exact covariance model, where the $d - q$ smallest eigenvalues of $\mathbf{S}$ are identical and equal to σ^2, $\mathbf{W}$ is identifiable since

$$\sigma^2\mathbf{I} + \mathbf{W}\mathbf{W}^{\mathrm{T}} = \mathbf{S},$$
$$\Rightarrow \mathbf{W} = \mathbf{U}(\mathbf{\Lambda} - \sigma^2\mathbf{I})^{1/2}\mathbf{R}, \tag{A.3}$$

   where $\mathbf{U}$ is a square matrix whose columns are the eigenvectors of $\mathbf{S}$, with $\mathbf{\Lambda}$ the corresponding diagonal matrix of eigenvalues, and $\mathbf{R}$ is an arbitrary orthogonal (i.e., rotation) matrix.

3. $\mathbf{S}\mathbf{C}^{-1}\mathbf{W} = \mathbf{W}$, with $\mathbf{W} \neq \mathbf{0}$ and $\mathbf{C} \neq \mathbf{S}$.

We are interested in case 3 where $C \neq S$ and the model covariance need not be equal to the sample covariance. First, we express the weight matrix W in terms of its singular value decomposition:

$$W = ULV^T, \tag{A.4}$$

where U is a $d \times q$ matrix of orthonormal column vectors, $L = \text{diag}(l_1, l_2, \ldots, l_q)$ is the $q \times q$ diagonal matrix of singular values, and V is a $q \times q$ orthogonal matrix. Now,

$$\begin{aligned} C^{-1}W &= (\sigma^2 I + WW^T)^{-1}W, \\ &= W(\sigma^2 I + W^T W)^{-1}, \\ &= UL(\sigma^2 I + L^2)^{-1}V^T. \end{aligned} \tag{A.5}$$

Then at the stationary points, $SC^{-1}W = W$ implies that

$$\begin{aligned} SUL(\sigma^2 I + L^2)^{-1}V^T &= ULV^T, \\ \Rightarrow \qquad\qquad SUL &= U(\sigma^2 I + L^2)L. \end{aligned} \tag{A.6}$$

For $l_j \neq 0$, equation A.6 implies that if $U = (u_1, u_2, \ldots, u_q)$, then the corresponding column vector u_j must be an eigenvector of S, with eigenvalue λ_j such that $\sigma^2 + l_j^2 = \lambda_j$, and so

$$l_j = (\lambda_j - \sigma^2)^{1/2}. \tag{A.7}$$

For $l_j = 0$, u_j is arbitrary (and if all l_j are zero, then we recover case 1). All potential solutions for W may thus be written as

$$W = U_q(K_q - \sigma^2 I)^{1/2}R, \tag{A.8}$$

where U_q is a $d \times q$ matrix comprising q column eigenvectors of S, and K_q is a $q \times q$ diagonal matrix with elements:

$$k_j = \begin{cases} \lambda_j, & \text{the corresponding eigenvalue to } u_j, \text{ or,} \\ \sigma^2, & \end{cases} \tag{A.9}$$

where the latter case may be seen to be equivalent to $l_j = 0$. Again, R is an arbitrary orthogonal matrix, equivalent to a rotation in the principal subspace.

A.2 The Global Maximum of the Likelihood. The matrix U_q may contain any of the eigenvectors of S, so to identify those that maximize the likelihood, the expression for $\mathbf{W}$ in equation A.8 is substituted into the log-likelihood function (see equation 3.8) to give

$$
\mathcal{L} = -\frac{N}{2}\left\{ d\ln(2\pi) + \sum_{j=1}^{q'}\ln(\lambda_j) + \frac{1}{\sigma^2}\sum_{j=q'+1}^{d}\lambda_j \right.
$$
$$
\left. + (d - q')\ln\sigma^2 + q' \right\},
\tag{A.10}
$$

where q' is the number of nonzero l_j, $\{\lambda_1, \ldots, \lambda_{q'}\}$ are the eigenvalues corresponding to those retained in $\mathbf{W}$, and $\{\lambda_{q'+1}, \ldots, \lambda_d\}$ are those discarded. Maximizing equation A.10 with respect to σ^2 gives

$$
\sigma^2 = \frac{1}{d - q'}\sum_{j=q'+1}^{d}\lambda_j,
\tag{A.11}
$$

and so

$$
\mathcal{L} = -\frac{N}{2}\left\{ \sum_{j=1}^{q'}\ln(\lambda_j) + (d - q')\ln\left(\frac{1}{d-q'}\sum_{j=q'+1}^{d}\lambda_j\right) \right.
$$
$$
\left. + d\ln(2\pi) + d \right\}.
\tag{A.12}
$$

Note that equation A.11 implies that $\sigma^2 > 0$ if rank($\mathbf{S}$) $> q$ as stated earlier. We wish to find the maximum of equation A.12 with respect to the choice of eigenvectors/eigenvalues to retain in $\mathbf{W}$, $j \in \{1, \ldots, q'\}$, and those to discard, $j \in \{q'+1, \ldots, d\}$. By exploiting the constancy of the sum of all eigenvalues with respect to this choice, the condition for maximization of the likelihood can be expressed equivalently as minimization of the quantity

$$
E = \ln\left(\frac{1}{d-q'}\sum_{j=q'+1}^{d}\lambda_j\right) - \frac{1}{d-q'}\sum_{j=q'+1}^{d}\ln(\lambda_j),
\tag{A.13}
$$

which conveniently depends on only the discarded values and is nonnegative (Jensen's inequality).

We consider minimization of E by first assuming that $d - q'$ discarded eigenvalues have been chosen arbitrarily and, by differentiation, consider how a single such value λ_k affects the value of E:

$$
\frac{\partial E}{\partial \lambda_k} = \frac{1}{\sum_{j=q'+1}^{d}\lambda_j} - \frac{1}{(d-q')\lambda_k}.
\tag{A.14}
$$

From equation A.14, it can be seen that $E(\lambda_k)$ is convex and has a single minimum when λ_k is equal to the mean of the discarded eigenvalues (including itself). The eigenvalue λ_k can only take discrete values, but if we consider exchanging λ_k for some retained eigenvalue λ_j, $j \in \{1, \ldots, q'\}$, then if λ_j lies between λ_k and the current mean discarded eigenvalue, swapping λ_j and λ_k must decrease E. If we consider that the eigenvalues of $\mathbf{S}$ are ordered, for any combination of discarded eigenvalues that includes a gap occupied by a retained eigenvalue, there will always be a sequence of adjacent eigenvalues with a lower value of E. It follows that to minimize E, the discarded eigenvalues $\lambda_{q'+1}, \ldots, \lambda_d$ must be chosen to be adjacent among the ordered eigenvalues of $\mathbf{S}$.

This alone is not sufficient to show that the smallest eigenvalues must be discarded in order to maximize the likelihood. However, a further constraint is available from equation A.7, since $l_j = (\lambda_j - \sigma^2)^{1/2}$ implies that there can be no real solution to the stationary equations of the log-likelihood if any retained eigenvalue $\lambda_j < \sigma^2$. Since, from equation A.11, σ^2 is the average of the discarded eigenvalues, this condition would be violated if the smallest eigenvalue were not discarded. Now, combined with the previous result, this indicates that E must be minimized when $\lambda_{q'+1}, \ldots, \lambda_d$ are the smallest $d - q'$ eigenvalues and so $\mathcal{L}$ is maximized when $\lambda_1, \ldots, \lambda_q$ are the principal eigenvalues of $\mathbf{S}$.

It should also be noted that the log-likelihood $\mathcal{L}$ is maximized, with respect to q', when there are fewest terms in the sum in equation A.13 that occurs when $q' = q$, and therefore no l_j is zero. Furthermore, $\mathcal{L}$ is minimized when $\mathbf{W} = 0$, which is equivalent to the case of $q' = 0$.

A.3 The Nature of Other Stationary Points.

If stationary points represented by minor (nonprincipal) eigenvector solutions are stable maxima of the likelihood, then local maximization (via an EM algorithm, for example) is not guaranteed to find the principal eigenvectors. We may show, however, that minor eigenvector solutions are in fact saddle points on the likelihood surface.

Consider a stationary point of the log-likelihood, given by equation A.8, at $\widehat{\mathbf{W}} = \mathbf{U}_q (\mathbf{K}_q - \sigma^2 \mathbf{I})^{1/2} \mathbf{R}$, where $\mathbf{U}_q$ may contain q arbitrary eigenvectors of $\mathbf{S}$ and $\mathbf{K}_q$ contains either the corresponding eigenvalue or σ^2. We examine the nature of this stationary point by considering a small perturbation of the form $\mathbf{W} = \widehat{\mathbf{W}} + \epsilon \mathbf{PR}$, where ϵ is an arbitrarily small, positive constant and $\mathbf{P}$ is a $d \times q$ matrix of zeroes except for column W, which contains a discarded eigenvector $\mathbf{u}_P$ not contained in $\mathbf{U}_q$. By considering each potential eigenvector $\mathbf{u}_P$ individually applied to each column W of $\widehat{\mathbf{W}}$, we may elucidate the nature of the stationary point by evaluating the inner product of the perturbation with the gradient at $\mathbf{W}$ (where we treat the parameter matrix $\mathbf{W}$ or its derivative as a single column vector). If this inner product is negative for all possible perturbations, then the stationary point will be stable and represent a (local) maximum.

So defining $\mathbf{G} = (\partial \mathcal{L} / \partial \mathbf{W}) / N$ evaluated at $\mathbf{W} = \widehat{\mathbf{W}} + \epsilon \mathbf{PR}$, then from equation A.1,

$$\begin{aligned}
\mathbf{CG} &= \mathbf{SC}^{-1}\mathbf{W} - \mathbf{W}, \\
&= \mathbf{SW}(\sigma^2\mathbf{I} + \mathbf{W}^T\mathbf{W})^{-1} - \mathbf{W}, \\
&= \mathbf{SW}(\sigma^2\mathbf{I} + \widehat{\mathbf{W}}^T\widehat{\mathbf{W}} + \epsilon^2\mathbf{R}^T\mathbf{P}^T\mathbf{P}\mathbf{R})^{-1} - \mathbf{W},
\end{aligned} \tag{A.15}$$

since $\mathbf{P}^T\widehat{\mathbf{W}} = 0$. Ignoring the term in ϵ^2 then gives:

$$\begin{aligned}
\mathbf{CG} &= \mathbf{S}(\widehat{\mathbf{W}} + \epsilon\mathbf{PR})(\sigma^2\mathbf{I} + \widehat{\mathbf{W}}^T\widehat{\mathbf{W}})^{-1} - (\widehat{\mathbf{W}} + \epsilon\mathbf{PR}), \\
&= \epsilon\mathbf{SPR}(\sigma^2\mathbf{I} + \widehat{\mathbf{W}}^T\widehat{\mathbf{W}})^{-1} - \epsilon\mathbf{PR},
\end{aligned} \tag{A.16}$$

since $\mathbf{S}\widehat{\mathbf{W}}(\sigma^2\mathbf{I} + \widehat{\mathbf{W}}^T\widehat{\mathbf{W}}) - \widehat{\mathbf{W}} = 0$ at the stationary point. Then substituting for $\widehat{\mathbf{W}}$ gives $\sigma^2\mathbf{I} + \widehat{\mathbf{W}}^T\widehat{\mathbf{W}} = \mathbf{R}^T\mathbf{K}_q\mathbf{R}$, and so

$$\begin{aligned}
\mathbf{CG} &= \epsilon\mathbf{SPR}(\mathbf{R}^T\mathbf{K}_q^{-1}\mathbf{R}) - \epsilon\mathbf{PR}, \\
\Rightarrow \mathbf{G} &= \epsilon\mathbf{C}^{-1}\mathbf{P}(\mathbf{\Lambda}\mathbf{K}_q^{-1} - \mathbf{I})\mathbf{R},
\end{aligned} \tag{A.17}$$

where $\mathbf{\Lambda}$ is a $d \times d$ matrix of zeros, except for the Wth diagonal element, which contains the eigenvalue corresponding to $\mathbf{u}_P$, such that $(\mathbf{\Lambda})_{WW} = \lambda_P$. Then the sign of the inner product of the gradient $\mathbf{G}$ and the perturbation $\epsilon\mathbf{PR}$ is given by

$$\begin{aligned}
\text{sign}\left\{\text{tr}\left(\mathbf{G}^T\mathbf{PR}\right)\right\} &= \text{sign}\left\{\epsilon\text{tr}\left[\mathbf{R}^T(\mathbf{\Lambda}\mathbf{K}_q^{-1} - \mathbf{I})\mathbf{P}^T\mathbf{C}^{-1}\mathbf{PR}\right]\right\}, \\
&= \text{sign}\left\{(\lambda_P/k_W - 1)\mathbf{u}_P^T\mathbf{C}^{-1}\mathbf{u}_P\right\}, \\
&= \text{sign}\left\{\lambda_P/k_W - 1\right\},
\end{aligned} \tag{A.18}$$

since $\mathbf{C}^{-1}$ is positive definite and where k_W is the Wth diagonal element value in $\mathbf{K}_q$, and thus in the corresponding position to λ_P in $\mathbf{\Lambda}$. When $k_W = \lambda_W$, the expression given by equation A.18 is negative (and the maximum a stable one) if $\lambda_P < \lambda_W$. For $\lambda_P > \lambda_W$, $\widehat{\mathbf{W}}$ must be a saddle point.

In the case that $k_W = \sigma^2$, the stationary point will generally not be stable since, from equation A.11, σ^2 is the average of $d - q'$ eigenvalues, and so $\lambda_P > \sigma^2$ for at least one of those eigenvalues, *except* when all those eigenvalues are identical. Such a case is considered shortly.

From this, by considering all possible perturbations $\mathbf{P}$, it can be seen that the only stable maximum occurs when $\mathbf{W}$ comprises the q principal eigenvectors, for which $\lambda_P < \lambda_W, \forall P \neq W$.

A.4 Equality of Eigenvalues. Equality of any of the q principal eigenvalues does not affect the maximum likelihood estimates. However, in terms of conventional PCA, consideration should be given to the instance when all the $d - q$ minor (discarded) eigenvalue(s) are equal and identical to at least one retained eigenvalue. (In practice, particularly in the case of sample covariance matrices, this is unlikely.)

To illustrate, consider the example of extracting two components from data with a covariance matrix possessing eigenvalues λ_1, λ_2 and λ_2, and $\lambda_1 > \lambda_2$. In this case, the second principal axis is not uniquely defined within the minor subspace. The spherical noise distribution defined by $\sigma^2 = \lambda_2$, in addition to explaining the residual variance, can also optimally explain the second principal component. Because $\lambda_2 = \sigma^2$, l_2 in equation A.7 is zero, and $\mathbf{W}$ effectively comprises only a single vector. The combination of this single vector and the noise distribution still represents the maximum of the likelihood, but no second eigenvector is defined.

A.5 An EM Algorithm for PPCA. In the EM approach to PPCA, we consider the latent variables $\{x_n\}$ to be "missing" data. If their values were known, estimation of $\mathbf{W}$ would be straightforward from equation 2.2 by applying standard least-squares techniques. However, for a given t_n, we do not know the value of x_n that generated it, but we do know the joint distribution of the observed and latent variables, $p(t, x)$, and we can calculate the expectation of the corresponding complete-data log-likelihood. In the E-step of the EM algorithm, this expectation, calculated with respect to the posterior distribution of x_n given the observed t_n, is computed. In the M-step, new parameter values $\widetilde{\mathbf{W}}$ and $\widetilde{\sigma}^2$ are determined that maximize the expected complete-data log-likelihood, and this is guaranteed to increase the likelihood of interest, $\prod_n p(t_n)$, unless it is already at a local maximum (Dempster, Laird, & Rubin, 1977).

The complete-data log-likelihood is given by:

$$\mathcal{L}_C = \sum_{n=1}^{N} \ln \left\{ p(t_n, x_n) \right\}, \tag{A.19}$$

where, in PPCA, from equations 3.1 and 3.4,

$$p(t_n, x_n) = (2\pi\sigma^2)^{-d/2} \exp\left\{-\frac{\|t_n - \mathbf{W}x_n - \mu\|^2}{2\sigma^2}\right\} (2\pi)^{-q/2}$$

$$\times \exp\left\{-\frac{1}{2}x_n^T x_n\right\}. \tag{A.20}$$

In the E-step, we take the expectation with respect to the distributions $p(x_n | t_n, \mathbf{W}, \sigma^2)$:

$$\langle \mathcal{L}_C \rangle = -\sum_{n=1}^{N} \left\{ \frac{d}{2} \ln \sigma^2 + \frac{1}{2} \mathrm{tr}\left(\langle x_n x_n^T \rangle\right) + \frac{1}{2\sigma^2} \|t_n - \mu\|^2 \right.$$

$$\left. -\frac{1}{\sigma^2} \langle x_n \rangle^T \mathbf{W}^T (t_n - \mu) + \frac{1}{2\sigma^2} \mathrm{tr}\left(\mathbf{W}^T \mathbf{W} \langle x_n x_n^T \rangle\right) \right\}, \tag{A.21}$$

where we have omitted terms independent of the model parameters and

$$\langle x_n \rangle = M^{-1} W^T (t_n - \mu), \tag{A.22}$$
$$\langle x_n x_n^T \rangle = \sigma^2 M^{-1} + \langle x_n \rangle \langle x_n \rangle^T, \tag{A.23}$$

with $M = (\sigma^2 I + W^T W)$. Note that these statistics are computed using the current (fixed) values of the parameters and that equation A.22 is simply the posterior mean from equation 3.6. Equation A.23 follows from this in conjunction with the posterior covariance of equation 3.7.

In the M-step, $\langle \mathcal{L}_C \rangle$ is maximized with respect to W and σ^2 by differentiating equation A.21 and setting the derivatives to zero. This gives:

$$\widetilde{W} = \left[\sum_n (t_n - \mu) \langle x_n^T \rangle \right] \left[\sum_n \langle x_n x_n^T \rangle \right]^{-1} \tag{A.24}$$

$$\widetilde{\sigma}^2 = \frac{1}{Nd} \sum_{n=1}^{N} \left\{ \| t_n - \mu \|^2 - 2 \langle x_n^T \rangle \widetilde{W}^T (t_n - \mu) \right.$$
$$\left. + \operatorname{tr} \left(\langle x_n x_n^T \rangle \widetilde{W}^T \widetilde{W} \right) \right\} \tag{A.25}$$

To maximize the likelihood then, the sufficient statistics of the posterior distributions are calculated from the E-step equations A.22 and A.23, followed by the maximizing M-step equations (A.24 and A.25). These four equations are iterated in sequence until the algorithm is judged to have converged.

We may gain considerable insight into the operation of equations A.24 and A.25 by substituting for $\langle x_n \rangle$ and $\langle x_n x_n^T \rangle$ from A.22 and A.23. Taking care not to confuse new and old parameters, some further manipulation leads to both the E-step and M-step's being combined and rewritten as:

$$\widetilde{W} = SW(\sigma^2 I + M^{-1} W^T SW)^{-1}, \text{ and} \tag{A.26}$$

$$\widetilde{\sigma}^2 = \frac{1}{d} \operatorname{tr} \left(S - SWM^{-1} \widetilde{W}^T \right), \tag{A.27}$$

where S is again given by

$$S = \frac{1}{N} \sum_{n=1}^{N} (t_n - \mu)(t_n - \mu)^T. \tag{A.28}$$

Note that the first instance of W in equation A.27 is the *old* value of the weights, while the second instance $\widetilde{W}$ is the *new* value calculated from equation A.26. Equations A.26, A.27, and A.28 indicate that the data enter into the EM formulation only through its covariance matrix S, as we would expect.

Although it is algebraically convenient to express the EM algorithm in terms of $\mathbf{S}$, care should be exercised in any implementation. When $q \ll d$, it is possible to obtain considerable computational savings by not explicitly evaluating the covariance matrix, computation of which is $O(Nd^2)$. This is because inspection of equations A.24 and A.25 indicates that complexity is only $O(Ndq)$, and is reflected in equations A.26 and A.27 by the fact that $\mathbf{S}$ appears only within the terms $\mathbf{SW}$ and tr $(\mathbf{S})$, which may be computed with $O(Ndq)$ and $O(Nd)$ complexity, respectively. That is, $\mathbf{SW}$ should be computed as $\sum_n (\mathbf{t}_n - \boldsymbol{\mu}) \{ (\mathbf{t}_n - \boldsymbol{\mu})^\mathsf{T} \mathbf{W} \}$, as that form is more efficient than $\{ \sum_n (\mathbf{t}_n - \boldsymbol{\mu})(\mathbf{t}_n - \boldsymbol{\mu})^\mathsf{T} \} \mathbf{W}$, which is equivalent to finding $\mathbf{S}$ explicitly. However, because $\mathbf{S}$ need only be computed once in the single model case and the EM algorithm is iterative, potential efficiency gains depend on the number of iterations required to obtain the desired accuracy of solution, as well as the ratio of d to q. For example, in our implementation of the model using $q = 2$ for data visualization, we found that an iterative approach could be more efficient for $d > 20$.

A.6 Rotational Ambiguity. If $\mathbf{W}$ is determined by the above algorithm, or any other iterative method that maximizes the likelihood (see equation 3.8), then at convergence, $\mathbf{W}_{\mathrm{ML}} = \mathbf{U}_q (\boldsymbol{\Lambda}_q - \sigma^2 \mathbf{I})^{1/2} \mathbf{R}$. If it is desired to find the true principal axes $\mathbf{U}_q$ (and not just the principal subspace) then the arbitrary rotation matrix $\mathbf{R}$ presents difficulty. This rotational ambiguity also exists in factor analysis, as well as in certain iterative PCA algorithms, where it is usually not possible to determine the actual principal axes if $\mathbf{R} \neq \mathbf{I}$ (although there are algorithms where the constraint $\mathbf{R} = \mathbf{I}$ is imposed and the axes may be found).

However, in probabilistic PCA, $\mathbf{R}$ may actually be found since

$$\mathbf{W}_{\mathrm{ML}}^\mathsf{T} \mathbf{W}_{\mathrm{ML}} = \mathbf{R}^\mathsf{T} (\boldsymbol{\Lambda}_q - \sigma^2 \mathbf{I}) \mathbf{R} \tag{A.29}$$

implies that $\mathbf{R}^\mathsf{T}$ may be computed as the matrix of eigenvectors of the $q \times q$ matrix $\mathbf{W}_{\mathrm{ML}}^\mathsf{T} \mathbf{W}_{\mathrm{ML}}$. Hence, both $\mathbf{U}_q$ and $\boldsymbol{\Lambda}_q$ may be found by inverting the rotation followed by normalization of $\mathbf{W}_{\mathrm{ML}}$. That the rotational ambiguity may be resolved in PPCA is a consequence of the scaling of the eigenvectors by $(\boldsymbol{\Lambda}_q - \sigma^2 \mathbf{I})^{1/2}$ prior to rotation by $\mathbf{R}$. Without this scaling, $\mathbf{W}_{\mathrm{ML}}^\mathsf{T} \mathbf{W}_{\mathrm{ML}} = \mathbf{I}$, and the corresponding eigenvectors remain ambiguous. Also, note that while finding the eigenvectors of $\mathbf{S}$ directly requires $O(d^3)$ operations, to obtain them from $\mathbf{W}_{\mathrm{ML}}$ in this way requires only $O(q^3)$.

Appendix B: Optimal Least-Squares Reconstruction ⸺⸺⸺⸺⸺

One of the motivations for adopting PCA in many applications, notably in data compression, is the property of optimal linear least-squares reconstruction. That is, for all orthogonal projections $\mathbf{x} = \mathbf{A}^\mathsf{T}\mathbf{t}$ of the data, the least-squares reconstruction error,

$$E_{\text{rec}}^2 = \frac{1}{N} \sum_{n=1}^{N} \| t_n - BA^T t_n \|^2, \tag{B.1}$$

is minimized when the columns of A span the principal subspace of the data covariance matrix, and $B = A$. (For simplification, and without loss of generality, we assume here that the data has zero mean.)

We can similarly obtain this property from our probabilistic formalism, without the need to determine the exact orthogonal projection W, by finding the optimal reconstruction of the posterior mean vectors $\langle x_n \rangle$. To do this we simply minimize

$$E_{\text{rec}}^2 = \frac{1}{N} \sum_{n=1}^{N} \| t_n - B \langle x_n \rangle \|^2, \tag{B.2}$$

over the reconstruction matrix B, which is equivalent to a linear regression problem giving

$$B = SW(W^T SW)^{-1} M, \tag{B.3}$$

where we have substituted for $\langle x_n \rangle$ from equation A.22. In general, the resulting projection $B \langle x_n \rangle$ of t_n is not orthogonal, except in the maximum likelihood case, where $W = W_{\text{ML}} = U_q (\Lambda_q - \sigma^2 I)^{1/2} R$, and the optimal reconstructing matrix becomes

$$B_{\text{ML}} = W(W^T W)^{-1} M, \tag{B.4}$$

and so

$$\hat{t}_n = W(W^T W)^{-1} M \langle x_n \rangle, \tag{B.5}$$
$$= W(W^T W)^{-1} W^T t_n, \tag{B.6}$$

which is the expected orthogonal projection. The implication is thus that in the data compression context, at the maximum likelihood solution, the variables $\langle x_n \rangle$ can be transmitted down the channel and the original data vectors optimally reconstructed using equation B.5 given the parameters W and σ^2. Substituting for B in equation B.2 gives $E_{\text{rec}}^2 = (d - q)\sigma^2$, and the noise term σ^2 thus represents the expected squared reconstruction error per "lost" dimension.

Appendix C: EM for Mixtures of Probabilistic PCA

In a mixture of probabilistic principal component analyzers, we must fit a mixture of latent variable models in which the overall model distribution takes the form

$$p(\mathbf{t}) = \sum_{i=1}^{M} \pi_i p(\mathbf{t}|i), \qquad (C.1)$$

where $p(\mathbf{t}|i)$ is a single probabilistic PCA model and π_i is the corresponding mixing proportion. The parameters for this mixture model can be determined by an extension of the EM algorithm. We begin by considering the standard form that the EM algorithm would take for this model and highlight a number of limitations. We then show that a two-stage form of EM leads to a more efficient algorithm.

We first note that in addition to a set of $\mathbf{x}_{ni}$ for each model i, the missing data include variables z_{ni} labeling which model is responsible for generating each data point $\mathbf{t}_n$. At this point we can derive a standard EM algorithm by considering the corresponding complete-data log-likelihood, which takes the form

$$\mathcal{L}_C = \sum_{n=1}^{N} \sum_{i=1}^{M} z_{ni} \ln\{\pi_i p(\mathbf{t}_n, \mathbf{x}_{ni})\}. \qquad (C.2)$$

Starting with "old" values for the parameters π_i, $\boldsymbol{\mu}_i$, $\mathbf{W}_i$, and σ_i^2, we first evaluate the posterior probabilities R_{ni} using equation 4.3 and similarly evaluate the expectations $\langle \mathbf{x}_{ni} \rangle$ and $\langle \mathbf{x}_{ni}\mathbf{x}_{ni}^T \rangle$:

$$\langle \mathbf{x}_{ni} \rangle = \mathbf{M}_i^{-1}\mathbf{W}_i^T(\mathbf{t}_n - \boldsymbol{\mu}_i), \qquad (C.3)$$

$$\langle \mathbf{x}_{ni}\mathbf{x}_{ni}^T \rangle = \sigma_i^2 \mathbf{M}_i^{-1} + \langle \mathbf{x}_{ni} \rangle \langle \mathbf{x}_{ni} \rangle^T, \qquad (C.4)$$

with $\mathbf{M}_i = \sigma_i^2\mathbf{I} + \mathbf{W}_i^T\mathbf{W}_i$.

Then we take the expectation of $\mathcal{L}_C$ with respect to these posterior distributions to obtain

$$\langle \mathcal{L}_C \rangle = \sum_{n=1}^{N} \sum_{i=1}^{M} R_{ni} \left\{ \ln \pi_i - \frac{d}{2} \ln \sigma_i^2 - \frac{1}{2}\text{tr}\left(\langle \mathbf{x}_{ni}\mathbf{x}_{ni}^T \rangle\right) \right.$$

$$- \frac{1}{2\sigma_i^2}\|\mathbf{t}_{ni} - \boldsymbol{\mu}_i\|^2 + \frac{1}{\sigma_i^2}\langle \mathbf{x}_{ni} \rangle^T \mathbf{W}_i^T(\mathbf{t}_n - \boldsymbol{\mu}_i)$$

$$\left. - \frac{1}{2\sigma_i^2}\text{tr}\left(\mathbf{W}_i^T\mathbf{W}_i\langle \mathbf{x}_{ni}\mathbf{x}_{ni}^T \rangle\right) \right\}, \qquad (C.5)$$

where $\langle \cdot \rangle$ denotes the expectation with respect to the posterior distributions of both $\mathbf{x}_{ni}$ and z_{ni} and terms independent of the model parameters have been omitted. The M-step then involves maximizing equation C.5 with respect to π_i, $\boldsymbol{\mu}_i$, σ_i^2, and $\mathbf{W}_i$ to obtain "new" values for these parameters. The maximization with respect to π_i must take account of the constraint that

$\sum_i \pi_i = 1$. This can be achieved with the use of a Lagrange multiplier λ (see Bishop, 1995) and maximizing

$$\langle \mathcal{L}_C \rangle + \lambda \left(\sum_{i=1}^{M} \pi_i - 1 \right). \tag{C.6}$$

Together with the results of maximizing equation C.5 with respect to the remaining parameters, this gives the following M-step equations:

$$\tilde{\pi}_i = \frac{1}{N} \sum_n R_{ni} \tag{C.7}$$

$$\tilde{\mu}_i = \frac{\sum_n R_{ni}(\mathbf{t}_{ni} - \tilde{\mathbf{W}}_i \langle \mathbf{x}_{ni} \rangle)}{\sum_n R_{ni}} \tag{C.8}$$

$$\tilde{\mathbf{W}}_i = \left[\sum_n R_{ni}(\mathbf{t}_n - \tilde{\mu}_i)\langle \mathbf{x}_{ni} \rangle^{\mathrm{T}} \right] \left[\sum_n R_{ni}\langle \mathbf{x}_{ni}\mathbf{x}_{ni}^{\mathrm{T}} \rangle \right]^{-1} \tag{C.9}$$

$$\tilde{\sigma}_i^2 = \frac{1}{d \sum_n R_{ni}} \left\{ \sum_n R_{ni}\|\mathbf{t}_n - \tilde{\mu}_i\|^2 - 2 \sum_n R_{ni}\langle \mathbf{x}_{ni} \rangle^{\mathrm{T}} \tilde{\mathbf{W}}_i^{\mathrm{T}}(\mathbf{t}_n - \tilde{\mu}_i) \right.$$
$$\left. + \sum_n R_{ni}\mathrm{tr}\left(\langle \mathbf{x}_{ni}\mathbf{x}_{ni}^{\mathrm{T}} \rangle \tilde{\mathbf{W}}_i^{\mathrm{T}} \tilde{\mathbf{W}}_i \right) \right\} \tag{C.10}$$

where the symbol $\tilde{\ }$ denotes "new" quantities that may be adjusted in the M-step. Note that the M-step equations for $\tilde{\mu}_i$ and $\tilde{\mathbf{W}}_i$, given by equations C.8 and C.9, are coupled, and so further (albeit straightforward) manipulation is required to obtain explicit solutions.

In fact, simplification of the M-step equations, along with improved speed of convergence, is possible if we adopt a two-stage EM procedure as follows. The likelihood function we wish to maximize is given by

$$\mathcal{L} = \sum_{n=1}^{N} \ln \left\{ \sum_{i=1}^{M} \pi_i p(\mathbf{t}_n | i) \right\}. \tag{C.11}$$

Regarding the component labels z_{ni} as missing data, and ignoring the presence of the latent $\mathbf{x}$ variables for now, we can consider the corresponding expected complete-data log-likelihood given by

$$\hat{\mathcal{L}}_C = \sum_{n=1}^{N} \sum_{i=1}^{M} R_{ni} \ln \left\{ \pi_i p(\mathbf{t}_n | i) \right\}, \tag{C.12}$$

where R_{ni} represent the posterior probabilities (corresponding to the expected values of z_{ni}) and are given by equation 4.2. Maximization of equation C.12 with respect to π_i, again using a Lagrange multiplier, gives the

M-step equation (4.4). Similarly, maximization of equation C.12 with respect to μ_i gives equation 4.5. This is the first stage of the combined EM procedure.

In order to update W_i and σ_i^2, we seek only to increase the value of $\widehat{\mathcal{L}}_C$, and not actually to maximize it. This corresponds to the generalized EM (or GEM) algorithm. We do this by considering $\widehat{\mathcal{L}}_C$ as our likelihood of interest and, introducing the missing x_{ni} variables, perform one cycle of the EM algorithm, now with respect to the parameters W_i and σ_i^2. This second stage is guaranteed to increase $\widehat{\mathcal{L}}_C$, and therefore $\mathcal{L}$ as desired.

The advantages of this approach are twofold. First, the new values $\tilde{\mu}_i$ calculated in the first stage are used to compute the sufficient statistics of the posterior distribution of x_{ni} in the second stage using equations C.3 and C.4. By using updated values of μ_i in computing these statistics, this leads to improved convergence speed.

A second advantage is that for the second stage of the EM algorithm, there is a considerable simplification of the M-step updates, since when equation C.5 is expanded for $\langle x_{ni} \rangle$ and $\langle x_{ni} x_{ni}^T \rangle$, only terms in $\tilde{\mu}_i$ (and not μ_i) appear. By inspection of equation C.5, we see that the expected complete-data log-likelihood now takes the form

$$\langle \mathcal{L}_C \rangle = \sum_{n=1}^{N} \sum_{i=1}^{M} R_{ni} \left\{ \ln \tilde{\pi}_i - \frac{d}{2} \ln \sigma_i^2 - \frac{1}{2} \mathrm{tr}\left(\langle x_{ni} x_{ni}^T \rangle \right) \right.$$
$$- \frac{1}{2\sigma_i^2} \|t_{ni} - \tilde{\mu}_i\|^2 + \frac{1}{\sigma_i^2} \langle x_{ni}^T \rangle W_i^T (t_n - \tilde{\mu}_i)$$
$$\left. - \frac{1}{2\sigma_i^2} \mathrm{tr}\left(W_i^T W_i \langle x_{ni} x_{ni}^T \rangle \right) \right\}. \tag{C.13}$$

Now when we maximize equation C.13 with respect to W_i and σ_i^2 (keeping $\tilde{\mu}_i$ fixed), we obtain the much simplified M-step equations:

$$\widetilde{W}_i = S_i W_i (\sigma_i^2 I + M_i^{-1} W_i^T S_i W_i)^{-1}, \tag{C.14}$$

$$\tilde{\sigma}_i^2 = \frac{1}{d} \mathrm{tr}\left(S_i - S_i W_i M_i^{-1} \widetilde{W}_i^T \right), \tag{C.15}$$

where

$$S_i = \frac{1}{\tilde{\pi}_i N} \sum_{n=1}^{N} R_{ni} (t_n - \tilde{\mu}_i)(t_n - \tilde{\mu}_i)^T. \tag{C.16}$$

Iteration of equations 4.3 through 4.5 followed by equations C.14 and C.15 in sequence is guaranteed to find a local maximum of the likelihood (see equation 4.1).

Comparison of equations C.14 and C.15 with equations A.26 and A.27 shows that the updates for the mixture case are identical to those of the single PPCA model, given that the local responsibility-weighted covariance matrix S_i is substituted for the global covariance matrix S. Thus, at stationary points, each weight matrix W_i contains the (scaled and rotated) eigenvectors of its respective S_i, the local covariance matrix. Each submodel is then performing a local PCA, where each data point is weighted by the responsibility of that submodel for its generation, and a soft partitioning, similar to that introduced by Hinton et al. (1997), is automatically effected.

Given the established results for the single PPCA model, there is no need to use the iterative updates (see equations C.14 and C.15) since W_i and σ_i^2 may be determined by eigendecomposition of S_i, and the likelihood must still increase unless at a maximum. However, as discussed in appendix A.5, the iterative EM scheme may offer computational advantages, particularly for $q \ll d$. In such a case, the iterative approach of equations C.14 and C.15 can be used, taking care to evaluate $S_i W_i$ efficiently as $\sum_n R_{ni}(t_n - \tilde{\mu}_i)\left\{(t_n - \tilde{\mu}_i)^T W_i\right\}$. In the mixture case, unlike for the single model, S_i must be recomputed at each iteration of the EM algorithm, as the responsibilities R_{ni} will change.

As a final computational note, it might appear that the necessary calculation of $p(t|i)$ would require inversion of the $d \times d$ matrix C, an $O(d^3)$ operation. However, $(\sigma^2 I + WW^T)^{-1} = \{I - W(\sigma^2 I + W^T W)^{-1}W^T\}/\sigma^2$ and so C^{-1} may be computed using the already calculated $q \times q$ matrix M^{-1}.

Acknowledgments

This work was supported by EPSRC contract GR/K51808: Neural Networks for Visualization of High Dimensional Data, at Aston University. We thank Michael Revow for supplying the handwritten digit data in its processed form.

References

Anderson, T. W. (1963). Asymptotic theory for principal component analysis. *Annals of Mathematical Statistics, 34*, 122–148.

Anderson, T. W., & Rubin, H. (1956). Statistical inference in factor analysis. In J. Neyman (Ed.), *Proceedings of the Third Berkeley Symposium on Mathematical Statistics and Probability* (Vol. 5, pp. 111–150). Berkeley: University of California, Berkeley.

Bartholomew, D. J. (1987). *Latent variable models and factor analysis*. London: Charles Griffin & Co. Ltd.

Basilevsky, A. (1994). *Statistical factor analysis and related methods*. New York: Wiley.

Bishop, C. M. (1995). *Neural networks for pattern recognition*. Oxford: Clarendon Press.

Bishop, C. M., Svensén, M., & Williams, C. K. I. (1998). GTM: The generative topographic mapping. *Neural Computation, 10*(1), 215–234.

Bishop, C. M., & Tipping, M. E. (1998). A hierarchical latent variable model for data visualization. *IEEE Transactions on Pattern Analysis and Machine Intelligence, 20*(3), 281–293.

Bregler, C., & Omohundro, S. M. (1995). Nonlinear image interpolation using manifold learning. In G. Tesauro, D. S. Touretzky, & T. K. Leen (Eds.), *Advances in neural information processing systems, 7* (pp. 973–980). Cambridge, MA: MIT Press.

Broomhead, D. S., Indik, R., Newell, A. C., & Rand, D. A. (1991). Local adaptive Galerkin bases for large-dimensional dynamical systems. *Nonlinearity, 4*(1), 159–197.

Dempster, A. P., Laird, N. M., & Rubin, D. B. (1977). Maximum likelihood from incomplete data via the EM algorithm. *Journal of the Royal Statistical Society, B39*(1), 1–38.

Dony, R. D., & Haykin, S. (1995). Optimally adaptive transform coding. *IEEE Transactions on Image Processing, 4*(10), 1358–1370.

Hastie, T., & Stuetzle, W. (1989). Principal curves. *Journal of the American Statistical Association, 84,* 502–516.

Hinton, G. E., Dayan, P., & Revow, M. (1997). Modelling the manifolds of images of handwritten digits. *IEEE Transactions on Neural Networks, 8*(1), 65–74.

Hinton, G. E., Revow, M., & Dayan, P. (1995). Recognizing handwritten digits using mixtures of linear models. In G. Tesauro, D. S. Touretzky, & T. K. Leen (Eds.), *Advances in neural information processing systems, 7* (pp. 1015–1022). Cambridge, MA: MIT Press.

Hotelling, H. (1933). Analysis of a complex of statistical variables into principal components. *Journal of Educational Psychology, 24,* 417–441.

Hull, J. J. (1994). A database for handwritten text recognition research. *IEEE Transactions on Pattern Analysis and Machine Intelligence, 16,* 550–554.

Japkowicz, N., Myers, C., & Gluck, M. (1995). A novelty detection approach to classification. In *Proceedings of the Fourteenth International Conference on Artificial Intelligence* (pp. 518–523).

Jolliffe, I. T. (1986). *Principal component analysis.* New York: Springer-Verlag.

Jordan, M. I., & Jacobs, R. A. (1994). Hierarchical mixtures of experts and the EM algorithm. *Neural Computation, 6*(2), 181–214.

Kambhatla, N. (1995). *Local models and gaussian mixture models for statistical data processing.* Unpublished doctoral dissertation, Oregon Graduate Institute, Center for Spoken Language Understanding.

Kambhatla, N., & Leen, T. K. (1997). Dimension reduction by local principal component analysis. *Neural Computation, 9*(7), 1493–1516.

Kramer, M. A. (1991). Nonlinear principal component analysis using autoassociative neural networks. *AIChE Journal, 37*(2), 233–243.

Krzanowski, W. J., & Marriott, F. H. C. (1994). *Multivariate analysis part 2: Classification, Covariance structures and repeated measurements.* London: Edward Arnold.

Lawley, D. N. (1953). A modified method of estimation in factor analysis and some large sample results. In *Uppsala Symposium on Psychological Factor Analysis.* Nordisk Psykologi Monograph Series (pp. 35–42). Uppsala: Almqvist and Wiksell.

Oja, E. (1983). *Subspace methods of pattern recognition*. New York: Wiley.

Ormoneit, D., & Tresp, V. (1996). Improved gaussian mixture density estimates using Bayesian penalty terms and network averaging. In D. S. Touretzky, M. C. Mozer, & M. E. Hasselmo (Eds.), *Advances in neural information processing systems, 8* (pp. 542–548). Cambridge, MA: MIT Press.

Pearson, K. (1901). On lines and planes of closest fit to systems of points in space. *London, Edinburgh and Dublin Philosophical Magazine and Journal of Science, Sixth Series, 2*, 559–572.

Petsche, T., Marcantonio, A., Darken, C., Hanson, S. J., Kuhn, G. M., & Santoso, I. (1996). A neural network autoassociator for induction motor failure prediction. In D. S. Touretzky, M. C. Mozer, & M. E. Hasselmo (Eds.), *Advances in neural information processing systems, 8* (pp. 924–930). Cambridge, MA: MIT Press.

Rao, C. R. (1955). Estimation and tests of significance in factor analysis. *Psychometrika, 20*, 93–111.

Rubin, D. B., & Thayer, D. T. (1982). EM algorithms for ML factor analysis. *Psychometrika, 47*(1), 69–76.

Tibshirani, R. (1992). Principal curves revisited. *Statistics and Computing, 2*, 183–190.

Tipping, M. E., & Bishop, C. M. (1997). Mixtures of principal component analysers. In *Proceedings of the IEE Fifth International Conference on Artificial Neural Networks, Cambridge* (pp. 13–18). London: IEE.

Titterington, D. M., Smith, A. F. M., & Makov, U. E. (1985). *The statistical analysis of finite mixture distributions*. New York: Wiley.

Webb, A. R. (1996). An approach to nonlinear principal components analysis using radially symmetrical kernel functions. *Statistics and Computing, 6*(2), 159–168.

Received June 19, 1997; accepted May 19, 1998.

Independent Factor Analysis

H. Attias
Sloan Center for Theoretical Neurobiology and W. M. Keck Foundation Center for Integrative Neuroscience, University of California at San Francisco, San Francisco, CA 94143-0444, U.S.A.

We introduce the independent factor analysis (IFA) method for recovering independent hidden sources from their observed mixtures. IFA generalizes and unifies ordinary factor analysis (FA), principal component analysis (PCA), and independent component analysis (ICA), and can handle not only square noiseless mixing but also the general case where the number of mixtures differs from the number of sources and the data are noisy. IFA is a two-step procedure. In the first step, the source densities, mixing matrix, and noise covariance are estimated from the observed data by maximum likelihood. For this purpose we present an expectation-maximization (EM) algorithm, which performs unsupervised learning of an associated probabilistic model of the mixing situation. Each source in our model is described by a mixture of gaussians; thus, all the probabilistic calculations can be performed analytically. In the second step, the sources are reconstructed from the observed data by an optimal nonlinear estimator. A variational approximation of this algorithm is derived for cases with a large number of sources, where the exact algorithm becomes intractable. Our IFA algorithm reduces to the one for ordinary FA when the sources become gaussian, and to an EM algorithm for PCA in the zero-noise limit. We derive an additional EM algorithm specifically for noiseless IFA. This algorithm is shown to be superior to ICA since it can learn arbitrary source densities from the data. Beyond blind separation, IFA can be used for modeling multidimensional data by a highly constrained mixture of gaussians and as a tool for nonlinear signal encoding.

1 Statistical Modeling and Blind Source Separation ————————

The blind source separation (BSS) problem presents multivariable data measured by L' sensors. These data arise from L source signals that are mixed together by some linear transformation corrupted by noise. Further, the sources are mutually statistically independent. The task is to obtain those source signals. However, the sources are not observable, and nothing is known about their properties beyond their mutual statistical independence or about the properties of the mixing process and the noise. In the absence of this information, one has to proceed "blindly" to recover the source signals from their observed noisy mixtures.

Despite its signal-processing appearance, BSS is a problem in statistical modeling of data. In this context, one wishes to describe the L' observed variables y_i, which are generally correlated, in terms of a smaller set of L unobserved variables x_j that are mutually independent. The simplest such description is given by a probabilistic linear model,

$$y_i = \sum_{j=1}^{L} H_{ij} x_j + u_i, \qquad i = 1, \ldots, L', \tag{1.1}$$

where y_i depends on linear combinations of the x_js with constant coefficients H_{ij}; the probabilistic nature of this dependence is modeled by the L' additive noise signals u_i. In general, the statistician's task is to estimate H_{ij} and x_j. The latter are regarded as the independent "causes" of the data in some abstract sense; their relation to the actual physical causes is often highly nontrivial. In BSS, on the other hand, the actual causes of the sensor signals y_i are the source signals x_j, and the model, equation 1.1, with H_{ij} being the mixing matrix, is known to be the correct description.

One might expect that since linear models have been analyzed and applied extensively for many years, the solution to the BSS problem can be found in some textbook or review article. This is not the case. Consider, for example, the close relation of equation 1.1 to the well-known factor analysis (FA) model (see Everitt, 1984). In the context of FA, the unobserved sources x_j are termed *common factors* (usually just *factors*), the noise u_i *specific factors*, and the mixing matrix elements H_{ij} *factor loadings*. The factor loadings and noise variances can be estimated from the data by, for example, maximum likelihood (there exists an efficient expectation-maximization algorithm for this purpose), leading to an optimal estimate of the factors. However, ordinary FA cannot perform BSS. Its inadequacy stems from using a gaussian model for the probability density $p(x_j)$ of each factor. This seemingly technical point turns out to have important consequences, since it implies that FA exploits only second-order statistics of the observed data to perform those estimates and hence, in effect, does not require the factors to be mutually independent but merely uncorrelated. As a result, the factors (and factor loading matrix) are not defined uniquely but only to within an arbitrary rotation, since the likelihood function is rotation invariant in factor space. Put in the context of BSS, the true sources and mixing matrix cannot be distinguished from any rotation thereof when only second-order statistics are used. More modern statistical analysis methods, such as projection pursuit (Friedman & Stuetzle, 1981; Huber, 1985) and generalized additive models (Hastie & Tibshirani, 1990), do indeed use nongaussian densities (modeled by nonlinear functions of gaussian variables), but the resulting models are quite restricted and unsuitable for solving the BSS problem.

Most of the work in the field of BSS since its emergence in the mid-1980s (see Jutten & Hérault, 1991; Comon, Jutten, & Hérault, 1991) aimed at a highly idealized version of the problem where the mixing is square ($L' = L$), invertible, instantaneous and noiseless. This version is termed *independent component analysis* (ICA) (Comon, 1994). A satisfactory solution for ICA was found only in the past few years (Bell & Sejnowski, 1995; Cardoso & Laheld, 1996; Pham, 1996; Pearlmutter & Parra, 1997; Hyvärinen & Oja, 1997). Contrary to FA, algorithms for ICA employ nongaussian models of the source densities $p(x_j)$. Consequently, the likelihood is no longer rotation invariant, and the maximum likelihood estimate of the mixing matrix is unique; for appropriately chosen $p(x_j)$ (see below), it is also correct.

Mixing in realistic situations, however, generally includes noise and different numbers of sources and sensors. As the noise level increases, the performance of ICA algorithms deteriorates and the separation quality decreases, as manifested by cross-talk and noisy outputs. More important, many situations have a relatively small number of sensors but many sources, and one would like to lump the low-intensity sources together and regard them as effective noise, while the separation focuses on the high-intensity ones. There is no way to accomplish this using ICA methods.

Another important problem in ICA is determining the source density model. The ability to learn the densities $p(x_j)$ from the observed data is crucial. However, existing algorithms usually employ a source model that is either fixed or has only limited flexibility. When the actual source densities in the problem are known in advance, this model can be tailored accordingly; otherwise an inaccurate model often leads to failed separation, since the global maximum of the likelihood shifts away from the one corresponding to the correct mixing matrix. In principle, one can use a flexible parametric density model whose parameters may also be estimated by maximum likelihood (MacKay, 1996; Pearlmutter & Parra, 1997). However, ICA algorithms use gradient-based maximization methods, which result in rather slow learning of the density parameters.

In this article we present a novel unsupervised learning algorithm for blind separation of nonsquare, noisy mixtures. The key to our approach lies in the introduction of a new probabilistic generative model, termed the *independent factor* (IF) model, described schematically in Figure 1. This model is defined by equation 1.1, associated with arbitrary nongaussian adaptive densities $p(x_j)$ for the factors. We define *independent factor analysis* (IFA) as the reconstruction of the unobserved factors x_j from the observed data y_i. Hence, performing IFA amounts to solving the BSS problem.

IFA is performed in two steps. The first consists of learning the IF model, parameterized by the mixing matrix, noise covariance, and source density parameters, from the data. To make the model analytically tractable while maintaining the ability to describe arbitrary sources, each source density is modeled by a mixture of one-dimensional gaussians. This enables us to derive an expectation-maximization (EM) algorithm, given by equations 3.12

and 3.13, which performs maximum likelihood estimation of all the parameters, the source densities included.

Due to the presence of noise, the sources can be recovered from the sensor signals only approximately. This is done in the second step of IFA using the posterior density of the sources given the data. Based on this posterior, we derive two different source estimators, which provide optimal source reconstructions using the parameters learned in the first step. Both estimators, the first given by equation 4.2 and the second found iteratively using equation 4.4, are nonlinear, but each satisfies a different optimality criterion.

As the number of sources increases, the E-step of this algorithm becomes increasingly computationally expensive. For such cases we derive an approximate algorithm that is shown to be quite accurate. The approximation is based on the variational approach introduced in the context of feedforward probabilistic networks by Saul et al. (1996).

Our IFA algorithm reduces to ordinary FA when the model sources become gaussian and performs principal component analysis (PCA) when used in the zero-noise limit. An additional EM algorithm, derived specifically for noiseless IFA, is also presented (see equations 7.8–7.10). A particular version of this algorithm, termed *Seesaw*, is composed of two alternating phases, as shown schematically in Figure 8. The first phase learns the unmixing matrix while keeping the source densities fixed; the second phase freezes the unmixing matrix and learns the source densities using EM. Its ability to learn the source densities from the data in an efficient manner makes Seesaw a powerful extension of Bell and Sejnowski's (1995) ICA algorithm, since it can separate mixtures that ICA fails to separate.

IFA therefore generalizes and unifies ordinary FA, PCA, and ICA and provides a new method for modeling multivariable data in terms of a small set of independent hidden variables. Furthermore, IFA amounts to fitting those data to a mixture model of coadaptive Gaussians (see Figure 3, bottom right), that is, the gaussians cannot adapt independently but are strongly constrained to move and expand together.

This article deals only with instantaneous mixing. Real-world mixing situations are generally not instantaneous but include propagation delays and reverberations (described mathematically by convolutions in place of matrix multiplication in equation 1.1). A significant step toward solving the convolutive BSS problem was taken by Attias and Schreiner (1998), who obtained a family of maximum-likelihood-based learning algorithms for separating noiseless convolutive mixtures; Torkkola (1996) and Lee, Bell, and Lambert (1997) derived one of those algorithms from information-maximization considerations. Algorithms for noisy convolutive mixing can be derived using an extension of the methods described here and will be presented elsewhere.

This article is organized as follows. Section 2 introduces the IF model. The EM algorithm for learning the generative model parameters is presented in section 3, and source reconstruction procedures are discussed in section 4. The performance of the IFA algorithm is demonstrated by its application to noisy mixtures of signals with arbitrary densities in section 5. The factorized variational approximation of IFA is derived and tested in section 6. The EM algorithm for noiseless IFA and its Seesaw version is presented and demonstrated in section 7. Most derivations are relegated to appendixes A–C.

Notation. Throughout this article, vectors are denoted by boldfaced lower-case letters and matrices by boldfaced upper-class letters. Vector and matrix elements are not boldfaced. The inverse of a matrix $\mathbf{A}$ is denoted by $\mathbf{A}^{-1}$ and its transposition by $\mathbf{A}^T$ ($A_{ij}^T = A_{ji}$).

To denote ensemble averaging we use the operator E. Thus, if $\mathbf{x}^{(t)}$, $t = 1, \dots, T$ are different observations of the random vector $\mathbf{x}$, then for any vector function $\mathbf{F}$ of $\mathbf{x}$,

$$EF(\mathbf{x}) = \frac{1}{T} \sum_{t=1}^{T} \mathbf{F}(\mathbf{x}^{(t)}). \tag{1.2}$$

The multivariable gaussian distribution for a random vector $\mathbf{x}$ with mean μ and covariance Σ is denoted by

$$\mathcal{G}(\mathbf{x} - \mu, \Sigma) = |\det(2\pi\Sigma)|^{-1/2} \exp\left[-(\mathbf{x} - \mu)^T \Sigma^{-1} (\mathbf{x} - \mu)/2\right], \tag{1.3}$$

implying $E\mathbf{x} = \mu$ and $E\mathbf{x}\mathbf{x}^T = \Sigma + \mu\mu^T$.

2 Independent Factor (IF) Generative Model

Independent factor analysis is a two-step method. The first step is concerned with the unsupervised learning task of a generative model (Everitt, 1984)—the IF model, which we introduce in the following. Let $\mathbf{y}$ be an $L' \times 1$ observed data vector. We wish to explain the correlated y_i in terms of L hidden variables x_j, referred to as factors, that are mutually statistically independent. Specifically, the data are modeled as dependent on linear combinations of the factors with constant coefficients H_{ij}, and an additive $L' \times 1$ random vector $\mathbf{u}$ makes this dependence nondeterministic:

$$\mathbf{y} = \mathbf{H}\mathbf{x} + \mathbf{u}. \tag{2.1}$$

In the language of BSS, the independent factors $\mathbf{x}$ are the unobserved source signals, and the data $\mathbf{y}$ are the observed sensor signals. The sources are mixed by the matrix $\mathbf{H}$. The resulting mixtures are corrupted by noise signals $\mathbf{u}$ originating in the sources, the mixing process (e.g., the propagation medium response), or the sensor responses.

In order to produce a generative model for the probability density of the sensor signals $p(\mathbf{y})$, we must first specify the density of the sources and the noise. We model the sources x_i as L independent random variables with arbitrary distributions $p(x_i \mid \theta_i)$, where the individual ith source density is parameterized by the parameter set θ_i.

The noise is assumed to be gaussian with mean zero and covariance matrix Λ, allowing correlations between sensors; even when the sensor noise signals are independent, correlations may arise due to source noise or propagation noise. Hence,

$$p(\mathbf{u}) = \mathcal{G}(\mathbf{u}, \Lambda). \tag{2.2}$$

Equations 2.1–2.2 define the IF generative model, which is parameterized by the source parameters θ, mixing matrix $\mathbf{H}$, and noise covariance Λ. We denote the IF parameters collectively by

$$W = (\mathbf{H}, \Lambda, \theta). \tag{2.3}$$

The resulting model sensor density is

$$p(\mathbf{y} \mid W) = \int d\mathbf{x}\, p(\mathbf{y} \mid \mathbf{x})\, p(\mathbf{x})$$

$$= \int d\mathbf{x}\, \mathcal{G}(\mathbf{y} - \mathbf{H}\mathbf{x}, \Lambda) \prod_{i=1}^{L} p(x_i \mid \theta_i), \tag{2.4}$$

where $d\mathbf{x} = \prod_i dx_i$. The parameters W should be adapted to minimize an error function that measures the distance between the model and observed sensor densities.

2.1 Source Model: Factorial Mixture of Gaussians. Although in principle $p(\mathbf{y})$ of equation 2.4 is a perfectly viable starting point and can be evaluated by numerical integration given a suitably chosen $p(x_i)$, this could become quite computationally intensive in practice. A better strategy is to choose a parametric form for $p(x_i)$ that is sufficiently general to model arbitrary source densities and allows performing the integral in equation 2.4 analytically. A form that satisfies both requirements is the mixture of gaussians (MOG) model.

In this article we describe the density of source i as a mixture of n_i gaussians $q_i = 1, \ldots, n_i$ with means μ_{i,q_i}, variances v_{i,q_i}, and mixing proportions w_{i,q_i}:

$$p(x_i \mid \theta_i) = \sum_{q_i=1}^{n_i} w_{i,q_i}\, \mathcal{G}(x_i - \mu_{i,q_i}, v_{i,q_i}), \qquad \theta_i = \{w_{i,q_i}, \mu_{i,q_i}, v_{i,q_i}\}, \tag{2.5}$$

where q_i runs over the gaussians of source i. For this mixture to be normalized, the mixing proportions for each source should sum to unity: $\sum_{q_i} w_{i,q_i} = 1$.

The parametric form (2.5) provides a probabilistic generative description of the sources in which the different gaussians play the role of hidden states. To generate the source signal x_i, we first pick a state q_i with probability $p(q_i) = w_{i,q_i}$ and then draw a number x_i from the corresponding gaussian density $p(x_i \mid q_i) = \mathcal{G}(x_i - \mu_{i,q_i}, v_{i,q_i})$.

Viewed in L-dimensional space, the joint source density $p(\mathbf{x})$ formed by the product of the one-dimensional MOGs (see equation 2.5) is itself an MOG. Its collective hidden states,

$$\mathbf{q} = (q_1, \ldots, q_L),\tag{2.6}$$

consist of all possible combinations of the individual source states q_i. As Figure 3 (upper right) illustrates for $L = 2$, each state $\mathbf{q}$ corresponds to an L-dimensional gaussian density whose mixing proportions $w_\mathbf{q}$, mean $\mu_\mathbf{q}$, and diagonal covariance matrix $\mathbf{V_q}$ are determined by those of the constituent source states,

$$w_\mathbf{q} = \prod_{i=1}^{L} w_{i,q_i} = w_{1,q_1}, \ldots, w_{L,q_L}, \qquad \mu_\mathbf{q} = (\mu_{1,q_1}, \ldots, \mu_{L,q_L}),$$

$$\mathbf{V_q} = \mathrm{diag}(v_{1,q_1}, \ldots, v_{L,q_L}).\tag{2.7}$$

Hence we have,

$$p(\mathbf{x} \mid \boldsymbol{\theta}) = \prod_{i=1}^{L} p(x_i \mid \theta_i) = \sum_\mathbf{q} w_\mathbf{q}\, \mathcal{G}(\mathbf{x} - \mu_\mathbf{q}, \mathbf{V_q}),\tag{2.8}$$

where the gaussians factorize, $\mathcal{G}(\mathbf{x} - \mu_\mathbf{q}, \mathbf{V_q}) = \prod_i \mathcal{G}(x_i - \mu_{i,q_i}, v_{i,q_i})$, and the sum over collective states $\mathbf{q}$ (see equation 2.6) represents summing over all the individual source states, $\sum_\mathbf{q} = \sum_{q_1}, \ldots, \sum_{q_L}$.

Contrary to ordinary MOG, the gaussians in equation 2.8 are not free to adapt independently but are rather strongly constrained. Modifying the mean and variance of a single-source state q_i would result in shifting a whole column of collective states $\mathbf{q}$. Our source model is therefore a mixture of coadaptive gaussians, termed *factorial MOG*. Hinton and Zemel (1994) proposed and studied a related generative model, which differed from this one in that all gaussians had the same covariance; an EM algorithm for their model was derived by Ghahramani (1995). Different forms of coadaptive MOG were used by Hinton, Williams, and Revow (1992) and by Bishop, Svensén, and Williams (1998).

2.2 Sensor Model. The source model in equation 2.8, combined by equation 2.1 with the noise model in equation 2.2, leads to a two-step generative model of the observed sensor signals. This model can be viewed as a hierarchical feedforward network with a visible layer and two hidden layers, as

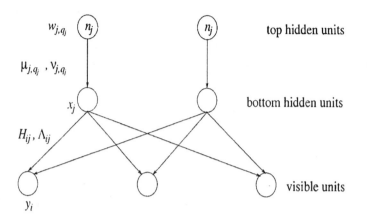

Figure 1: Feedforward network representation of the IF generative model. Each source signal x_j is generated by an independent n_j-state MOG model (see equation 2.5). The sensor signals y_i are generated from a gaussian model (see equation 2.11) whose mean depends linearly on the sources.

shown in Figure 1. To generate sensor signals $\mathbf{y}$, first pick a unit q_i for each source i with probability

$$p(\mathbf{q}) = w_{\mathbf{q}} \tag{2.9}$$

from the top hidden layer of source states. This unit has a top-down generative connection with weight μ_{j,q_j} to each of the units j in the bottom hidden layer. When activated, it causes unit j to produce a sample x_j from a gaussian density centered at μ_{j,q_j} with variance v_{j,q_j}; the probability of generating a particular source vector $\mathbf{x}$ in the bottom hidden layer is

$$p(\mathbf{x} \mid \mathbf{q}) = \mathcal{G}(\mathbf{x} - \boldsymbol{\mu}_{\mathbf{q}}, \mathbf{V}_{\mathbf{q}}). \tag{2.10}$$

Second, each unit j in the bottom hidden layer has a top-down generative connection with weight H_{ij} to each unit i in the visible layer. Following the generation of $\mathbf{x}$, unit i produces a sample y_i from a gaussian density centered at $\sum_j H_{ij}x_j$. In case of independent sensor noise, the variance of this density is Λ_{ii}; generally the noise is correlated across sensors, and the probability for generating a particular sensor vector $\mathbf{y}$ in the visible layer is

$$p(\mathbf{y} \mid \mathbf{x}) = \mathcal{G}(\mathbf{y} - \mathbf{Hx}, \mathbf{\Lambda}). \tag{2.11}$$

It is important to emphasize that our IF generative model is probabilistic: it describes the *statistics* of the unobserved source and observed sensor signals, that is, the densities $p(\mathbf{x})$ and $p(\mathbf{y})$ rather than the actual signals $\mathbf{x}$ and $\mathbf{y}$. This model is fully described by the joint density of the visible layer and the two hidden layers,

$$p(\mathbf{q}, \mathbf{x}, \mathbf{y} \mid W) = p(\mathbf{q})\, p(\mathbf{x} \mid \mathbf{q})\, p(\mathbf{y} \mid \mathbf{x}). \tag{2.12}$$

Notice from equation 2.12 that since the sensor signals depend on the sources but not on the source states, that is, $p(\mathbf{y} \mid \mathbf{x}, \mathbf{q}) = p(\mathbf{y} \mid \mathbf{x})$ (once $\mathbf{x}$ is produced, the identity of the state $\mathbf{q}$ that generated it becomes irrelevant), the IF network layers form a top-down first-order Markov chain.

The generative model attributes a probability $p(\mathbf{y})$ for each observed sensor data vector $\mathbf{y}$. We are now able to return to equation 2.4 and express $p(\mathbf{y})$ in a closed form. From equation 2.12, we have

$$p(\mathbf{y} \mid W) = \sum_{\mathbf{q}} \int d\mathbf{x}\, p(\mathbf{q})\, p(\mathbf{x} \mid \mathbf{q})\, p(\mathbf{y} \mid \mathbf{x}) = \sum_{\mathbf{q}} p(\mathbf{q})\, p(\mathbf{y} \mid \mathbf{q}), \tag{2.13}$$

where, thanks to the gaussian forms (see equations 2.10 and 2.11), the integral over the sources in equation 2.13 can be performed analytically to yield

$$p(\mathbf{y} \mid \mathbf{q}) = \mathcal{G}(\mathbf{y} - H\mu_{\mathbf{q}},\ HV_{\mathbf{q}}H^{T} + \Lambda). \tag{2.14}$$

Thus, like the source density, our sensor density model is a coadaptive (although not factorial) MOG, as is illustrated in Figure 3 (bottom right). Changing one element of the mixing matrix would result in a rigid rotation and scaling of a whole line of states. Learning the IF model therefore amounts to fitting the sensor data by a mixture of coadaptive gaussians, then using them to deduce the model parameters.

3 Learning the IF Model

3.1 Error Function and Maximum Likelihood.
To estimate the IF model parameters, we first define an error function that measures the difference between our model sensor density $p(\mathbf{y} \mid W)$ (see equation 2.13) and the observed one $p^{o}(\mathbf{y})$. The parameters W are then adapted iteratively to minimize this error. We choose the Kullback-Leibler (KL) distance function (Cover & Thomas, 1991), defined by

$$\mathcal{E}(W) = \int d\mathbf{y}\, p^{o}(\mathbf{y}) \log \frac{p^{o}(\mathbf{y})}{p(\mathbf{y} \mid W)} = -E\left[\log p(\mathbf{y} \mid W)\right] - H_{p^{o}}, \tag{3.1}$$

where the operator E performs averaging over the observed $\mathbf{y}$. As is well known, the KL distance $\mathcal{E}$ is always nonnegative and vanishes when $p(\mathbf{y}) = p^{o}(\mathbf{y})$.

This error consists of two terms. The first is the negative log-likelihood of the observed sensor signals given the model parameters W. The second term is the sensor entropy, which is independent of W and will henceforth be dropped. Minimizing $\mathcal{E}$ is thus equivalent to maximizing the likelihood of the data with respect to the model.

The KL distance has an interesting relation also to the mean square point-by-point distance. To see it, we define the relative error of $p(\mathbf{y} \mid W)$ with respect to the true density $p^o(\mathbf{y})$ by

$$e(\mathbf{y}) = \frac{p(\mathbf{y}) - p^o(\mathbf{y})}{p^o(\mathbf{y})} \tag{3.2}$$

at each $\mathbf{y}$, omitting the dependence on W. When $p(\mathbf{y})$ in equation 3.1 is expressed in terms of $e(\mathbf{y})$, we obtain

$$\mathcal{E}(W) = -\int d\mathbf{y}\, p^o(\mathbf{y}) \log\left[1 + e(\mathbf{y})\right] \approx \frac{1}{2} \int d\mathbf{y}\, p^o(\mathbf{y})\, e^2(\mathbf{y}), \tag{3.3}$$

where the approximation $\log e \approx e - e^2/2$, valid in the limit of small $e(\mathbf{y})$, was used. Hence, in the parameter regime where the model $p(\mathbf{y} \mid W)$ is "near" the observed density, minimizing $\mathcal{E}$ amounts to minimizing the mean square relative error of the model density. This property, however, has little computational significance.

A straightforward way to minimize the error in equation 3.1 would be to use the gradient-descent method where, starting from random values, the parameters are incremented at each iteration by a small step in the direction of the gradient $\partial \mathcal{E}/\partial W$. However, this results in rather slow learning. Instead, we shall employ the EM approach to develop an efficient algorithm for learning the IF model.

3.2 An Expectation-Maximization Algorithm. Expectation-maximization (Dempster, Laird, & Rubin, 1977; Neal & Hinton, 1998) is an iterative method to maximize the log-likelihood of the observed data with respect to the parameters of the generative model describing those data. It is obtained by noting that, in addition to the likelihood $E[\log p(\mathbf{y} \mid W)]$ of the observed sensor data (see equation 3.1), one may consider the likelihood $E[\log p(\mathbf{y}, \mathbf{x}, \mathbf{q} \mid W)]$ of the "complete" data, composed of both the observed and the "missing" data, that is, the unobserved source signals and states. For each observed $\mathbf{y}$, this complete-data likelihood as a function of $\mathbf{x}, \mathbf{q}$ is a random variable. Each iteration then consists of two steps:

1. (E) Calculate the expected value of the complete data likelihood, given the observed data and the current model. That is, calculate

$$\mathcal{F}(W', W) = -E\left[\log p(\mathbf{q}, \mathbf{x}, \mathbf{y} \mid W)\right] + \mathcal{F}_H(W'), \tag{3.4}$$

where, for each observed $\mathbf{y}$, the average in the first term on the right-hand side (r.h.s.) is taken over the unobserved $\mathbf{x}, \mathbf{q}$ using the source posterior $p(\mathbf{x}, \mathbf{q} \mid \mathbf{y}, W')$; W' are the parameters obtained in the previous iteration, and $\mathcal{F}_H(W')$ is the entropy of the posterior (see equation 3.10). The result is then averaged over all the observed $\mathbf{y}$. The second term on the r.h.s. is W-independent and has no effect on the following.

2. (M) Minimize $\mathcal{F}(W', W)$ (i.e., maximize the corresponding averaged likelihood) with respect to W to obtain the new parameters:

$$W = \arg \min_{W''} \mathcal{F}(W', W''). \tag{3.5}$$

In the following we develop the EM algorithm for our IF model. First, we show that $\mathcal{F}$ (see equation 3.4) is bounded from below by the error $\mathcal{E}$ (see equation 3.1), following Neal and Hinton (1998). Dropping the average over the observed $\mathbf{y}$, we have

$$\mathcal{E}(W) = -\log p(\mathbf{y} \mid W) = -\log \sum_{\mathbf{q}} \int d\mathbf{x}\, p(\mathbf{q}, \mathbf{x}, \mathbf{y} \mid W)$$

$$\leq -\sum_{\mathbf{q}} \int d\mathbf{x}\, p'(\mathbf{q}, \mathbf{x} \mid \mathbf{y})\, \log \frac{p(\mathbf{q}, \mathbf{x}, \mathbf{y} \mid W)}{p'(\mathbf{q}, \mathbf{x} \mid \mathbf{y})} \equiv \mathcal{F}, \tag{3.6}$$

where the second line follows from Jensen's inequality (Cover & Thomas, 1991) and holds for any conditional density p'. In EM, we choose p' to be the source posterior computed using the parameters from the previous iteration,

$$p'(\mathbf{q}, \mathbf{x} \mid \mathbf{y}) = p(\mathbf{q}, \mathbf{x} \mid \mathbf{y}, W'), \tag{3.7}$$

which is obtained directly from equation 2.12 with $W = W'$.

Hence, after the previous iteration we have an approximate error function $\mathcal{F}(W', W)$, which, due to the Markov property (see equation 2.12) of the IF model, is obtained by adding up four terms,

$$\mathcal{E}(W) \leq \mathcal{F}(W', W) = \mathcal{F}_V + \mathcal{F}_B + \mathcal{F}_T + \mathcal{F}_H, \tag{3.8}$$

to be defined shortly. A closer inspection reveals that although they all depend on the model parameters W, each of the first three terms involves only the parameters of a single layer (see Figure 1). Thus, $\mathcal{F}_V$ depends on only the parameters $\mathbf{H}, \Lambda$ of the visible layer, whereas $\mathcal{F}_B$ and $\mathcal{F}_T$ depend on the parameters $\{\mu_{i,q_i}, \nu_{i,q_i}\}$ and $\{w_{i,q_i}\}$ of the bottom and top hidden layers, respectively; they also depend on all the previous parameters W'. From equations 2.12 and 3.6, the contributions of the different layers are given by

$$\mathcal{F}_V(W', \mathbf{H}, \Lambda) = -\int d\mathbf{x}\, p(\mathbf{x} \mid \mathbf{y}, W')\, \log p(\mathbf{y} \mid \mathbf{x}),$$

$$\mathcal{F}_B(W', \{\mu_{i,q_i}, v_{i,q_i}\}) = -\sum_{i=1}^{L}\sum_{q_i=1}^{n_i} p(q_i \mid \mathbf{y}, W')$$

$$\times \int dx_i \, p(x_i \mid q_i, \mathbf{y}, W') \, \log p(x_i \mid q_i),$$

$$\mathcal{F}_T(W', \{w_{i,q_i}\}) = -\sum_{i=1}^{L}\sum_{q_i=1}^{n_i} p(q_i \mid \mathbf{y}, W') \, \log p(q_i), \tag{3.9}$$

and the last contribution is the negative entropy of the source posterior,

$$\mathcal{F}_H(W') = \sum_{\mathbf{q}} \int d\mathbf{x} \, p(\mathbf{q}, \mathbf{x} \mid \mathbf{y}, W') \, \log p(\mathbf{q}, \mathbf{x} \mid \mathbf{y}, W'). \tag{3.10}$$

To get $\mathcal{F}_B$ (the second line in equation 3.9) we used $p(\mathbf{q} \mid \mathbf{x})p(\mathbf{x} \mid \mathbf{y}) = p(\mathbf{q} \mid \mathbf{y})p(\mathbf{x} \mid \mathbf{q}, \mathbf{y})$, which can be obtained using equation 2.12.

The EM procedure now follows by observing that equation 3.8 becomes an equality when $W = W'$, thanks to the choice in equation 3.7. Hence, given the parameter values W' produced by the previous iteration, the E-step (see equation 3.4) results in the approximate error coinciding with the true error, $\mathcal{F}(W', W') = \mathcal{E}(W')$. Next, we consider $\mathcal{F}(W', W)$ and minimize it with respect to W. From equation 3.8, the new parameters obtained from the M-step (see equation 3.5) satisfy

$$\mathcal{E}(W) \leq \mathcal{F}(W', W) \leq \mathcal{F}(W', W') = \mathcal{E}(W'), \tag{3.11}$$

proving that the current EM step does not increase the error.

The EM algorithm for learning the IF model parameters is derived from equations 3.8 and 3.9 in appendix A, where the new parameters W at each iteration are obtained in terms of the old ones W'. The learning rules for the mixing matrix and noise covariance are given by

$$\mathbf{H} = E\mathbf{y}\langle \mathbf{x}^T \mid \mathbf{y}\rangle \left(E\langle \mathbf{x}\mathbf{x}^T \mid \mathbf{y}\rangle\right)^{-1},$$

$$\Lambda = E\mathbf{y}\mathbf{y}^T - E\mathbf{y}\langle \mathbf{x}^T \mid \mathbf{y}\rangle \mathbf{H}^T, \tag{3.12}$$

whereas the rules for the source MOG parameters are

$$\mu_{i,q_i} = \frac{E p(q_i \mid \mathbf{y})\langle x_i \mid q_i, \mathbf{y}\rangle}{E p(q_i \mid \mathbf{y})},$$

$$v_{i,q_i} = \frac{E p(q_i \mid \mathbf{y})\langle x_i^2 \mid q_i, \mathbf{y}\rangle}{E p(q_i \mid \mathbf{y})} - \mu_{i,q_i}^2,$$

$$w_{i,q_i} = E p(q_i \mid \mathbf{y}). \tag{3.13}$$

Notation. $\langle \mathbf{x} \mid \mathbf{y} \rangle$ is an $L \times 1$ vector denoting the conditional mean of the sources given the sensors; the $L \times L$ matrix $\langle \mathbf{x}\mathbf{x}^T \mid \mathbf{y} \rangle$ is the source covariance conditioned on the sensors. Similarly, $\langle x_i \mid q_i, \mathbf{y} \rangle$ denotes the mean of sensor i conditioned on both the hidden state q_i of this source, and the observed sensors. $p(q_i \mid \mathbf{y})$ is the probability of the state q_i of source i conditioned on the sensors. The conditional averages are defined in equations A.2 and A.4. Both the conditional averages and the conditional probabilities depend on the observed sensor signals $\mathbf{y}$ and on the parameters W', and are computed during the E-step. Finally, the operator E performs averaging over the observed $\mathbf{y}$.

Scaling. In the BSS problem, the sources are defined only to within an order permutation and scaling. This ambiguity is implied by equation 2.1: the effect of an arbitrary permutation of the sources can be cancelled by a corresponding permutation of the columns of $\mathbf{H}$, leaving the observed $\mathbf{y}$ unchanged. Similarly, scaling source x_j by a factor σ_j would not affect $\mathbf{y}$ if the jth column of $\mathbf{H}$ is scaled by $1/\sigma_j$ at the same time. Put another way, the error function cannot distinguish between the true $\mathbf{H}$ and a scaled and permuted version of it, and thus possesses multiple continuous manifolds of global minima. Whereas each point on those manifolds corresponds to a valid solution, their existence may delay convergence and cause numerical problems (e.g., H_{ij} may acquire arbitrarily large values). To minimize the effect of such excessive freedom, we maintain the variance of each source at unity by performing the following scaling transformation at each iteration:

$$\sigma_j^2 = \sum_{q_j=1}^{n_j} w_{j,q_j}(\nu_{j,q_j} + \mu_{j,q_j}^2) - \left(\sum_{q_j=1}^{n_j} w_{j,q_j}\mu_{j,q_j} \right)^2,$$

$$\mu_{j,q_j} \to \frac{\mu_{j,q_j}}{\sigma_j}, \qquad \nu_{j,q_j} \to \frac{\nu_{j,q_j}}{\sigma_j^2}, \qquad H_{ij} \to H_{ij}\sigma_j. \tag{3.14}$$

This transformation amounts to scaling each source j by its standard deviation

$$\sigma_j = \sqrt{Ex_j^2 - (Ex_j)^2}$$

and compensating the mixing matrix appropriately. It is easy to show that this scaling leaves the error function unchanged.

3.3 Hierarchical Interpretation. The above EM algorithm can be given a natural interpretation in the context of our hierarchical generative model (see Figure 1). From this point of view, it bears some resemblance to the mixture of experts algorithm of Jordan and Jacobs (1994). Focusing first on the learning rules (see equation 3.13) for the top hidden-layer parameters, one notes their similarity to the usual EM rules for fitting an MOG model. To make the connection explicit we rewrite the rules on the left column below,

$$\mu_{i,q_i} = \frac{E \int dx_i \, p(x_i \mid \mathbf{y}) \left[p(q_i \mid x_i, \mathbf{y}) \, x_i\right]}{E \int dx_i \, p(x_i \mid \mathbf{y}) \left[p(q_i \mid x_i, \mathbf{y})\right]} \quad \longleftrightarrow \quad \frac{E \, p(q_i \mid x_i) \, x_i}{E \, p(q_i \mid x_i)},$$

$$v_{i,q_i} = \frac{E \int dx_i \, p(x_i \mid \mathbf{y}) \left[p(q_i \mid x_i, \mathbf{y}) \, x_i^2\right]}{E \int dx_i \, p(x_i \mid \mathbf{y}) \left[p(q_i \mid x_i, \mathbf{y})\right]} - \mu_{i,q_i}^2$$

$$\longleftrightarrow \quad \frac{E \, p(q_i \mid x_i) \, x_i^2}{E \, p(q_i \mid x_i)} - \mu_{i,q_i}^2,$$

$$w_{i,q_i} = E \int dx_i \, p(x_i \mid \mathbf{y}) \left[p(q_i \mid x_i, \mathbf{y})\right] \longleftrightarrow E \, p(q_i \mid x_i), \tag{3.15}$$

where to go from equation 3.13 to the left column of equation 3.15 we used $p(q_i \mid \mathbf{y}) = \int dx_i \, p(x_i, q_i \mid \mathbf{y})$ and $p(q_i \mid \mathbf{y})\langle m(x_i) \mid q_i, \mathbf{y}\rangle = \int dx_i \, m(x_i) \, p(x_i, q_i \mid \mathbf{y})$ (see equation A.4). Note that each p in equation 3.15 should be read as p'.

Shown on the right column of equation 3.15 are the standard EM rules for learning a one-dimensional MOG model parameterized by μ_{i,q_i}, v_{i,q_i}, and w_{i,q_i} for each source x_i, assuming the source signals were directly observable. A comparison with the square-bracketed expressions on the left column shows that the EM rules in equation 3.13 for the IF source parameters are precisely the rules for learning a separate MOG model for each source i, with the actual x_i replaced by all values x_i that are possible given the observed sensor signals $\mathbf{y}$, weighted by their posterior $p(x_i \mid \mathbf{y})$.

The EM algorithm for learning the IF model can therefore be viewed hierarchically: the visible layer learns a noisy linear model for the sensor data, parameterized by $\mathbf{H}$ and $\mathbf{\Lambda}$. The hidden layers learn an MOG model for each source. Since the actual sources are not available, all possible source signals are used, weighted by their posterior given the observed data; this couples the visible and hidden layers since all the IF parameters participate in computing that posterior.

3.4 Relation to Ordinary Factor Analysis. Ordinary FA uses a generative model of independent gaussian sources with zero mean and unit variance, $p(x_i) = \mathcal{G}(x_i, 1)$, mixed (see equation 2.1) by a linear transformation with added gaussian noise whose covariance matrix $\mathbf{\Lambda}$ is diagonal. This is a special case of our IF model obtained when each source has a single state ($n_i = 1$ in equation 2.5). From equations 2.13 and 2.14, the resulting sensor density is

$$p(\mathbf{y} \mid W) = \mathcal{G}(\mathbf{y}, \mathbf{H}\mathbf{H}^T + \mathbf{\Lambda}), \tag{3.16}$$

since we now have only one collective source state $\mathbf{q} = (1, 1, \ldots, 1)$ with $w_{\mathbf{q}} = 1$, $\mu_{\mathbf{q}} = 0$, and $\mathbf{V_q} = \mathbf{I}$ (see equations 2.6 and 2.7).

The invariance of FA under factor rotation mentioned in section 1 is manifested in the FA model density (equation 3.16). For any $L \times L'$ matrix $\mathbf{P}$ whose rows are orthonormal (i.e., $\mathbf{PP}^T = \mathbf{I}$ – a rotation matrix), we can define a new mixing matrix $\mathbf{H}' = \mathbf{HP}$. However, the density in equation 3.16 does not discriminate between $\mathbf{H}'$ and the true $\mathbf{H}$ since $\mathbf{H}'\mathbf{H}'^T = \mathbf{HH}^T$, rendering FA unable to identify the true mixing matrix. Notice from equation 2.1 that the factors corresponding to $\mathbf{H}'$ are obtained from the true sources by that rotation: $\mathbf{x}' = \mathbf{P}^T\mathbf{x}$. In contrast, our IF model density (see equations 2.13 and 2.14) is, in general, not invariant under the transformation $\mathbf{H} \to \mathbf{H}'$; the rotational symmetry is broken by the MOG source model. Hence the true $\mathbf{H}$ can, in principle, be identified.

For square mixing ($L' = L$) the symmetry of the FA density is even larger: for an arbitrary diagonal noise covariance Λ', the transformation $\Lambda \to \Lambda'$, $\mathbf{H} \to \mathbf{H}' = (\mathbf{HH}^T + \Lambda - \Lambda')^{1/2}\mathbf{P}$ leaves equation 3.16 invariant. Hence neither the mixing nor the noise can be identified in this case.

The well-known EM algorithm for FA (Rubin & Thayer, 1982) is obtained as a special case of our IFA algorithm, by freezing the source parameters at their values under equation 3.16 and using only the learning rules in equation 3.12. Given the observed sensors $\mathbf{y}$, the source posterior now becomes simply a gaussian, $p(\mathbf{x} \mid \mathbf{y}) = \mathcal{G}(\mathbf{x} - \rho, \Sigma)$, whose covariance and data-dependent mean are given by

$$\Sigma = \left(\mathbf{H}^T\Lambda^{-1}\mathbf{H} + \mathbf{I}\right)^{-1}, \qquad \rho(\mathbf{y}) = \Sigma\,\mathbf{H}^T\Lambda^{-1}\mathbf{y}, \qquad (3.17)$$

rather than the MOG implied by equations A.6 through A.8. Consequently, the conditional source mean and covariance (see equation A.10) used in equation 3.12 become $\langle \mathbf{x} \mid \mathbf{y} \rangle = \rho(\mathbf{y})$ and $\langle \mathbf{xx}^T \mid \mathbf{y} \rangle = \Sigma + \rho(\mathbf{y})\rho(\mathbf{y})^T$.

4 Recovering the Sources

Once the IF generative model parameters have been estimated, the sources can be reconstructed from the sensor signals. A complete reconstruction is possible only when noise is absent and the mixing is invertible, that is, if $\Lambda = 0$ and rank $\mathbf{H} \geq L$; in this case, the sources are given by the pseudo-inverse of $\mathbf{H}$ via the linear relation $\mathbf{x} = (\mathbf{H}^T\mathbf{H})^{-1}\mathbf{H}^T\mathbf{y}$.

In general, however, an estimate $\hat{\mathbf{x}}(\mathbf{y})$ of the sources must be found. There are many ways to obtain a parametric estimator of an unobserved signal from data. In the following we discuss two of them: the least mean squares (LMS) and maximum a posteriori probability (MAP) source estimators. Both are nonlinear functions of the data, but each satisfies a different optimality criterion. It is easy to show that for gaussian sources, both reduce to the same linear estimator of ordinary FA, given by $\hat{\mathbf{x}}(\mathbf{y}) = \rho(\mathbf{y})$ in equation 3.17. For nongaussian sources, however, the LMS and MAP estimators differ, and neither has an a priori advantage over the other. For either choice, obtaining the source estimate $\{\hat{x}(y)\}$ for a given sensor data set $\{y\}$ completes the IFA of these data.

4.1 LMS Estimator. As is well known, the optimal estimate in the least-square sense of minimizing $E(\hat{x} - x)^2$ is given by the conditional mean of the sources given the observed sensors,

$$\hat{x}^{LMS}(y) = \langle x \mid y \rangle = \int dx\, x\, p(x \mid y, W), \tag{4.1}$$

where $p(x \mid y, W) = \sum_q p(q \mid y)p(x \mid q, y)$ (see equations A.6–A.8) is the source posterior and depends on the generative parameters. This conditional mean has already been calculated for the E-step of our EM algorithm; as shown in appendix A, it is given by a weighted sum of terms that are linear in the data y,

$$\hat{x}^{LMS}(y) = \sum_q p(q \mid y)\, \left(A_q\, y + b_q\right), \tag{4.2}$$

where $A_q = \Sigma_q H^T \Lambda^{-1}$, $b_q = \Sigma_q V_q^{-1} \mu_q$, and Σ_q is given in terms of the generative parameters in equation A.7. Notice that the weighting coefficients themselves depend nonlinearly on the data via $p(q \mid y) = p(y \mid q)p(q)/\sum_{q'} p(y \mid q')p(q')$ and equations 2.9 and 2.14.

4.2 MAP Estimator. The MAP optimal estimator maximizes the source posterior $p(x \mid y)$. For a given y, maximizing the posterior is equivalent to maximizing the joint $p(x, y)$ or its logarithm, hence

$$\hat{x}^{MAP}(y) = \arg\max_x \left[\log p(y \mid x) + \sum_{i=1}^{L} \log p(x_i) \right]. \tag{4.3}$$

A simple way to compute this estimator is to maximize the quantity on the r.h.s. of equation 4.3 iteratively using the method of gradient ascent for each data vector y. After initialization, $\hat{x}(y)$ is incremented at each iteration by

$$\delta\hat{x} = \eta H^T \Lambda^{-1}(y - H\hat{x}) - \eta\phi(\hat{x}), \tag{4.4}$$

where η is the learning rate and $\phi(x)$ is an $L \times 1$ vector given by the logarithmic derivative of the source density (see equation 2.5),

$$\phi(x_i) = -\frac{\partial \log p(x_i)}{\partial x_i} = -\sum_{q_i=1}^{n_i} p(q_i \mid x_i)\frac{x_i - \mu_{i,q_i}}{v_{i,q_i}}. \tag{4.5}$$

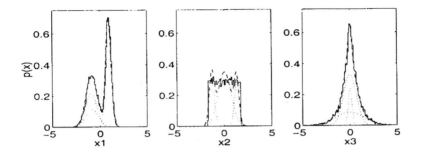

Figure 2: Source density histograms (solid lines) and their MOG models learned by IFA (dashed lines). Each model is a sum of three weighted gaussian densities (dotted lines). Shown are bimodal (left) and uniform (middle) synthetic signals and an actual speech signal (right).

A good initialization is provided by the pseudo-inverse relation $\hat{x}(y) = (H^T H)^{-1} H^T y$. However, since the posterior may have multiple maxima, several initial values should be used in order to identify the highest maximum.

Notice that $\hat{x}^{MAP}$ is a fixed point of the equation $\delta \hat{x} = 0$. This equation is nonlinear, reflecting the nongaussian nature of the source densities. A simple analysis shows that this fixed point is stable when $| \det H^T \Lambda^{-1} H | > | \prod_i \phi'(\hat{x}_i^{MAP}) |$, and the equation can then be solved by iterating over $\hat{x}$ rather than using the slower gradient ascent. For gaussian sources with unit covariance, $\phi(x) = x$ and the MAP estimator reduces to the ordinary FA one $\rho(y)$ (see equation 3.17).

5 IFA: Simulation Results

Here we demonstrate the performance of our EM algorithm for IFA on mixtures of sources corrupted by gaussian noise at different intensities. We used 5 sec-long speech and music signals obtained from commercial CDs at the original sampling rate of 44.1 kHz, that were down-sampled to $f_s = 8.82$ kHz, resulting in $T = 44,100$ sample points. These signals are characterized by peaky unimodal densities, as shown in Figure 2 (right). We also used synthetic signals obtained by a random number generator. These signals had arbitrary densities, two examples of which are shown in Figure 2 (left, middle).

All signals were scaled to have unit variance and mixed by a random $L' \times L$ mixing matrix H^0 with varying number of sensors L'. L' white gaussian signals with covariance matrix Λ^0 were added to these mixtures. Different noise levels were used (see below). The learning rules in equations 3.12 and 3.13 were iterated in batch mode, starting from random parameter values.

In all our experiments, we modeled each source density by a $n_i = 3$-state MOG, which provided a sufficiently accurate description of the signals we used, as Figure 2 (dashed and dotted lines) shows. In principle, prior knowledge of the source densities can be exploited by freezing the source parameters at the values corresponding to an MOG fit to their densities, and learning only the mixing matrix and noise covariance, which would result in faster convergence. However, we allowed the source parameters to adapt as well, starting from random values. Learning the source densities is illustrated in Figure 3.

Figure 4 (top, solid lines) shows the convergence of the estimated mixing matrix $\mathbf{H}$ toward the true one $\mathbf{H}^0$, for $L' = 3, 8$ mixtures of the $L = 3$ sources whose densities are histogrammed in Figure 2. Plotted are the matrix elements of the product

$$\mathbf{J} = (\mathbf{H}^T\mathbf{H})^{-1}\mathbf{H}^T\mathbf{H}^0. \tag{5.1}$$

Notice that for the correct estimate $\mathbf{H} = \mathbf{H}^0$, $\mathbf{J}$ becomes the unit matrix $\mathbf{I}$. Recall that the effect of source scaling is eliminated by equation 3.14; to prevent possible source permutations from affecting this measure, we permuted the columns of $\mathbf{H}$ such that the largest element (in absolute value) in column i of $\mathbf{J}$ would be J_{ii}. Indeed, this product is shown to converge to $\mathbf{I}$ in both cases.

To observe the convergence of the estimated noise covariance matrix Λ toward the true one Λ^0, we measured the KL distance between the corresponding noise densities. Since both densities are gaussian (see equation 2.2), it is easy to calculate this distance analytically:

$$K_n = \int d\mathbf{u}\, \mathcal{G}(\mathbf{u}, \Lambda^0)\, \log \frac{\mathcal{G}(\mathbf{u}, \Lambda^0)}{\mathcal{G}(\mathbf{u}, \Lambda)}$$
$$= \frac{1}{2}\mathrm{Tr}\,\Lambda^{-1}\Lambda^0 - \frac{L'}{2} - \frac{1}{2}\log|\det \Lambda^{-1}\Lambda^0|. \tag{5.2}$$

We recall that the KL distance is always nonnegative; notice from equation 5.2 that $K_n = 0$ when $\Lambda = \Lambda^0$. Differentiating with respect to Λ shows that this is the only minimum point. As shown in Figure 4 (bottom, dashed line), K_n approaches zero in both cases.

The convergence of the estimated source densities $p(x_i)$ (see equation 2.5) was quantified by measuring their KL distance from the true densities $p^0(x_i)$. For this purpose, we first fitted an MOG model, $p^0(x_i) = \sum_{q_i} w^0_{i,q_i}\mathcal{G}(x_i - \mu^0_{i,q_i}, v^0_{i,q_i})$, to each source i and obtained the parameters $w^0_{i,q_i}, \mu^0_{i,q_i}, v^0_{i,q_i}$ for

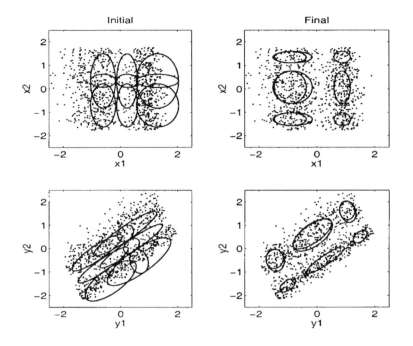

Figure 3: IFA learns a coadaptive MOG model of the data. (Top) Joint density of sources x_1, x_2 (dots) whose individual densities are shown in Figure 2. (Bottom) Observed sensor density (dots) resulting from a linear 2×2 mixing of the sources contaminated by low noise. The MOG source model (see equation 2.8) is represented by ellipsoids centered at the means μ_q of the source states; same for the corresponding MOG sensor model (see equations 2.13 and 2.14). Note that the mixing affects a rigid rotation and scaling of the states. Starting from random source parameters (left), as well as random mixing matrix noise covariance, IFA learns their actual values (right).

$q_i = 1, 2, 3$. The KL distance at each EM step was then estimated via

$$K_i = \int dx_i \, p^0(x_i) \, \log \frac{p^0(x_i)}{p(x_i)} \approx \sum_{t=1}^{T} \log \frac{p^0(x_i^{(t)})}{p(x_i^{(t)})}, \qquad (5.3)$$

where $p(x_i)$ was computed using the parameters values w_{i,q_i}, μ_{i,q_i}, v_{i,q_i} obtained by IFA at that step; $x_i^{(t)}$ denotes the value of source i at time point t. Figure 4 (bottom, solid lines) shows the convergence of K_i toward zero for $L' = 3, 8$ sensors.

Figure 2 illustrates the accuracy of the source densities $p(x_i)$ learned by IFA. The histogram of the three sources used in this experiment is compared

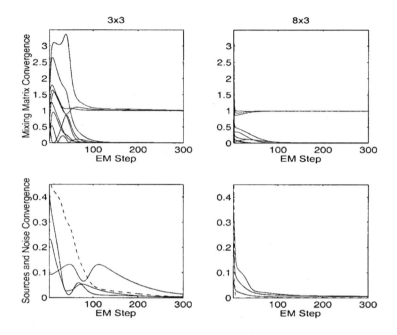

Figure 4: (Top) Convergence of the mixing matrix **H** with $L = 3$ sources, for $L' = 3$ (left) and $L' = 8$ (right) sensors and SNR = 5dB. Plotted are the matrix elements of **J** (see equation 5.1) (solid lines) against the EM step number. (Bottom) Convergence of the noise and source densities. Plotted are the KL distance K_n (see equation 5.2) between the estimated and true noise densities (dashed line) and the KL distances K_i (see equation 5.3) between the estimated source densities $p(x_i)$ and the true ones (solid lines).

to its MOG description, obtained by adding up the corresponding three weighted gaussians using the final IFA estimates of their parameters. The agreement is very good, demonstrating that the IFA algorithm successfully learned the source densities.

Figure 5 examines more closely the precision of the IFA estimates as the noise level increases. The mixing matrix error ϵ_H quantifies the distance of the final value of **J** (see equation 5.1) from **I**; we define it as the mean square nondiagonal elements of **J** normalized by its mean square diagonal elements:

$$\epsilon_H = \left(\frac{1}{L^2 - L} \sum_{i \neq j=1}^{L} J_{ij}^2 \right) \left(\frac{1}{L} \sum_{i=1}^{L} J_{ii}^2 \right)^{-1}. \tag{5.4}$$

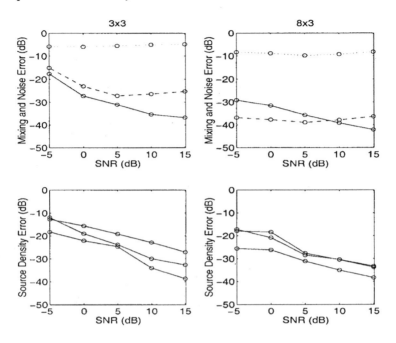

Figure 5: (Top) Estimate errors of the mixing matrix, ϵ_H (see equation 5.4) (solid line), and noise covariance, K_n (see equation 5.2) (dashed line), against the signal-to-noise ratio (see equation 5.5), for $L' = 3$ (left) and $L' = 8$ (right). For reference, the errors of the ICA estimate of the mixing matrix (dotted line) are also plotted. (Bottom) Estimate errors K_i (see equation 5.3) of the source densities.

The signal-to-noise ratio (SNR) is obtained by noting that the signal level in sensor i is $E(\sum_j H_{ij}^0 x_j)^2 = \sum_j (H_{ij}^0)^2$ (recall that $Exx^T = I$), and the corresponding noise level is $Eu_i^2 = \Lambda_{ii}^0$. Averaging over the sensors, we get

$$\text{SNR} = \frac{1}{L'} \sum_{i=1}^{L'} \left[\sum_{j=1}^{L} (H_{ij}^0)^2 \right] / \Lambda_{ii}^0. \tag{5.5}$$

We plot the mixing matrix error against the SNR in Figure 5 (top, solid line), both measured in dB (i.e., $10 \log_{10} \epsilon_H$ versus $10 \log_{10} \text{SNR}$), for $L' = 3, 8$ sensors. For reference, we also plot the error of the ICA (Bell & Sejnowski, 1995) estimate of the mixing matrix (top, dotted line). Since ICA is formulated for the square ($L' = L$) noiseless case, we employed a two-step procedure: (1) the first L principal components (PC's) $y_1 = P_1^T y$ of the sensor data

y are obtained; (2) ICA is applied to yield $\hat{x}^{ICA} = \mathbf{G}\mathbf{y}_1$. The resulting estimate of the mixing matrix is then $\mathbf{H}^{ICA} = \mathbf{P}_1\mathbf{G}^{-1}$. Notice that this procedure is exact for zero noise, since in that case the first L PCs are the only nonzero ones and the problem reduces to one of square noiseless mixing, described by $\mathbf{y}_1 = \mathbf{P}_1\mathbf{H}\mathbf{x}$ (see also the discussion at the end of section 7.1).

Also plotted in Figure 5 is the error in the estimated noise covariance $\mathbf{\Lambda}$ (top, dashed line), given by the KL distance K_n (see equation 5.2) for the final value of $\mathbf{\Lambda}$. (Measuring the KL distance in dB is suggested by its mean-square-error interpretation; see equation 3.3). Figure 5 (bottom) shows the estimate errors of the source densities $p(x_i)$, given by their KL distance (see equation 5.3) from the true densities after the IFA was completed.

As expected, these errors decrease with increasing SNR and also with increasing L'. The noise error K_n forms an exception, however, by showing a slight increase with the SNR, reflecting the fact that a lower noise level is harder to estimate to a given precision. In general, convergence is faster for larger L'.

We conclude that the estimation errors for the IF model parameters are quite small, usually falling in the range of 20 to 40 dB, and never larger than 15 dB as long as the noise level is not higher than the signal level (SNR ≥ 0 dB). Similar results were obtained in other simulations we performed. The small values of the estimate errors suggest that those errors originate from the finite sample size rather than from convergence to undesired local minima.

Finally, we studied how the noise level affects the separation performance, as measured by the quality of source reconstructions obtained from $\hat{x}^{LMS}$ (see equation 4.2) and $\hat{x}^{MAP}$ (see equation 4.4). We quantified it by the mean square reconstruction error ϵ^{rec}, which measures how close the reconstructed sources are to the original ones. This error is composed of two components, one arising from the presence of noise and the other from interference of the other sources (cross-talk); the additional component arising from IF parameter estimation errors is negligible in comparison. The amount of cross-talk is measured by ϵ^{xtalk}:

$$\epsilon^{rec} = \frac{1}{L}\sum_{i=1}^{L} E(\hat{x}_i - x_i)^2, \qquad \epsilon^{xtalk} = \frac{1}{L^2 - L}\sum_{i\neq j=1}^{L} |E\hat{x}_i x_j|. \qquad (5.6)$$

Note that for zero noise and perfect separation ($\hat{x}_i = x_i$), both quantities approach zero in the infinite sample limit.

The reconstruction error (which is normalized since $Ex_i^2 = 1$) and the cross-talk level are plotted in Figure 6 against the SNR for both the LMS (solid lines) and MAP (dashed lines) source estimators. For reference, we also plot the ICA results (dotted lines). As expected, ϵ^{rec} and ϵ^{xtalk} decrease with increasing SNR and are significantly higher for ICA. Notice that the LMS reconstruction error is always lower than the MAP one, since it is

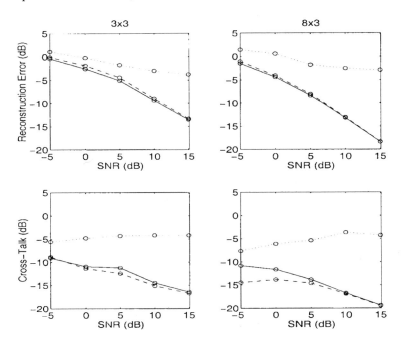

Figure 6: Source reconstruction quality with $L = 3$ sources for $L' = 3$ (left) and $L' = 8$ (right) sensors. Plotted are the reconstruction error ϵ^{rec} (top) and the cross-talk level ϵ^{xtalk} (see equation 5.6) (bottom) versus signal-to-noise ratio, for the LMS (solid lines), MAP (dashed lines), and ICA (dotted lines) estimators.

derived by demanding that it minimizes precisely ϵ^{rec}. In contrast, the MAP estimator has a lower cross-talk level.

6 IFA with Many Sources: The Factorized Variational Approximation

Whereas the EM algorithm (equations 3.12 and 3.13) is exact and all the required calculations can be done analytically, it becomes intractable as the number of sources in the IF model increases. This is because the conditional means computed in the E-step (see equations A.10–A.12) involve summing over all $\prod_i n_i$ possible configurations of the source states, that is $\sum_q = \sum_{q_1} \sum_{q_2} \cdots \sum_{q_L}$, whose number grows exponentially with the number of sources. As long as we focus on separating a small number L of sources (treating the rest as noise) and describe each source by a small number n_i of states, the E-step is tractable, but separating, for example, $L = 13$ sources with $n_i = 3$ states each would involve $3^{13} \approx 1.6 \times 10^6$ element sums at each iteration.

The intractability of exact learning is a problem not unique to the IF model but is shared by many probabilistic models. In general, approximations must be made. A suitable starting point for approximations is the function $\mathcal{F}$ of equation 3.6, which is bounded from below by the exact error $\mathcal{E}$ for an arbitrary p'.

The density p' is a posterior over the hidden variables of our generative model, given the values of the visible variables. The root of the intractability of EM is the choice (see equation 3.7) of p' as the exact posterior, which is derived from p via Bayes' rule and is parameterized by the generative parameters W. Several approximation schemes were proposed in other contexts (Hinton, Dayan, Neal, & Frey, 1995; Dayan, Hinton, Neal, & Zemel, 1995; Saul & Jordan, 1995; Saul, Jaakkola, & Jordan, 1996; Ghahramani & Jordan, 1997) where p' has a form that generally differs from that of the exact posterior and has its own set of parameters τ, which are learned separately from W by an appropriate procedure. Of crucial significance is the functional form of p', which should be chosen so as to make the E-step tractable, while still providing a reasonable approximation of the exact posterior. The parameters τ are then optimized to minimize the distance between p' and the exact posterior.

In the case of the IF model, we consider the function

$$\mathcal{F}(\tau, W) = -\sum_q \int dx\, p'(q, x \mid y, \tau)\, \log \frac{p(q, x, y \mid W)}{p'(q, x \mid y, \tau)} \geq \mathcal{E}(W), \quad (6.1)$$

where averaging over the data is implied. We shall use a variational approach, first formulated in the context of feedforward probabilistic models by Saul and Jordan (1995). Given the chosen form of the posterior p' (see below), $\mathcal{F}$ will be minimized iteratively with respect to both W and the variational parameters τ.

This minimization leads to the following approximate EM algorithm for IFA, which we derive in this section. Assume that the previous iteration produced W'. The E-step of the current iteration consists of determining the values of τ in terms of W' by solving a pair of coupled "mean-field" equations (see equations 6.8 and 6.9). It is straightforward to show that this step minimizes the KL distance between the variational and exact posteriors, $KL[p'(q, x \mid y, \tau), p(q, x \mid y, W')]$. In fact, this distance equals the difference $\mathcal{F}(\tau, W') - \mathcal{E}(W')$. Hence, this E-step approximates the exact one in which this distance actually vanishes.

Once the variational parameters have been determined, the new generative parameters W are obtained in the M-step using equations 3.12 and 3.13, where the conditional source means can be readily computed in terms of τ.

6.1 Factorized Posterior. We begin with the observation that whereas the sources in the IF model are independent, the sources conditioned on a data vector are correlated. This is clear from the fact that the conditional source correlation matrix $\langle \mathbf{x}\mathbf{x}^T \mid \mathbf{q}, \mathbf{y} \rangle$ (see equation A.9) is nondiagonal. More generally, the joint source posterior density $p(\mathbf{q}, \mathbf{x} \mid \mathbf{y})$ given by equations A.6 and A.8 does not factorize; it cannot be expressed as a product over the posterior densities of the individual sources.

In the factorized variational approximation, we assume that even when conditioned on a data vector, the sources are independent. Our approximate posterior source density is defined as follows. Given a data vector $\mathbf{y}$, the source x_i at state q_i is described by a gaussian distribution with a $\mathbf{y}$-dependent mean ψ_{i,q_i} and variance ξ_{i,q_i}, weighted by a mixing proportion κ_{i,q_i}. The posterior is defined simply by the product

$$p'(\mathbf{q}, \mathbf{x} \mid \mathbf{y}, \tau) = \prod_{i=1}^{L} \kappa_{i,q_i}(\mathbf{y}) \, \mathcal{G}\left[x_i - \psi_{i,q_i}(\mathbf{y}), \xi_{i,q_i}\right]$$

$$\tau_i = \{\kappa_{i,q_i}, \psi_{i,q_i}, \xi_{i,q_i}\}. \tag{6.2}$$

As alluded to by equation 6.2, the variances ξ_{i,q_i} will turn out to be $\mathbf{y}$-independent.

To gain some insight into the approximation, notice first that it implies an MOG form for the posterior of x_i,

$$p'(x_i \mid \mathbf{y}, \tau_i) = \sum_{q_i=1}^{n_i} \kappa_{i,q_i}(\mathbf{y}) \, \mathcal{G}(x_i - \psi_{i,q_i}(\mathbf{y}), \xi_{i,q_i}), \tag{6.3}$$

which is in complete analogy with its *prior* (see equation 2.5). Thus, conditioning the sources on the data is approximated simply by allowing the variational parameters to depend on $\mathbf{y}$. Next, compare equation 6.2 to the exact posterior $p(\mathbf{q}, \mathbf{x} \mid \mathbf{y}, W)$ (see equation A.6 and A.8). The latter also implies an MOG form for $p(x_i \mid \mathbf{y})$, but one that differs from equation 6.2; and in contrast with our approximate posterior, the exact one implies an MOG form for $p(x_i \mid q_i, \mathbf{y})$ as well, reflecting the fact that the source states and signals are all correlated given the data.

Therefore, the approximation (see equation 6.2) can be viewed as the result of shifting the source prior toward the true posterior for each data vector, with the variational parameters τ assuming the shifted values of the source parameters θ. Whereas this shift cannot capture correlations between the sources, it can be optimized to allow equation 6.2 to best approximate the true posterior while maintaining a factorized form. A procedure for determining the optimal values of τ is derived in the next section.

The factorized posterior of equation 6.2 is advantageous since it facilitates performing the E-step calculations in polynomial time. Once the variational parameters have been determined, the data-conditioned mean and covariance of the sources, required for the EM learning rule in equation 3.12, are

$$\langle x_i \mid \mathbf{y} \rangle = \sum_{q_i=1}^{n_i} \kappa_{i,q_i} \psi_{i,q_i},$$

$$\langle x_i^2 \mid \mathbf{y} \rangle = \sum_{q_i=1}^{n_i} \kappa_{i,q_i} (\psi_{i,q_i}^2 + \xi_{i,q_i}), \qquad \langle x_i x_{j \neq i} \mid \mathbf{y} \rangle = \sum_{q_i q_j} \kappa_{i,q_i} \kappa_{j,q_j} \psi_{i,q_i} \psi_{j,q_j}, \quad (6.4)$$

whereas those required for the rules in equation 3.13, which are further conditioned on the source states, are given by

$$p(q_i \mid \mathbf{y}) = \kappa_{i,q_i}, \qquad \langle x_i \mid q_i, \mathbf{y} \rangle = \psi_{i,q_i}, \qquad \langle x_i^2 \mid q_i, \mathbf{y} \rangle = \psi_{i,q_i}^2 + \xi_{i,q_i}. \quad (6.5)$$

Recovering the sources. In section 4, the LMS (see equations 4.1 and 4.2) and MAP (see equations 4.3 and 4.4) source estimators were given for exact IFA. Notice that being part of the E-step, computing the LMS estimator exactly quickly becomes intractable as the number of sources increases. In the variational approximation, it is replaced by $\hat{x}_i^{LMS}(\mathbf{y}) = \langle x_i \mid \mathbf{y} \rangle$ (see equation 6.4), which depends on the variational parameters and avoids summing over all source state configurations. In contrast, the MAP estimator remains unchanged (but the parameters W on which it depends are now learned by variational IFA); note that its computational cost is only weakly dependent on L.

6.2 Mean-Field Equations. For fixed τ, the learning rules for W (equations 3.12 and 3.13) follow from $\mathcal{F}(\tau, W)$ (equation 6.1) by solving the equations $\partial \mathcal{F}/\partial W = 0$. These equations are linear, as is evident from the gradients given in section A.2, and their solution $W = W(\tau)$ is given in closed form.

The learning rules for τ are similarly derived by fixing $W = W'$ and solving $\partial \mathcal{F}/\partial \tau = 0$. Unfortunately, examining the gradients given in appendix B shows that these equations are nonlinear and must be solved numerically. We choose to find their solution $\tau = \tau(W')$ by iteration.

Define the $L \times L$ matrix $\bar{\mathbf{H}}$ by

$$\bar{\mathbf{H}} = \mathbf{H}^T \Lambda^{-1} \mathbf{H}. \tag{6.6}$$

The equation for the variances ξ_{i,q_i} does not involve $\mathbf{y}$ and can easily be solved:

$$\xi_{i,q_i} = \left(\bar{H}_{ii} + \frac{1}{v_{i,q_i}} \right)^{-1}. \tag{6.7}$$

The means $\psi_{i,q_i}(\mathbf{y})$ and mixing proportions $\kappa_{i,q_i}(\mathbf{y})$ are obtained by iterating the following mean-field equations for each data vector $\mathbf{y}$:

$$\sum_{j \neq i} \sum_{q_j=1}^{n_j} \bar{H}_{ij} \kappa_{j,q_j} \psi_{j,q_j} + \frac{1}{\xi_{i,q_i}} \psi_{i,q_i} = (\mathbf{H}^T \mathbf{\Lambda}^{-1} \mathbf{y})_i + \frac{\mu_{i,q_i}}{\nu_{i,q_i}}, \tag{6.8}$$

$$\log \kappa_{i,q_i} = \log w_{i,q_i} + \frac{1}{2}\left(\log \xi_{i,q_i} + \frac{\psi_{i,q_i}^2}{\xi_{i,q_i}}\right) - \frac{1}{2}\left(\log \nu_{i,q_i} + \frac{\mu_{i,q_i}^2}{\nu_{i,q_i}}\right) + z_i$$

$$\equiv \alpha_{i,q_i} + z_i, \tag{6.9}$$

where the z_i are Lagrange multipliers that enforce the normalization conditions $\sum_{q_i} \kappa_{i,q_i} = 1$. Note that equation 6.8 depends nonlinearly on $\mathbf{y}$ due to the nonlinear $\mathbf{y}$ dependence of κ_{i,q_i}.

To solve these equations, we first initialize $\kappa_{i,q_i} = w_{i,q_i}$. Equation 6.8 is a linear $(\sum_i n_i) \times (\sum_i n_i)$ system and can be solved for ψ_{i,q_i} using standard methods. The new κ_{i,q_i} are then obtained from equation 6.9 via

$$\kappa_{i,q_i} = \frac{e^{\alpha_{i,q_i}}}{\sum_{q_i'} e^{\alpha_{i,q_i'}}}. \tag{6.10}$$

These values are substituted back into equation 6.8, and the procedure is repeated until convergence.

Data-independent approximation. A simpler approximation results from setting $\kappa_{i,q_i}(\mathbf{y}) = w_{i,q_i}$ for all data vectors $\mathbf{y}$. The means ψ_{i,q_i} can then be obtained from equation 6.8 in a single iteration for all data vectors at once, since this equation becomes linear in $\mathbf{y}$. This approximation is much less expensive computationally, with a corresponding reduction in accuracy, as shown below.

6.3 Variational IFA: Simulation Results.

Whereas the factorized form of the true posterior (see equation 6.2) and its data-independent simplification are not exact, the mean-field equations optimize the variational parameters τ to make the approximate posterior as accurate as possible. Here we assess the quality of this approximation.

First, we studied the accuracy of the approximate error function $\mathcal{F}$ (equation 6.1). For this purpose we considered a small data set with 100 $L' \times 1$ vectors $\mathbf{y}$ generated independently from a gaussian distribution. The approximate log-likelihood $-\mathcal{F}(\tau, W)$ of these data were compared to the exact log-likelihood $-\mathcal{E}(W)$, with respect to 5000 IF models with random parameters W. Each realization of W was obtained by sampling the parameters from uniform densities defined over the appropriate intervals, followed by scaling the source parameters according to equation 3.14. In the case of

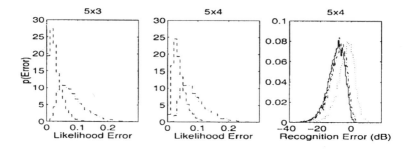

Figure 7: (Left, middle) Histogram of the relative error in the log-likelihood ϵ^{like} (see equation 6.11) of 100 random data vectors, for the factorized variational approximation (dashed line; mean error = 0.021 (left), 0.025 (middle)) and its data-independent simplification (dashed-dotted line; mean = 0.082, 0.084). The likelihoods were computed with respect to 5000 random IF model parameters with $L' = 5$ sensors and $L = 3$ (left) and $L = 4$ (middle) sources. (Right) Histogram of the reconstruction error ϵ^{rec} (5.6) at SNR = 10 dB for exact IFA (solid line; mean = −10.2 dB), the factorized (dashed line; mean = −10.1 dB) and data-independent (dashed-dotted line; mean = −8.9 dB) variational approximations, and ICA (dotted line; mean = −3.66 dB). The LMS source estimator was used.

the mixing proportions, $\bar{w}_{i,q_i}$ were sampled and w_{i,q_i} were obtained via equation A.15. $n_i = 3$-state MOG densities were used. The relative error in the log-likelihood,

$$\epsilon^{like} = \frac{\mathcal{F}(\tau, W)}{\mathcal{E}(W)} - 1, \tag{6.11}$$

was then computed for the factorized and data-independent approximations. Its histogram is displayed in Figure 7 for the case $L' = 5$, with $L = 3$ (left) and $L = 4$ (middle) sources.

In these examples, as well as in other simulations we performed, the mean error in the factorized approximation is under 3%. The data-independent approximation, as expected, is less accurate and increases the mean error above 8%.

Next, we investigated whether the variational IFA algorithm learns appropriate values for the IF model parameters W. The answer is quantified below in terms of the resulting reconstruction error. Five-second-long source signals, sampled from different densities (like those displayed in Figure 2) at a rate of 8.82 kHz, were generated. Noisy linear mixtures of these sources were used as data for the exact IFA algorithm and to its approximations. After learning, the source signals were reconstructed from the data by the LMS source estimator (see the discussion at the end of section 6.1). For each data vector, the reconstruction error ϵ^{rec} (see equation 5.6) was computed. The histograms of $10 \log_{10} \epsilon^{rec}$ (dB units) for the exact IFA and its approximations in a case with $L' = 5, L = 4$, SNR $= 10$ dB are displayed in Figure 7 (right). For reference, the ICA error histogram in this case is also plotted. Note that the variational histogram is very close to the exact one, whereas the data-independent histogram has a larger mean error. The ICA mean error is the largest, consistent with the results of Figure 6 (top).

We conclude that the factorized variational approximation of IFA is quite accurate. Of course, the real test is in its application to cases with large numbers of sources where exact IFA can no longer be used. In addition, other variational approximations can also be defined. A thorough assessment of the factorial and other variational approximations and their applications is somewhat beyond the scope of this article and will be published separately.

7 Noiseless IFA

We now consider the IF model (see equation 2.1) in the noiseless case $\Lambda = 0$. Here the sensor data depend deterministically on the sources,

$$\mathbf{y} = \mathbf{Hx}; \tag{7.1}$$

hence, once the mixing matrix $\mathbf{H}$ is found, the latter can be recovered exactly (rather than estimated) from the observed data using the pseudo-inverse of $\mathbf{H}$ via

$$\mathbf{x} = (\mathbf{H}^T\mathbf{H})^{-1}\mathbf{H}^T\mathbf{y}, \tag{7.2}$$

which reduces to $\mathbf{x} = \mathbf{H}^{-1}\mathbf{y}$ for square invertible mixing. Hence, vanishing noise level results in a linear source estimator that is independent of the source parameters.

One might expect that our EM algorithm (see equations 3.12 and 3.13) for the noisy case can also be applied to noiseless mixing, with the only consequence being that the noise covariance Λ would acquire very small values. This, however, is not the case, as we shall show. It turns out that in the zero-noise limit, that algorithm actually performs PCA; consequently, for low noise, convergence from the PCA to IFA solution is very slow. The root of the problem is that in the noiseless case we have only one type of "missing data," the source states $\mathbf{q}$; the source signals $\mathbf{x}$ are no longer missing, being given directly by the observed sensors via equation 7.2. We shall therefore proceed to derive an EM algorithm specifically for this case. This algorithm will turn out to be a powerful extension of Bell and Sejnowski's (1995) ICA algorithm.

7.1 An Expectation-Maximization Algorithm. We first focus on the square invertible mixing ($L' = L$, rank $\mathbf{H} = L$), and write equation 2.1 as

$$\mathbf{x} = \mathbf{Gy}, \tag{7.3}$$

where the unmixing (separating) matrix $\mathbf{G}$ is given by $\mathbf{H}^{-1}$ with its columns possibly scaled and permuted.

Unlike the noisy case, here there is only one type of "missing data," the source states $\mathbf{q}$, since the stochastic dependence of the sensor data on the sources becomes deterministic. Hence, the conditional density $p(\mathbf{y} \mid \mathbf{x})$ (see equation 2.11) must be replaced by $p(\mathbf{y}) = |\det \mathbf{G}| p(\mathbf{x})$ as implied by equation 7.3. Together with the factorial MOG model for the sources $\mathbf{x}$ (equation 2.8), the error function (see equation 3.6) becomes

$$\mathcal{E}(W) = -\log p(\mathbf{y} \mid W) = -\log |\det \mathbf{G}| - \log p(\mathbf{x} \mid W)$$

$$\leq -\log |\det \mathbf{G}| - \sum_{\mathbf{q}} p(\mathbf{q} \mid \mathbf{x}, W') \log \frac{p(\mathbf{x}, \mathbf{q} \mid W)}{p(\mathbf{q} \mid \mathbf{x}, W')}. \tag{7.4}$$

As in the noisy case (see equation 3.8), we have obtained an approximated error $\mathcal{F}(W', W)$ that is bounded from below by the true error and is given by a sum over the individual layer contributions (see Figure 1),

$$\mathcal{E}(W) \leq \mathcal{F}(W', W) = \mathcal{F}_V + \mathcal{F}_B + \mathcal{F}_T + \mathcal{F}_H. \tag{7.5}$$

Here, however, the contributions of both the visible and bottom hidden layers depend on the visible layer parameters $\mathbf{G}$,

$$\mathcal{F}_V(W', \mathbf{G}) = -\log |\det \mathbf{G}|,$$

$$\mathcal{F}_B(W', \mathbf{G}, \{\mu_{i,q_i}, v_{i,q_i}\}) = -\sum_{i=1}^{L} \sum_{q_i=1}^{n_i} p(q_i \mid x_i, W') \log p(x_i \mid q_i),$$

$$\mathcal{F}_T(W', \mathbf{G}, \{w_{i,q_i}\}) = -\sum_{i=1}^{L} \sum_{q_i=1}^{n_i} p(q_i \mid x_i, W') \log p(q_i), \tag{7.6}$$

whereas the top layer contribution remains separated (compare with equation 3.9, noting that $p(\mathbf{q} \mid \mathbf{y}) = p(\mathbf{q} \mid \mathbf{x})$ due to equation 7.3). The entropy term,

$$\mathcal{F}_H(W') = \sum_{\mathbf{q}} p(\mathbf{q} \mid \mathbf{x}, W') \log p(\mathbf{q} \mid \mathbf{x}, W'), \tag{7.7}$$

is W-independent. The complete form of the expressions in equation 7.6 includes replacing $\mathbf{x}$ by $\mathbf{Gy}$ and averaging over the observed $\mathbf{y}$.

The EM learning algorithm for the IF model parameters is derived in appendix C. A difficulty arises from the fact that the M-step equation $\partial \mathcal{F} / \partial \mathbf{G} = 0$, whose solution is the new value $\mathbf{G}$ in terms of the parameters W' obtained at the previous EM step, is nonlinear and cannot be solved analytically. Instead we solve it iteratively, so that each EM step $W' \to W$ is composed of a sequence of iterations on W with W' held fixed.

The noiseless IFA learning rule for the separating matrix is given by

$$\delta \mathbf{G} = \eta \mathbf{G} - \eta E \phi'(\mathbf{x}) \mathbf{x}^T \mathbf{G}, \tag{7.8}$$

where $\eta > 0$ determines the learning rate and its value should be set empirically. $\phi'(\mathbf{x})$ is an $L \times 1$ vector, which depends on the posterior $p'(q_i \mid x_i) \equiv p(q_i \mid x_i, W')$ (see equation C.3) computed using the parameters from the previous iteration; its ith coordinate is given by a weighted sum over the states q_i of source i,

$$\phi'(x_i) = \sum_{q_i=1}^{n_i} p'(q_i \mid x_i) \frac{x_i - \mu_{i,q_i}}{v_{i,q_i}}. \tag{7.9}$$

The rules for the source MOG parameters are

$$\mu_{i,q_i} = \frac{E p'(q_i \mid x_i) x_i}{E p'(q_i \mid x_i)},$$

$$v_{i,q_i} = \frac{E p'(q_i \mid x_i) x_i^2}{E p'(q_i \mid x_i)} - \mu_{i,q_i}^2,$$

$$w_{i,q_i} = E p'(q_i \mid x_i). \tag{7.10}$$

Recall that $\mathbf{x}$ is linearly related to $\mathbf{y}$ and the operator E averages over the observed $\mathbf{y}$.

The noiseless IFA learning rules (see equations 7.8–7.10) should be used as follows. Having obtained the parameters W' in the previous EM step, the new step starts with computing the posterior $p'(q_i \mid x_i)$ and setting the initial values of the new parameters W to W', except for w_{i,q_i} which can be set to its final value $E p'(q_i \mid x_i)$. Then a sequence of iterations begins, where each iteration consists of three steps: (1) computing the sources by $\mathbf{x} = \mathbf{G}\mathbf{y}$ using the current $\mathbf{G}$; (2) computing the new μ_{i,q_i}, v_{i,q_i} from equation 7.10 using the sources obtained in step 1; and (3) computing the new $\mathbf{G}$ from equations 7.8 and 7.9 using the sources obtained in step 1 and the means and variances obtained in step 2.

The iterations continue until some convergence criterion is satisfied. During this process, both $\mathbf{x}$ and W change, but $p'(q_i \mid x_i)$ are frozen. Achieving convergence completes the current EM step; the next step starts with updating those posteriors.

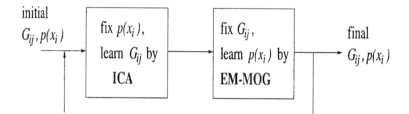

initial
$G_{ij}, p(x_i)$

| fix $p(x_i)$,
learn G_{ij} by
ICA | fix G_{ij},
learn $p(x_i)$ by
EM-MOG |

final
$G_{ij}, p(x_i)$

Figure 8: Seesaw GEM algorithm for noiseless IFA.

We recognize the learning rules for the source densities (equation 7.10) as precisely the standard EM rules for learning a separate MOG model for each source i, shown on the right column of equation 3.15. Hence, our noiseless IFA algorithm combines separating the sources, by learning G using the rule in equation 7.8, with simultaneously learning their densities by EM-MOG. These two processes are coupled by the priors $p'(q_i \mid x_i)$. We shall show in the next section that the two can decouple, and consequently the separating matrix rule in equation 7.8 becomes Bell and Sejnowski's (1995) ICA rule, producing the algorithm shown schematically in Figure 8.

We also point out that the MOG learning rules for the noiseless case in equation 7.10 can be obtained from those for the noisy case in equation 3.13 by replacing the conditional source means $\langle x_i \mid q_i, \mathbf{y} \rangle$ by $x_i = \sum_j G_{ij} y_j$, and replacing the source state posteriors $p(q_i \mid \mathbf{y})$ by $p(q_i \mid x_i)$. Both changes arise from the vanishing noise level, which makes the source-sensor dependence deterministic.

7.1.1 Scaling. As in the noisy case (see equation 3.14), noiseless IFA is augmented by the following scaling transformation at each iteration:

$$
\sigma_i^2 = \sum_{q_i=1}^{n_i} w_{i,q_i}(v_{i,q_i} + \mu_{i,q_i}^2) - \left(\sum_{q_i=1}^{n_i} w_{i,q_i} \mu_{i,q_i} \right)^2 ,
$$

$$
\mu_{i,q_i} \rightarrow \frac{\mu_{i,q_i}}{\sigma_i}, \qquad v_{i,q_i} \rightarrow \frac{v_{i,q_i}}{\sigma_i^2}, \qquad G_{ij} \rightarrow \frac{1}{\sigma_i} G_{ij}. \tag{7.11}
$$

7.1.2 More Sensors Than Sources. The noiseless IFA algorithm given above assumes that $\mathbf{H}$ is a square invertible $L \times L$ mixing matrix. The more general case of an $L' \times L$ mixing with $L' \geq L$ can be treated as follows.

We start with the observation that in this case, the $L' \times L'$ sensor covariance matrix $\mathbf{C_y} = E\mathbf{y}\mathbf{y}^T$ is of rank L. Let the columns of $\mathbf{P}$ contain the eigenvectors of $\mathbf{C_y}$, so that $\mathbf{P}^T \mathbf{C_y} \mathbf{P} = \mathbf{D}$ is diagonal. Then $\mathbf{P}^T \mathbf{y}$ are the L' principal components of the sensor data, and only L of them are nonzero.

The latter are denoted by $y_1 = P_1^T y$, where P_1 is formed by those columns of P corresponding to nonzero eigenvalues.

The algorithm (see equations 7.8–7.10) should now be applied to y_1 to find an $L \times L$ separating matrix, denoted G_1. Finally, the $L \times L'$ separating matrix G required for recovering the sources from sensors via equation 7.3 is simply $G = G_1 P_1^T$.

It remains to find P_1. This can be done using matrix diagonalization methods. Alternatively, observing that its columns are not required to be the first L eigenvectors of C_y but only to span the same subspace, the PCA learning rule (see equation 7.18) (with H replaced by P_1) may be used for this purpose.

7.2 Generalized EM and the Relation to Independent Component Analysis. Whereas the procedure described for using the noiseless IFA rules (equations 7.8–7.10) is a strictly EM algorithm (for a sufficiently small η), it is also possible to use them in a different manner. An alternative procedure can be defined by making either or both of the following changes: (1) complete each EM step and update the posteriors $p'(q_i \mid x_i)$ after some fixed number S of iterations, regardless of whether convergence has been achieved; (2) for a given EM step, select some parameters from the set W and freeze them during that step, while updating the rest; the choice of frozen parameters may vary from one step to the next.

Any procedure that incorporates either of these does not minimize the approximate error $\mathcal{F}$ at each M-step (unless S is sufficiently large) but merely reduces it. Of course, the EM convergence proof remains valid in this case. Such a procedure is termed a *generalized EM* (GEM) algorithm (Dempster et al., 1977; Neal & Hinton, 1998). Clearly there are many possible GEM versions of noiseless IFA. Two particular versions are defined below:

- *Chase.* Obtained from the EM version simply by updating the posteriors at each iteration. Each GEM step consists of (1) a single iteration of the separating matrix rule (equation 7.8), (2) a single iteration of the MOG rules (equation 7.10), and (3) updating the posteriors $p'(q_i \mid x_i)$ using the new parameter values. Hence, the source densities follow G step by step.

- *Seesaw.* Obtained by breaking the EM version into two phases and alternating between them. First, freeze the MOG parameters; each GEM step consists of a single iteration of the separating matrix rule (equation 7.8), followed by updating the posteriors using the new value of G. Second, freeze the separating matrix; each GEM step consists of a single iteration of the MOG rule (equation 7.10), followed by updating the posteriors using the new values of the MOG parameters. The sequence of steps in each phase terminates after making S steps or upon satisfying a convergence criterion. Hence, we switch back and forth between learning G and learning the source densities.

Both the Chase and Seesaw GEM algorithms were found to converge faster than the original EM one. Both require updating the posteriors at each step; this operation is not computationally expensive since each source posterior $p(q_i \mid x_i)$ (see equation C.3) is computed individually and requires summing only over its own n_i states, making the total cost linearly dependent on L. In our noisy IFA algorithm, in contrast, updating the source state posteriors $p(q \mid y)$ (see equation A.8) requires summing over the $\prod_i n_i$ collective source states q, and the total cost is exponential in L.

We now show that Seesaw combines two well-known algorithms in an intuitively appealing manner. Since the source density learning rules (equation 7.10) are the EM rules for fitting an MOG model to each source, as discussed in the previous section, the second phase of Seesaw is equivalent to EM-MOG. It will be shown below that its first phase is equivalent to Bell and Sejnowski's (1995) ICA algorithm, with their sigmoidal nonlinearity replaced by a function related to our MOG source densities. Therefore, Seesaw amounts to learning G_{ij} by applying ICA to the observed sensors y_j while the densities $p(x_i)$ are kept fixed, then fixing G_{ij} and learning the new $p(x_i)$ by applying EM-MOG to the reconstructed sources $x_i = \sum_j G_{ij} y_j$, and repeat. This algorithm is described schematically in Figure 8.

In the context of BSS, the noiseless IFA problem for an equal number of sensors and sources had already been formulated before as the problem of ICA by Comon (1994). An efficient ICA algorithm was first proposed by Bell and Sejnowski (1995) from an information-maximization viewpoint; it was soon observed (MacKay, 1996; Pearlmutter & Parra, 1997; Cardoso, 1997) that this algorithm was in fact performing a maximum-likelihood (or, equivalently, minimum KL distance) estimation of the separating matrix using a generative model of linearly mixed sources with nongaussian densities. In ICA, these densities are fixed throughout.

The derivation of ICA, like that of our noiseless IFA algorithm, starts from the KL error function $\mathcal{E}(W)$ (equation 7.4). However, rather than approximating it, ICA minimizes the exact error by the steepest descent method using its gradient $\partial \mathcal{E} / \partial G = -(G^T)^{-1} + \varphi(x)y^T$, where $\varphi(x)$ is an $L \times 1$ vector whose ith coordinate is related to the density $p(x_i)$ of source i via $\varphi(x_i) = -\partial \log p(x_i)/\partial x_i$. The separating matrix G is incremented at each iteration in the direction of the relative gradient (Cardoso & Laheld, 1996; Amari, Cichocki, & Yang, 1996; MacKay, 1996) of $\mathcal{E}(W)$ by $\delta G = -\eta(\partial \mathcal{E}/\partial G)G^T G$, resulting in the learning rule

$$\delta G = \eta G - \eta E\varphi(x)x^T G, \qquad (7.12)$$

where the sources are computed from the sensors at each iteration via $x = Gy$.

Now, the ICA rule in equation 7.12 has the form of our noiseless IFA separating matrix rule (equation 7.8) with $\phi(x_i)$ (equation 7.9) replaced by $\varphi(x_i)$ defined above. Moreover, whereas the original Bell and Sejnowski

(1995) algorithm used the source densities $p(x_i) = \cosh^{-2}(x_i)$, it can be shown that using our MOG form for $p(x_i)$ (see equation 2.5) produces

$$\varphi(x_i) = \sum_{q_i=1}^{n_i} p(q_i \mid x_i) \frac{x_i - \mu_{i,q_i}}{v_{i,q_i}}, \qquad (7.13)$$

which has the same form as $\phi(x_i)$ of equation 7.9; they become identical, $\varphi(x_i) = \phi(x_i)$, when noiseless IFA is used with the source state posteriors updated at each iteration ($S = 1$). We therefore conclude that the first phase of Seesaw is equivalent to ICA.

Although ICA can sometimes accomplish separation using an inaccurate source density model (e.g., speech signals with a Laplacian density $p(x_i) \approx e^{-|x_i|}$ are successfully separated using the model $p(x_i) = \cosh^{-2}(x_i)$), model inaccuracies often lead to failure. For example, a mixture of negative-kurtosis signals (e.g., with a uniform distribution) could not be separated using the $\cosh^{-2}$ model whose kurtosis is positive. Thus, when the densities of the sources at hand are not known in advance, the algorithm's ability to learn them becomes crucial.

A parametric source model can, in principle, be directly incorporated into ICA (MacKay, 1996; Pearlmutter & Parra, 1997) by deriving gradient-descent learning rules for its parameters θ_i via $\delta\theta_i = -\eta \partial \mathcal{E}/\partial \theta_i$, in addition to the rule for **G**. Unfortunately, the resulting learning rate is quite low, as is also the case when nonparametric density estimation methods are used (Pham, 1996). Alternatively, the source densities may be approximated using cumulant methods such as the Edgeworth or Gram-Charlier expansions (Comon, 1994; Amari et al., 1996; Cardoso & Laheld, 1996); this approach produces algorithms that are less robust since the approximations are not true probability densities, being nonnormalizable and sometimes negative.

In contrast, our noiseless IFA algorithm, and in particular its Seesaw GEM version, resolves these problems by combining ICA with source density learning rules in a manner that exploits the efficiency offered by the EM technique.

7.3 Noiseless IFA: Simulation Results. In this section we demonstrate and compare the performance of the Chase and Seesaw GEM algorithms on noiseless mixtures of $L = 3$ sources. We used 5-sec-long speech and music signals obtained from commercial CDs, as well as synthetic signals produced by a random number generator at a sampling rate of $f_s = 8.82$ kHz. The source signal densities used in the following example are shown in Figure 2. Those signals were scaled to unit variance and mixed by a random $L \times L$ mixing matrix $\mathbf{H}^0$. The learning rules (equations 7.8–7.10), used in the manner required by either the Chase or Seesaw procedures, were iterated in batch mode, starting from random parameter values. We used a fixed learning rate $\eta = 0.05$.

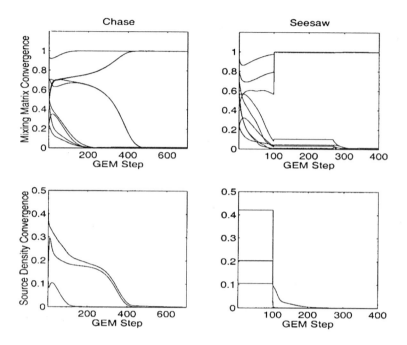

Figure 9: (Top) Convergence of the separating matrix $\mathbf{G}$ (left) and the source densities $p(x_i)$ (right) for the Chase algorithm with $L = 3$ sources. For $\mathbf{G}$ we plot the matrix elements of $\mathbf{J}$ (see equation 7.14) against GEM step number, whereas for $p(x_i)$ we plot their KL distance K_i (see equation 5.3) from the true densities. (Bottom) Same for the Seesaw algorithm.

Figure 9 shows the convergence of the estimated separating matrix $\mathbf{G}$ (left) and the source densities $p(x_i)$ (right) for Chase (top) and Seesaw (bottom). The distance of $\mathbf{G}^{-1}$ from the true mixing matrix $\mathbf{H}^0$ is quantified by the matrix elements of

$$\mathbf{J} = \mathbf{G}\mathbf{H}^0. \tag{7.14}$$

Notice that for the correct estimate $\mathbf{G}^{-1} = \mathbf{H}^0$, $\mathbf{J}$ becomes the unit matrix $\mathbf{I}$. Recall that the effect of source scaling is eliminated by equation 7.11; to prevent possible source permutations from affecting this measure, we permuted the columns of $\mathbf{G}$ such that the largest element (in absolute value) in column i of $\mathbf{J}$ would be J_{ii}. Indeed, this product is shown to converge to $\mathbf{I}$ in both cases. For the source densities, we plot their KL distances K_i (see equation 5.3) from the true densities $p^0(x_i)$, which approach zero as the learning proceeds. Notice that Seesaw required a smaller number of steps to converge; similar results were observed in other simulations we performed.

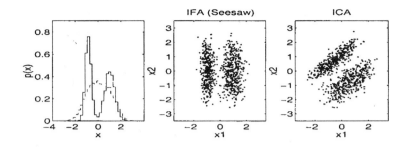

Figure 10: Noiseless IFA versus ICA. (Left) Source densities histograms. These sources were mixed by a random 2×2 matrix. (Middle) Joint density of the sources recovered from the mixtures by Seesaw. (Right) Same for ICA.

Seesaw was used in the following manner: After initializing the parameters, the MOG parameters were frozen and the first phase proceeded for $S = 100$ iterations on $\mathbf{G}$. Then $\mathbf{G}$ was frozen (except for the scaling (equation 7.11)), and the second phase proceeded until the maximal relative increment of the MOG parameters decreased below 5×10^{-4}. This phase alternation is manifested in Figure 9 by K_i being constant as $\mathbf{J}$ changes, and vice versa. In particular, the upward jump of one of the elements of $\mathbf{J}$ after $S = 100$ iterations is caused by the scaling, which is performed only in the second phase.

To demonstrate the advantage of noiseless IFA over Bell and Sejnowski's (1995) ICA, we applied both algorithms to a mixture of $L = 2$ sources whose densities are plotted in Figure 10 (left). The Seesaw version of IFA was used. After learning, the recovered sources were obtained; their joint densities are displayed in Figure 10 for IFA (middle) and ICA (right). The sources recovered by ICA are clearly correlated, reflecting the fact that this algorithm uses a nonadaptive source density model that is unsuitable for the present case.

7.4 Relation to Principal Component Analysis. The EM algorithm for IFA presented in section 3.2 fails to identify the mixing matrix $\mathbf{H}$ in the noiseless case. This can be shown by taking the zero-noise limit,

$$\Lambda = \eta \mathbf{I}, \qquad \eta \to 0, \tag{7.15}$$

where $\mathbf{I}$ is the $L \times L$ unit matrix, and examine the learning rule for $\mathbf{H}$ (first line in equation 3.12). Using equation 7.15 in equations A.6 and A.7, the source posterior becomes singular,

$$p(\mathbf{x} \mid \mathbf{q}, \mathbf{y}) = \delta \left[\mathbf{x} - \rho(\mathbf{y}) \right], \qquad \rho(\mathbf{y}) = (\mathbf{H}^T \mathbf{H})^{-1} \mathbf{H}^T \mathbf{y}, \tag{7.16}$$

and loses its dependence of the source states $\mathbf{q}$. This simply expresses the fact that for a given observation $\mathbf{y}$, the sources $\mathbf{x}$ are given by their conditional mean $\langle \mathbf{x} \mid \mathbf{y} \rangle$ with zero variance,

$$\langle \mathbf{x} \mid \mathbf{y} \rangle = \rho(\mathbf{y}), \qquad \langle \mathbf{x}\mathbf{x}^T \mid \mathbf{y} \rangle = \rho(\mathbf{y})\rho(\mathbf{y})^T, \tag{7.17}$$

as indeed is expected for zero noise.

The rule for $\mathbf{H}$ (see equation 3.12) now becomes

$$\mathbf{H} = \mathbf{C_y}\mathbf{H}'(\mathbf{H}'^T\mathbf{C_y}\mathbf{H}')^{-1}\mathbf{H}'^T\mathbf{H}', \tag{7.18}$$

where $\mathbf{H}'$ is the mixing matrix obtained in the previous iteration and $\mathbf{C_y} = E\mathbf{y}\mathbf{y}^T$ is the covariance matrix of the observed sensor data. This rule contains no information about the source parameters; in effect, the vanishing noise disconnected the bottom hidden layer from the top one. The bottom and visible layers now form together a separate generative model of *gaussian* sources (since the only source property used is their vanishing correlations) that are mixed linearly without noise.

In fact, if the columns of $\mathbf{H}$ are L of the orthogonal L' directions defined by the principal components of the observed data (recall that this matrix is $L' \times L$), the algorithm will stop. To see that, assume $\mathbf{H}^T\mathbf{C_y}\mathbf{H} = \mathbf{D}$ is diagonal and the columns of $\mathbf{H}$ are orthonormal (namely, $\mathbf{H}^T\mathbf{H} = \mathbf{I}$). Then $\mathbf{D}$ contains L eigenvalues of the data covariance matrix, which itself can be expressed as $\mathbf{C_y} = \mathbf{H}\mathbf{D}\mathbf{H}^T$. By direct substitution, the rule in equation 7.18 reduces to $\mathbf{H} = \mathbf{H}'$. Hence, the M-step contributes nothing toward minimizing the error since $W = W'$ is already a minimum of $\mathcal{F}(W', W)$ (see equation 3.5), so $\mathcal{F}(W', W) = \mathcal{F}(W', W')$ in equation 3.11. Mathematically, the origin of this phenomenon lies in the sensor density conditioned on the sources (see equation 2.11) becoming nonanalytic, that is, $p(\mathbf{y} \mid \mathbf{x}) = \delta(\mathbf{y} - \mathbf{H}\mathbf{x})$.

A more complete analysis of the generative model formed by linearly mixing uncorrelated gaussian variables (Tipping & Bishop, 1997) shows that any $\mathbf{H}$, whose columns span the L-dimensional space defined by any L principal directions of the data, is a stationary point of the corresponding likelihood; in particular, when the spanned space is defined by the first L principal directions, the likelihood is maximal at that point.

We conclude that in the zero-noise case, the EM algorithm (equations 3.12 and 3.13) performs PCA rather than IFA, with the top layer learning a factorial MOG model for some linear combinations of the first L principal components. For nonzero but very low noise, convergence from the PCA to IFA solution will therefore be rather slow, and the noiseless IFA algorithm may become preferable.

It is also interesting to point out that the rule in equation 7.18, obtained as a special case of noiseless IFA, has been discovered quite recently by Tipping and Bishop (1997) and independently by Roweis (1998) as an EM algorithm for PCA.

8 Conclusion

This article introduced the concept of independent factor analysis, a new method for statistical analysis of multivariable data. By performing IFA, the data are interpreted as arising from independent, unobserved sources that are mixed by a linear transformation with added noise. In the context of the blind source separation problem, IFA separates nonsquare, noisy mixtures where the sources, mixing process, and noise properties are all unknown.

To perform IFA, we introduced the hierarchical IF generative model of the mixing situation and derived an EM algorithm that learns the model parameters from the observed sensor data; the sources are then reconstructed by an optimal nonlinear estimator. Our IFA algorithm reduces to the well-known EM algorithm for ordinary FA when the model sources become gaussian. In the noiseless limit, it reduces to the EM algorithm for PCA. As the number of sources increases, the exact algorithm becomes intractable; an approximate algorithm, based on a variational approach, has been derived and its accuracy demonstrated.

An EM algorithm specifically for noiseless IFA, associated with a linear source estimator, has also been derived. This algorithm, and in particular its generalized EM versions, combines separating the sources by Bell and Sejnowski's (1995) ICA with learning their densities using the EM rules for mixtures of gaussians. In the Chase version, the source densities are learned simultaneously with the separating matrix, whereas the Seesaw version learns the two parameter sets in alternating phases. Hence, an efficient solution is provided for the problem of incorporating adaptive source densities into ICA.

A generative model similar to IF was recently proposed by Lewicki and Sejnowski (1998). In fact, their model was implicit in Olshausen and Field's (1996) algorithm, as exposed in Olshausen (1996). This model uses a Laplacian source prior $p(x_i) \propto e^{-|x_i|}$, and the integral over the sources required to obtain $p(\mathbf{y})$ in equation 2.4 is approximated by the value of the integrand at its maximum; this approximation can be improved on by incorporating gaussian corrections (Lewicki & Sejnowski, 1998). The resulting algorithm was used to derive efficient codes for images and sounds (Lewicki & Olshausen, 1998) and was put forth as a computational model for interpreting neural responses in V1 in the efficient coding framework (Olshausen & Field, 1996, 1997). In contrast with IFA, this algorithm use a nonadaptive source density model and may perform poorly on non-Laplacian sources; it uses gradient ascent rather than the efficient EM method, and the approximations involved in its derivation must be made even for a small number of sources, where exact IFA is available. It will be interesting to compare the performance of this algorithm with variational IFA on mixtures of many sources with arbitrary densities.

An EM algorithm for noisy BSS, which was restricted to discrete sources whose distributions are known in advance, was developed in Belouchrani and Cardoso (1994). Moulines, Cardoso, and Gassiat (1997) proposed an EM approach to noisy mixing of continuous sources. They did not discuss source reconstruction, and their method was restricted to a small number of sources and did not extend to noiseless mixing; nevertheless, they had essentially the same insight as the present article regarding the advantage of mixture source models. A related idea was discussed in Roweis and Ghahramani (1997).

An important issue that deserves a separate discussion is the determination of the number L of hidden sources, assumed known throughout this article. L is not a simple parameter since increasing the number of sources increases the number of model parameters, resulting, in effect, in a different generative model. Hence, to determine L, one should use model comparison methods, on which extensive literature is available (see, e.g., MacKay's 1992 discussion of Bayesian model comparison using the evidence framework). A much simpler but imprecise method would exploit the data covariance matrix $C_y = Eyy^T$ and fix the number of sources at the number of its "significant" (with respect to some threshold) eigenvalues. This method is suggested by the fact that in the zero-noise case, the number of positive eigenvalues is precisely L; however, for the noisy case, the result will depend strongly on the threshold (which there is no systematic way to determine), and the accuracy of this method is expected to decrease with increasing noise level.

Viewed as a data modeling tool, IFA provides an alternative to factor analysis on the one hand and to mixture models on the other by suggesting a description of the data in terms of a highly constrained mixture of coadaptive gaussians and simultaneously in terms of independent underlying sources that may reflect the actual generating mechanism of those data. In this capacity, IFA may be used for noise removal and completion of missing data. It is also related to the statistical methods of projection pursuit (Friedman & Stuetzle, 1981; Huber, 1985) and generalized additive models (Hastie & Tibshirani, 1990); a comparative study of IFA and those techniques would be of great interest.

Viewed as a compression tool, IFA constitutes a new method for redundancy reduction of correlated multichannel data into a factorial few-channel representation given by the reconstructed sources. It is well known that the optimal linear compression is provided by PCA and is characterized by the absence of second-order correlations among the new channels. In contrast, the compressed IFA representation is a nonlinear function of the original data, where the nonlinearity is effectively optimized to ensure the absence of correlations of arbitrarily high orders.

Finally, viewed as a tool for source separation in realistic situations, IFA is currently being extended to handle noisy convolutive mixing, where H becomes a matrix of filters. This extension exploits spatiotemporal generative models introduced by Attias and Schreiner (1998), where they served as a basis for deriving gradient-descent algorithms for convolutive noiseless mixtures. A related approach to this problem is outlined in Moulines et al. (1997). In addition to more complicated mixing models, IFA allows the use of complex models for the source densities, resulting in source estimators that are optimized to the properties of the sources and can thus reconstruct them more faithfully from the observed data. A simple extension of the source model used in this article could incorporate the source autocorrelations, following Attias and Schreiner (1998); this would produce a nonlinear, multichannel generalization of the Wiener filter. More powerful models may include useful high-order source descriptions.

Appendix A: IFA: Derivation of the EM Algorithm ⎯⎯⎯⎯⎯⎯⎯⎯⎯⎯

Here we provide the derivation of the EM learning rules (equations 3.12 and 3.13) from the approximate error (equation 3.9).

A.1 E-Step. To obtain $\mathcal{F}$ in terms of the IF model parameters W, we first substitute $p(\mathbf{y} \mid \mathbf{x}) = \mathcal{G}(\mathbf{y} - H\mathbf{x}, \Lambda)$ (see equation 2.11) in equation 3.9 and obtain, with a bit of algebra,

$$\mathcal{F}_V = \frac{1}{2} \log |\det \Lambda| + \frac{1}{2} \mathrm{Tr}\, \Lambda^{-1} (\mathbf{y}\mathbf{y}^T - 2\mathbf{y}\langle \mathbf{x}^T \mid \mathbf{y}\rangle H^T$$

$$+ H\langle \mathbf{x}\mathbf{x}^T \mid \mathbf{y}\rangle H^T). \tag{A.1}$$

The integration over the sources $\mathbf{x}$ required to compute $\mathcal{F}_V$ (see equation 3.9) appears in equation A.1 via the conditional mean and covariance of the sources given the observed sensor signals, defined by

$$\langle m(\mathbf{x}) \mid \mathbf{y}, W' \rangle = \int d\mathbf{x}\, p(\mathbf{x} \mid \mathbf{y}, W')\, m(\mathbf{x}), \tag{A.2}$$

where we used $m(\mathbf{x}) = \mathbf{x}, \mathbf{x}\mathbf{x}^T$. Note that these conditional averages depend on the parameters W' produced by the previous iteration. We point out that for a given $\mathbf{y}$, $\langle \mathbf{x} \mid \mathbf{y}\rangle$ is an $L \times 1$ vector and $\langle \mathbf{x}\mathbf{x}^T \mid \mathbf{y}\rangle$ is an $L \times L$ matrix.

Next, we substitute $p(x_i \mid q_i) = \mathcal{G}(x_i - \mu_{i,q_i}, \nu_{i,q_i})$ in equation 3.9 to get

$$\mathcal{F}_B = \sum_{i=1}^{L} \sum_{q_i=1}^{n_i} p(q_i \mid \mathbf{y}, W')$$

$$\times \left[\frac{1}{2} \log \nu_{i,q_i} + \frac{1}{2\nu_{i,q_i}} (\langle x_i^2 \mid q_i, \mathbf{y}\rangle - 2\langle x_i \mid q_i, \mathbf{y}\rangle \mu_{i,q_i} + \mu_{i,q_i}^2) \right], \tag{A.3}$$

where the integration over the source x_i indicated in $\mathcal{F}_B$ (equation 3.9) enters via the conditional mean and variance of this source given both the observed sensor signals and the hidden state of this source, defined by

$$\langle m(x_i) \mid q_i, \mathbf{y}, W' \rangle = \int dx_i \, p(x_i \mid q_i, \mathbf{y}, W') \, m(x_i), \qquad (A.4)$$

and we used $m(x_i) = x_i, x_i^2$. Note from equation A.3 that the quantity we are actually calculating is the joint conditional average of the source signal x_i and state q_i, that is, $\langle x_i, q_i \mid \mathbf{y}, W' \rangle = p(q_i \mid \mathbf{y}, W') \langle m(x_i) \mid q_i, \mathbf{y}, W' \rangle = \int dx_i \, p(x_i, q_i \mid \mathbf{y}, W') \, m(x_i)$. We broke the posterior over those hidden variables as in equation A.3 for computational convenience.

Finally, for the top layer we have

$$\mathcal{F}_T = -\sum_{i=1}^{L} \sum_{q_i=1}^{n_i} p(q_i \mid \mathbf{y}, W') \, \log w_{i,q_i}. \qquad (A.5)$$

To complete the E-step we must express the conditional averages (see equations A.2 and A.4) explicitly in terms of the parameters W'. The key to this calculation is the conditional densities $p(\mathbf{x} \mid \mathbf{q}, \mathbf{y}, W')$ and $p(\mathbf{q} \mid \mathbf{y}, W')$, whose product is the posterior density of the unobserved source signals and states given the observed sensor signals, $p(\mathbf{x}, \mathbf{q} \mid \mathbf{y}, W')$. Starting from the joint in equation 2.12, it is straightforward to show that had both the sensor signals and the state from which each source is drawn been known, the sources would have a gaussian density,

$$p(\mathbf{x} \mid \mathbf{q}, \mathbf{y}) = \mathcal{G} \left[\mathbf{x} - \rho_{\mathbf{q}}(\mathbf{y}), \Sigma_{\mathbf{q}} \right], \qquad (A.6)$$

with covariance matrix and mean given by

$$\Sigma_{\mathbf{q}} = (H^T \Lambda^{-1} H + V_{\mathbf{q}}^{-1})^{-1}, \quad \rho_{\mathbf{q}}(\mathbf{y}) = \Sigma_{\mathbf{q}} (H^T \Lambda^{-1} \mathbf{y} + V_{\mathbf{q}}^{-1} \mu_{\mathbf{q}}). \quad (A.7)$$

Note that the mean depends linearly on the data.

The posterior probability of the source states given the sensor data can be obtained from equations 2.9 and 2.14 via

$$p(\mathbf{q} \mid \mathbf{y}) = \frac{p(\mathbf{q}) p(\mathbf{y} \mid \mathbf{q})}{\sum_{\mathbf{q}'} p(\mathbf{q}') p(\mathbf{y} \mid \mathbf{q}')}. \qquad (A.8)$$

We are now able to compute the conditional source averages. From equation A.6, we have

$$\langle \mathbf{x} \mid \mathbf{q}, \mathbf{y} \rangle = \rho_{\mathbf{q}}(\mathbf{y}), \qquad \langle \mathbf{x}\mathbf{x}^T \mid \mathbf{q}, \mathbf{y} \rangle = \Sigma_{\mathbf{q}} + \rho_{\mathbf{q}}(\mathbf{y}) \rho_{\mathbf{q}}(\mathbf{y})^T. \qquad (A.9)$$

To obtain the conditional averages given only the sensors (see equation A.2), we sum equation A.9 over the states $\mathbf{q}$ with probabilities $p(\mathbf{q} \mid \mathbf{y})$

(see equation A.8) to get

$$\langle m(\mathbf{x}) \mid \mathbf{y} \rangle = \sum_{\mathbf{q}} p(\mathbf{q} \mid \mathbf{y}) \langle m(\mathbf{x}) \mid \mathbf{q}, \mathbf{y} \rangle, \tag{A.10}$$

taking $m(\mathbf{x}) = \mathbf{x}, \mathbf{x}\mathbf{x}^T$. We point out that the corresponding source posterior density, given by $p(\mathbf{x} \mid \mathbf{y}) = \sum_{\mathbf{q}} p(\mathbf{q} \mid \mathbf{y}) p(\mathbf{x} \mid \mathbf{q}, \mathbf{y})$, is a coadaptive MOG, just like the sensor density $p(\mathbf{y})$ (see equation 2.13). Notice that the sums over $\mathbf{q}$ in equations A.8 and A.10 mean $\sum_{q_1} \sum_{q_2} \cdots \sum_{q_L}$.

Individual source averages (in equation A.4) appear in equation A.3 together with the corresponding state posterior, and their product is given by summing over all the other sources,

$$p(q_i \mid \mathbf{y}) \langle m(x_i) \mid q_i, \mathbf{y} \rangle = \sum_{\{q_j\}_{j \neq i}} p(\mathbf{q} \mid \mathbf{y}) \langle m(x_i) \mid \mathbf{q}, \mathbf{y} \rangle, \tag{A.11}$$

and using the results of equations A.8 and A.9.

Finally, the individual state posterior appearing in equation A.5 is similarly obtained from equation A.8:

$$p(q_i \mid \mathbf{y}) = \sum_{\{q_j\}_{j \neq i}} p(\mathbf{q} \mid \mathbf{y}). \tag{A.12}$$

We emphasize that all the parameters appearing in equations A.6 through A.12 belong to W'. Substituting these expressions in equations A.1, A.3, and A.5 and adding them up completes the E-step, which yields $\mathcal{F}(W', W)$.

A.2 M-Step. To derive the EM learning rules we must minimize $\mathcal{F}(W', W)$ obtained above with respect to W. This can be done by first computing its gradient $\partial \mathcal{F} / \partial W$ layer by layer. For the visible-layer parameters we have

$$\frac{\partial \mathcal{F}_V}{\partial \mathbf{H}} = \mathbf{\Lambda}^{-1} \mathbf{y} \langle \mathbf{x}^T \mid \mathbf{y} \rangle - \mathbf{\Lambda}^{-1} \mathbf{H} \langle \mathbf{x}\mathbf{x}^T \mid \mathbf{y} \rangle,$$

$$\frac{\partial \mathcal{F}_V}{\partial \mathbf{\Lambda}} = -\frac{1}{2} \mathbf{\Lambda}^{-1}$$

$$+ \frac{1}{2} \mathbf{\Lambda}^{-1} \left(\mathbf{y}\mathbf{y}^T - 2\mathbf{y}\langle \mathbf{x}^T \mid \mathbf{y} \rangle \mathbf{H}^T + \mathbf{H}\langle \mathbf{x}\mathbf{x}^T \mid \mathbf{y} \rangle \mathbf{H}^T \right) \mathbf{\Lambda}^{-1}, \tag{A.13}$$

whereas for the bottom hidden layer, we have

$$\frac{\partial \mathcal{F}_B}{\partial \mu_{i,q_i}} = -\frac{1}{v_{i,q_i}} p(q_i \mid \mathbf{y}) \left(\langle x_i \mid q_i, \mathbf{y} \rangle - \mu_{i,q_i} \right),$$

$$\frac{\partial \mathcal{F}_B}{\partial v_{i,q_i}} = -\frac{1}{2 v_{i,q_i}^2} p(q_i \mid \mathbf{y}) (\langle x_i^2 \mid q_i, \mathbf{y} \rangle - 2 \langle x_i \mid q_i, \mathbf{y} \rangle \mu_{i,q_i}$$

$$+ \mu_{i,q_i}^2 - v_{i,q_i}). \tag{A.14}$$

In computing the gradient with respect to the top hidden-layer parameters, we should ensure that being probabilities $w_{i,q_i} = p(q_i)$, they satisfy the nonnegativity $w_{i,q_i} \geq 0$ and normalization $\sum_{q_i} w_{i,q_i} = 1$ constraints. Both can be enforced automatically by working with new parameters $\bar{w}_{i,q_i}$, related to the mixing proportions through

$$w_{i,q_i} = \frac{e^{\bar{w}_{i,q_i}}}{\sum\limits_{q_i'} e^{\bar{w}_{i,q_i'}}}. \tag{A.15}$$

The gradient is then taken with respect to the new parameters:

$$\frac{\partial \mathcal{F}_T}{\partial \bar{w}_{i,q_i}} = -p(q_i \mid \mathbf{y}) + w_{i,q_i}. \tag{A.16}$$

Recall that the conditional source averages and state probabilities depend on W' and that the equations A.13 through A.16 include averaging over the observed $\mathbf{y}$. We now set the new parameters W to the values that make the gradient vanish, obtaining the IF learning rules (see equations 3.12 and 3.13).

Appendix B: Variational IFA: Derivation of the Mean-Field Equations

To derive the mean-field equations 6.7 through 6.9 we start from the approximate error $\mathcal{F}(\tau, W)$ (equation 6.1) using the factorial posterior (equation 6.2). The approximate error is composed of the three-layer contributions and the negative entropy of the posterior, as in equation 3.8. $\mathcal{F}_V$, $\mathcal{F}_B$, and $\mathcal{F}_T$ are given by equations A.1, A.3, and A.5, with the conditional source means and densities expressed in terms of the variational parameters τ via equations 6.4 and 6.5.

The last term in $\mathcal{F}$ is given by

$$\mathcal{F}_H(\tau) = \sum_{i=1}^{L} \sum_{q_i=1}^{n_i} \kappa_{i,q_i} \left(\frac{1}{2} \log \xi_{i,q_i} - \log \kappa_{i,q_i} \right) + Const., \tag{B.1}$$

where *Const.* reflects the fact that the source posterior is normalized. $\mathcal{F}_H$ is obtained by using the factorial posterior (see equation 6.2) in equation 3.10. Since this term does not depend on the generative parameters W, it did not contribute to the exact EM algorithm but is crucial for the variational approximation.

To minimize $\mathcal{F}$ with respect to τ we compute its gradient $\partial \mathcal{F} / \partial \tau$:

$$\frac{\partial \mathcal{F}}{\partial \xi_{i,q_i}} = -\frac{1}{2} \left(\bar{H}_{ii} + \frac{1}{v_{i,q_i}} - \frac{1}{\xi_{i,q_i}} \right) \kappa_{i,q_i},$$

$$\frac{\partial \mathcal{F}}{\psi_{i,q_i}} = \left[(\mathbf{H}^T \mathbf{\Lambda}^{-1}\mathbf{y})_i + \frac{\mu_{i,q_i}}{v_{i,q_i}} - \sum_{j \neq i} \sum_{q_j=1}^{n_j} \bar{H}_{ij}\kappa_{i,q_j}\psi_{j,q_j} \right.$$

$$\left. - \left(\bar{H}_{ii} + \frac{1}{v_{i,q_i}} \right) \psi_{i,q_i} \right] \kappa_{i,q_i},$$

$$\frac{\partial \mathcal{F}}{\kappa_{i,q_i}} = -\log \kappa_{i,q_i} + \log w_{i,q_i} + \frac{1}{2}\left(\log \xi_{i,q_i} + \frac{\psi_{i,q_i}^2}{\xi_{i,q_i}} \right)$$

$$- \frac{1}{2}\left(\log v_{i,q_i} + \frac{\mu_{i,q_i}^2 + \xi_{i,q_i}}{v_{i,q_i}} \right) - \frac{1}{2}\bar{H}_{ii}\xi_{i,q_i} + z_i. \tag{B.2}$$

The first equation leads directly to equation 6.7. The second and third equations, after a bit of simplification using equation 6.7, lead to equations 6.8 and 6.9. The z_i reflect the normalization of the mixing proportions κ_{i,q_i}: to impose normalization, we actually minimize $\mathcal{F} + \sum_i z_i(\sum_{q_i} \kappa_{i,q_i} - 1)$ using the method of Lagrange multipliers.

Appendix C: Noiseless IFA: Derivation of the GEM Algorithm

In this appendix we derive the GEM learning rules for the noiseless case (see equation 7.1). This derivation follows the same steps as the one in appendix A.

C.1 E-Step. By substituting $p(x_i \mid q_i) = \mathcal{G}(x_i - \mu_i, v_i)$ in equation 7.6, we get for the bottom layer

$$\mathcal{F}_B = \sum_{i=1}^{L} \sum_{q_i=1}^{n_i} p(q_i \mid x_i, W') \left[\frac{1}{2}\log v_{i,q_i} + \frac{(x_i - \mu_{i,q_i})^2}{2v_{i,q_i}} \right], \tag{C.1}$$

whereas for the top layer we have

$$\mathcal{F}_T = -\sum_{i=1}^{L} \sum_{q_i=1}^{n_i} p(q_i \mid x_i, W') \log w_{i,q_i}. \tag{C.2}$$

Note that unlike $\mathcal{F}_B$ in the noisy case, no conditional source means should be computed. The posterior probability of the ith source states is obtained from Bayes' rule:

$$p(q_i \mid x_i) = \frac{p(x_i \mid q_i)p(q_i)}{\sum_{q_i'} p(x_i \mid q_i')p(q_i')}. \tag{C.3}$$

C.2 M-Step. To derive the learning rule for the unmixing matrix $\mathbf{G}$, we use the error gradient

$$\frac{\partial \mathcal{F}}{\partial \mathbf{G}} = -\left(\mathbf{G}^T\right)^{-1} + \phi(\mathbf{x})\mathbf{y}^T, \tag{C.4}$$

where $\phi(\mathbf{x})$ is given by equation 7.9. To determine the increment of $\mathbf{G}$ we use the relative gradient of the approximate error,

$$\delta \mathbf{G} = -\eta \frac{\partial \mathcal{F}}{\partial \mathbf{G}} \mathbf{G}^T \mathbf{G} = \eta \mathbf{G} - \eta \phi(\mathbf{x})\mathbf{x}^T \mathbf{G}. \tag{C.5}$$

Since the extremum condition $\delta \mathbf{G} = 0$, implying $E\phi(\mathbf{Gy})\mathbf{y}^T\mathbf{G}^T = \mathbf{I}$, is not analytically solvable, equation C.5 leads to the iterative rule of equation 7.8.

As explained in Amari et al. (1996), Cardoso and Laheld (1996), and MacKay (1996), the relative gradient has an advantage over the ordinary gradient since the algorithm it produces is equivariant; its performance is independent of the rank of the mixing matrix, and its computational cost is lower since it does not require matrix inversion.

The learning rules (see equation 3.13) for the MOG source parameters are obtained from the gradient of the bottom- and top-layer contributions,

$$\frac{\partial \mathcal{F}_B}{\partial \mu_{i,q_i}} = -\frac{1}{v_{i,q_i}} p(q_i \mid x_i)(x_i - \mu_{i,q_i}),$$

$$\frac{\partial \mathcal{F}_B}{\partial v_{i,q_i}} = -\frac{1}{2v_{i,q_i}} p(q_i \mid x_i)\left[(x_i - \mu_{i,q_i})^2 - v_{i,q_i}\right],$$

$$\frac{\partial \mathcal{F}_T}{\partial \bar{w}_{i,q_i}} = -p(q_i \mid x_i) + w_{i,q_i}, \tag{C.6}$$

where the last line was obtained using equation A.15.

Acknowledgments

I thank B. Bonham, K. Miller, S. Nagarajan, T. Troyer, and especially V. deSa, for useful discussions. Thanks are also due to two anonymous referees for very helpful suggestions. Research was supported by the Office of Naval Research (N00014-94-1-0547), NIDCD (R01-02260), and the Sloan Foundation.

References

Amari, S., Cichocki, A., & Yang, H. H. (1996). A new learning algorithm for blind signal separation. In D. S. Touretzky, M. C. Mozer, & M. E. Hasselmo (Eds.), *Advances in neural information processing systems, 8* (pp. 757–763). Cambridge, MA: MIT Press.

Attias, H., & Schreiner, C. E. (1998). Blind source separation and deconvolution: The dynamic component analysis algorithm. *Neural Computation 10*, 1373–1424.

Bell, A. J., & Sejnowski, T. J. (1995). An information-maximization approach to blind separation and blind deconvolution. *Neural Computation, 7*, 1129–1159.

Belouchrani, A., & Cardoso, J.-F. (1994). Maximum likelihood source separation for discrete sources. In *Proc. EUSIPCO*, 768–771.

Bishop, C. M., Svensén, M., & Williams, C. K. I. (1998). GTM: The generative topographic mapping. *Neural Computation, 10*, 215–234.

Cardoso, J.-F. (1997). Infomax and maximum likelihood for source separation. *IEEE Signal Processing Letters, 4*, 112–114.

Cardoso, J.-F., & Laheld, B. H. (1996). Equivariant adaptive source separation. *IEEE Transactions on Signal Processing, 44*, 3017–3030.

Comon, P., Jutten, C., & Hérault, J. (1991). Blind separation of sources, Part II: Problem statement. *Signal Processing, 24*, 11–20.

Comon, P. (1994). Independent component analysis: a new concept? *Signal Processing, 36*, 287–314.

Cover, T.M., & Thomas, J. A. (1991). *Elements of information theory.* New York: Wiley.

Dayan, P., Hinton, G., Neal, R., & Zemel, R. (1995). The Helmholtz machine. *Neural Computation, 7*, 889–904.

Dempster, A. P., Laird, N. M., & Rubin, D. B. (1977). Maximum likelihood from incomplete data via the EM algorithm (with discussion). *Journal of the Royal Statistical Society B, 39*, 1–38.

Everitt, B. S. (1984). *An introduction to latent variable models.* London: Chapman & Hall.

Friedman, J. H., & Stuetzle, W. (1981). Projection pursuit regression. *Journal of the American Statistical Association, 76*, 817–823.

Ghahramani, Z. (1995). Factorial learning and the EM algorithm. In G. Tesauro, D. S. Touretzky, & J. Alspector (Eds.), *Advances in neural information processing systems, 7* (pp. 617–624). San Mateo, CA: Morgan Kaufmann.

Ghahramani, Z., & Jordan, M. I. (1997). Factorial hidden Markov models. *Machine Learning, 29*, 245–273.

Hastie, T. J., & Tibshirani, R. J. (1990). *Generalized additive models.* London: Chapman & Hall.

Hinton, G. E., Dayan, P., Frey, B. J., & Neal, R. M. (1995). The "wake-sleep" algorithm for unsupervised neural networks. *Science, 268*, 1158–1161.

Hinton, G. E., Williams, C. K. I., & Revow, M. D. (1992). Adaptive elastic models for hand-printed character recognition. In J. E. Moody, S. J. Hanson, & P. P. Lippmann (Eds.), *Advances in neural information processing systems, 4* (pp. 512–519). San Mateo, CA: Morgan Kaufmann.

Hinton, G. E., & Zemel, R. S. (1994). Autoencoders, minimum description length, and Helmholtz free energy. In J. D. Cowan, G. Tesauro, & J. Alspector (Eds.), *Advances in neural information processing systems, 6* (pp. 3–10). San Mateo, CA: Morgan Kaufmann.

Huber, P. J. (1985). Projection pursuit. *Annals of Statistics, 13*, 435–475.

Hyvärinen, A., & Oja, E. (1997). A fast fixed-point algorithm for independent component analysis. *Neural Computation, 9*, 1483–1492.

Jordan, M. I., & Jacobs, R. A. (1994). Hierarchical mixtures of experts and the EM algorithm. *Neural Computation, 6*, 181–214.

Jutten, C., and Hérault, J. (1991). Blind separation of sources, part I: An adaptive algorithm based on neuromimetic architecture. *Signal Processing, 24*, 1–10.

Lee, T.-W., Bell, A. J., & Lambert, R. (1997). Blind separation of delayed and convolved sources. In M. C. Mozer, M. I. Jordan, & T. Petsche (Eds.), *Advances in neural information processing systems, 9* (pp. 758–764). Cambridge, MA: MIT Press.

Lewicki, M. S., & Sejnowski, T. J. (1998). Learning nonlinear overcomplete representations for efficient coding. In M. Kearns, M. Jordan, & S. Solla (Eds.), *Advances in neural information processing systems, 10* (pp. 556–562). Cambridge, MA: MIT Press.

Lewicki, M. S., & Olshausen, B. A. (1998). Inferring sparse, overcomplete image codes using an efficient coding framework. In M. Kearns, M. Jordan, & S. Solla (Eds.), *Advances in neural information processing systems, 10* (pp. 815–821). Cambridge, MA: MIT Press.

MacKay, D. J. C. (1992). Bayesian interpolation. *Neural Computation, 4*, 415–447.

MacKay, D. J. C. (1996). *Maximum likelihood and covariant algorithms for independent component analysis* (Tech. Rep.) Cambridge: Cavendish Laboratory, Cambridge University.

Moulines, E., Cardoso, J.-P., & Gassiat, E. (1997). Maximum likelihood for blind separation and deconvolution of noisy signals using mixture models. In *Proceedings of IEEE Conference on Acoustics, Speech, and Signal Processing 1997* (Vol. 5, pp. 3617–3620). New York: IEEE.

Neal, R. M., and Hinton, G. E. (1998). A view of the EM algorithm that justifies incremental, sparse, and other variants. In M. I. Jordan (Ed.), *Learning in graphical models*, pp. 355–368. Norwell, MA: Kluwer Academic Press.

Olshausen, B. A. (1996). *Learning linear, sparse, factorial codes.* (Tech. Rep. AI Memo 1580, CBCL 138). Cambridge, MA: Artificial Intelligence Lab, MIT.

Olshausen, B. A., & Field, D. J. (1996). Emergence of simple-cell receptive field properties by learning a sparse code for natural images. *Nature, 381* 607–609.

Olshausen, B. A., & Field, D. J. (1997). Sparse coding with an overcomplete basis set: A strategy employed by V1? *Vision Research, 37*, 3311–3325.

Pearlmutter, B. A., & Parra, L. C. (1997). Maximum likelihood blind source separation: A context-sensitive generalization of ICA. In M. C. Mozer, M. I. Jordan, & T. Petsche (Eds.), *Advances in neural information processing systems, 9* (pp. 613–619). Cambridge, MA: MIT Press. .

Pham, D. T. (1996). Blind separation of instantaneous mixture of sources via an independent component analysis. *IEEE Transactions on Signal Processing, 44*, 2768–2779.

Roweis, S. (1998). EM algorithms for PCA and SPCA. In M. Kearns, M. Jordan, & S. Solla (Eds.), *Advances in neural information processing systems, 10* (pp. 626–632). Cambridge, MA: MIT Press.

Roweis, S., & Ghahramani, Z. (1997). *A unifying review of linear gaussian models.*

Neural Computation 11, 297–337.

Rubin, D., & Thayer, D. (1982). EM algorithms for ML factor analysis. *Psychometrika, 47*, 69–76.

Saul, L., & Jordan, M. I. (1995). Exploiting tractable structures in intractable networks. In D. S. Touretzky, M. C. Mozer, & M. E. Hasselmo (Eds.), *Advances in neural information processing systems, 8* (pp. 486–492). Cambridge, MA: MIT Press.

Saul, L. K., Jaakkola, T., & Jordan, M. I. (1996). Mean field theory of sigmoid belief networks. *Journal of Artificial Intelligence Research, 4*, 61–76.

Tipping, M. E., and Bishop, C. M. (1997). *Probabilistic principal component analysis* (Tech. Report NCRG/97/010). Aston University, U.K.

Torkkola, K. (1996). Blind separation of convolved sources based on information maximization. In *Neural Networks for Signal Processing VI*. New York: IEEE.

11

Hierarchical Mixtures of Experts and the EM Algorithm

Michael I. Jordan
Department of Brain and Cognitive Sciences,
Massachusetts Institute of Technology, Cambridge, MA 02139 USA

Robert A. Jacobs
Department of Psychology, University of Rochester,
Rochester, NY 14627 USA

We present a tree-structured architecture for supervised learning. The statistical model underlying the architecture is a hierarchical mixture model in which both the mixture coefficients and the mixture components are generalized linear models (GLIM's). Learning is treated as a maximum likelihood problem; in particular, we present an Expectation–Maximization (EM) algorithm for adjusting the parameters of the architecture. We also develop an on-line learning algorithm in which the parameters are updated incrementally. Comparative simulation results are presented in the robot dynamics domain.

1 Introduction

The principle of divide-and-conquer is a principle with wide applicability throughout applied mathematics. Divide-and-conquer algorithms attack a complex problem by dividing it into simpler problems whose solutions can be combined to yield a solution to the complex problem. This approach can often lead to simple, elegant, and efficient algorithms. In this paper we explore a particular application of the divide-and-conquer principle to the problem of learning from examples. We describe a network architecture and a learning algorithm for the architecture, both of which are inspired by the philosophy of divide-and-conquer.

In the statistical literature and in the machine learning literature, divide-and-conquer approaches have become increasingly popular. The CART algorithm of Breiman *et al.* (1984), the MARS algorithm of Friedman (1991), and the ID3 algorithm of Quinlan (1986) are well-known examples. These algorithms fit surfaces to data by explicitly dividing the input space into a nested sequence of regions, and by fitting simple surfaces (e.g., constant functions) within these regions. They have convergence times that are often orders of magnitude faster than gradient-based neural network algorithms.

Although divide-and-conquer algorithms have much to recommend them, one should be concerned about the statistical consequences of dividing the input space. Dividing the data can have favorable consequences for the bias of an estimator, but it generally increases the variance. Consider linear regression, for example, in which the variance of the estimates of the slope and intercept depends quadratically on the spread of data on the x-axis. The points that are the most peripheral in the input space are those that have the maximal effect in decreasing the variance of the parameter estimates.

The foregoing considerations suggest that divide-and-conquer algorithms generally tend to be variance-increasing algorithms. This is indeed the case and is particularly problematic in high-dimensional spaces where data become exceedingly sparse (Scott 1992). One response to this dilemma—that adopted by CART, MARS, and ID3, and also adopted here—is to utilize piecewise constant or piecewise linear functions. These functions minimize variance at a cost of increased bias. We also make use of a second variance-decreasing device; a device familiar in the neural network literature. We make use of "soft" splits of data (Bridle 1989; Nowlan 1991; Wahba *et al.* 1993), allowing data to lie simultaneously in multiple regions. This approach allows the parameters in one region to be influenced by data in neighboring regions. CART, MARS, and ID3 rely on "hard" splits, which, as we remarked above, have particularly severe effects on variance. By allowing soft splits the severe effects of lopping off distant data can be ameliorated. We also attempt to minimize the bias that is incurred by using piecewise linear functions, by allowing the splits to be formed along hyperplanes at arbitrary orientations in the input space. This lessens the bias due to high-order interactions among the inputs and allows the algorithm to be insensitive to the particular choice of coordinates used to encode the data (an improvement over methods such as MARS and ID3, which are coordinate-dependent).

The work that we describe here makes contact with a number of branches of statistical theory. First, as in our earlier work (Jacobs *et al.* 1991), we formulate the learning problem as a mixture estimation problem (cf. Cheeseman *et al.* 1988; Duda and Hart 1973; Nowlan 1991; Redner and Walker 1984; Titterington *et al.* 1985). We show that the algorithm that is generally employed for the *unsupervised* learning of mixture parameters—the Expectation–Maximization (EM) algorithm of Dempster *et al.* (1977)—can also be exploited for *supervised* learning. Second, we utilize generalized linear model (GLIM) theory (McCullagh and Nelder 1983) to provide the basic statistical structure for the components of the architecture. In particular, the "soft splits" referred to above are modeled as *multinomial logit* models—a specific form of GLIM. We also show that the algorithm developed for fitting GLIMs—the iteratively reweighted least squares (IRLS) algorithm—can be usefully employed in our model, in particular as the M step of the EM algorithm. Finally, we show that these ideas can be developed in a recursive manner, yielding a tree-structured approach to estimation that is reminiscent of CART, MARS, and ID3.

The remainder of the paper proceeds as follows. We first introduce the hierarchical mixture-of-experts architecture and present the likelihood function for the architecture. After describing a gradient descent algorithm, we develop a more powerful learning algorithm for the architecture that is a special case of the general Expectation–Maximization (EM) framework of Dempster *et al.* (1977). We also describe a least-squares version of this algorithm that leads to a particularly efficient implementation. Both of the latter algorithms are batch learning algorithms. In the final section, we present an on-line version of the least-squares algorithm that in practice appears to be the most efficient of the algorithms that we have studied.

2 Hierarchical Mixtures of Experts

The algorithms that we discuss in this paper are supervised learning algorithms. We explicitly address the case of regression, in which the input vectors are elements of $\Re^m$ and the output vectors are elements of $\Re^n$. We also consider classification models and counting models in which the outputs are integer-valued. The data are assumed to form a countable set of paired observations $\mathcal{X} = \{(\mathbf{x}^{(t)}, \mathbf{y}^{(t)})\}$. In the case of the *batch* algorithms discussed below, this set is assumed to be finite; in the case of the *on-line* algorithms, the set may be infinite.

We propose to solve nonlinear supervised learning problems by dividing the input space into a nested set of regions and fitting simple surfaces to the data that fall in these regions. The regions have "soft" boundaries, meaning that data points may lie simultaneously in multiple regions. The boundaries between regions are themselves simple parameterized surfaces that are adjusted by the learning algorithm.

The hierarchical mixture-of-experts (HME) architecture is shown in Figure 1.[1] The architecture is a tree in which the *gating networks* sit at the nonterminals of the tree. These networks receive the vector $\mathbf{x}$ as input and produce scalar outputs that are a partition of unity at each point in the input space. The *expert networks* sit at the leaves of the tree. Each expert produces an output vector $\mathbf{\mu}_{ij}$ for each input vector. These output vectors proceed up the tree, being blended by the gating network outputs.

All of the expert networks in the tree are linear with a single output nonlinearity. We will refer to such a network as "generalized linear," borrowing the terminology from statistics (McCullagh and Nelder 1983).

---

[1]To simplify the presentation, we restrict ourselves to a two-level hierarchy throughout the paper. All of the algorithms that we describe, however, generalize readily to hierarchies of arbitrary depth. See Jordan and Xu (1993) for a recursive formalism that handles arbitrary hierarchies.

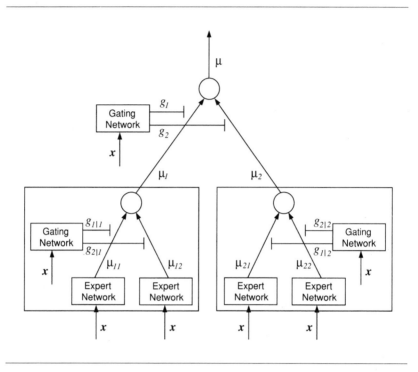

Figure 1: A two-level hierarchical mixture of experts. To form a deeper tree, each expert is expanded recursively into a gating network and a set of subexperts.

Expert network (i, j) produces its output μ_{ij} as a generalized linear function of the input **x**:

$$\mu_{ij} = f(U_{ij}\mathbf{x}) \tag{2.1}$$

where U_{ij} is a weight matrix and f is a fixed continuous nonlinearity. The vector **x** is assumed to include a fixed component of one to allow for an intercept term.

For regression problems, $f(\cdot)$ is generally chosen to be the identity function (i.e., the experts are linear). For binary classification problems, $f(\cdot)$ is generally taken to be the logistic function, in which case the expert outputs are interpreted as the log odds of "success" under a Bernoulli probability model (see below). Other models (e.g., multiway classification, counting, rate estimation, and survival estimation) are handled by making other choices for $f(\cdot)$. These models are smoothed piecewise analogs of the corresponding GLIM models (cf. McCullagh and Nelder 1983).

The gating networks are also generalized linear. Define intermediate variables ξ_i as follows:

$$\xi_i = \mathbf{v}_i^T \mathbf{x} \tag{2.2}$$

where $\mathbf{v}_i$ is a weight vector. Then the ith output of the top-level gating network is the "softmax" function of the ξ_i (Bridle 1989; McCullagh and Nelder 1983):

$$g_i = \frac{e^{\xi_i}}{\sum_k e^{\xi_k}} \tag{2.3}$$

Note that the g_i are positive and sum to one for each $\mathbf{x}$. They can be interpreted as providing a "soft" partitioning of the input space.

Similarly, the gating networks at lower levels are also generalized linear systems. Define ξ_{ij} as follows:

$$\xi_{ij} = \mathbf{v}_{ij}^T \mathbf{x} \tag{2.4}$$

Then

$$g_{j|i} = \frac{e^{\xi_{ij}}}{\sum_k e^{\xi_{ik}}} \tag{2.5}$$

is the output of the jth unit in the ith gating network at the second level of the architecture. Once again, the $g_{j|i}$ are positive and sum to one for each $\mathbf{x}$. They can be interpreted as providing a "soft" sub-partition of the input space nested within the partitioning providing by the higher-level gating network.

The output vector at each nonterminal of the tree is the weighted output of the experts below that nonterminal. That is, the output at the ith nonterminal in the second layer of the two-level tree is

$$\mu_i = \sum_j g_{j|i} \mu_{ij}$$

and the output at the top level of the tree is

$$\mu = \sum_i g_i \mu_i$$

Note that both the g's and the μ's depend on the input $\mathbf{x}$, thus the total output is a nonlinear function of the input.

2.1 Regression Surface. Given the definitions of the expert networks and the gating networks, the regression surface defined by the hierarchy is a piecewise blend of the regression surfaces defined by the experts. The gating networks provide a nested, "soft" partitioning of the input space and the expert networks provide local regression surfaces within the partition. There is overlap between neighboring regions. To understand the nature of the overlap, consider a one-level hierarchy with two expert networks. In this case, the gating network has two outputs, g_1 and g_2. The gating output g_1 is given by

$$g_1 = \frac{e^{\xi_1}}{e^{\xi_1} + e^{\xi_2}} \tag{2.6}$$

$$= \frac{1}{1 + e^{-(\mathbf{v}_1 - \mathbf{v}_2)^T \mathbf{x}}} \tag{2.7}$$

which is a logistic ridge function whose orientation is determined by the direction of the vector $\mathbf{v}_1 - \mathbf{v}_2$. The gating output g_2 is equal to $1 - g_1$. For a given $\mathbf{x}$, the total output μ is the convex combination $g_1\mu_1 + g_2\mu_2$. This is a weighted average of the experts, where the weights are determined by the values of the ridge function. Along the ridge, $g_1 = g_2 = 1/2$, and both experts contribute equally. Away from the ridge, one expert or the other dominates. The amount of smoothing across the ridge is determined by the magnitude of the vector $\mathbf{v}_2 - \mathbf{v}_1$. If $\mathbf{v}_2 - \mathbf{v}_1$ is large, then the ridge function becomes a sharp split and the weighted output of the experts becomes piecewise (generalized) linear. If $\mathbf{v}_2 - \mathbf{v}_1$ is small, then each expert contributes to a significant degree on each side of the ridge, thereby smoothing the piecewise map. In the limit of a zero difference vector, $g_1 = g_2 = 1/2$ for all $\mathbf{x}$, and the total output is the same fixed average of the experts on both sides of the fictitious "split."

In general, a given gating network induces a smoothed planar partitioning of the input space. Lower-level gating networks induce a partition within the partition induced by higher-level gating networks. The weights in a given gating network determine the amount of smoothing across the partition at that particular level of resolution: large weight vectors imply sharp changes in the regression surface across a ridge and small weights imply a smoother surface. In the limit of zero weights in all gating networks, the entire hierarchy reduces to a fixed average (a linear system in the case of regression).

2.2 A Probability Model. The hierarchy can be given a probabilistic interpretation. We suppose that the mechanism by which data are generated by the environment involves a nested sequence of decisions that terminates in a regressive process that maps $\mathbf{x}$ to $\mathbf{y}$. The decisions are modeled as multinomial random variables. That is, for each $\mathbf{x}$, we interpret the values $g_i(\mathbf{x}, \mathbf{v}_i^0)$ as the multinomial probabilities associated with the first decision and the $g_{j|i}(\mathbf{x}, \mathbf{v}_{ij}^0)$ as the (conditional) multinomial probabilities associated with the second decision, where the superscript "0" refers to the "true" values of the parameters. The decisions form a decision tree. We use a statistical model to model this decision tree; in particular, our choice of parameterization (cf. Equations 2.2, 2.3, 2.4, and 2.5) corresponds to a *multinomial logit* probability model at each nonterminal of the tree (see Appendix B). A multinomial logit model is a special case of a GLIM that is commonly used for "soft" multiway classification (McCullagh and Nelder 1983). Under the multinomial logit model, we interpret the gating networks as modeling the input-dependent, multi-nomial probabilities associated with decisions at particular levels of res-olution in a tree-structured model of the data.

Once a particular sequence of decisions has been made, resulting in a choice of regressive process (i,j), output $\mathbf{y}$ is assumed to be generated according to the following statistical model. First, a linear predictor η_{ij} is formed:

$$\eta_{ij}^0 = U_{ij}^0 \mathbf{x}$$

The expected value of $\mathbf{y}$ is obtained by passing the linear predictor through the *link function* f:[2]

$$\mu_{ij}^0 = f(\eta_{ij}^0)$$

The output $\mathbf{y}$ is then chosen from a probability density P, with mean μ_{ij}^0 and "dispersion" parameter ϕ_{ij}^0. We denote the density of $\mathbf{y}$ as

$$P(\mathbf{y}|\mathbf{x}, \theta_{ij}^0)$$

where the parameter vector θ_{ij}^0 includes the weights U_{ij}^0 and the dispersion parameter ϕ_{ij}^0:

$$\theta_{ij}^0 = \left[\begin{array}{c} U_{ij}^0 \\ \phi_{ij}^0 \end{array} \right]$$

We assume the density P to be a member of the exponential family of densities (McCullagh and Nelder 1983). The interpretation of the disper-sion parameter depends on the particular choice of density. For example, in the case of the n-dimensional gaussian, the dispersion parameter is the covariance matrix Σ_{ij}^0.[3]

Given these assumptions, the total probability of generating $\mathbf{y}$ from $\mathbf{x}$ is the mixture of the probabilities of generating $\mathbf{y}$ from each of the com-ponent densities, where the mixing proportions are multinomial proba-bilities:

$$P(\mathbf{y}|\mathbf{x}, \theta^0) = \sum_i g_i(\mathbf{x}, \mathbf{v}_i^0) \sum_j g_{j|i}(\mathbf{x}, \mathbf{v}_{ij}^0) P(\mathbf{y}|\mathbf{x}, \theta_{ij}^0) \qquad (2.8)$$

Note that θ^0 includes the expert network parameters θ_{ij}^0 as well as the gating network parameters $\mathbf{v}_i^0$ and $\mathbf{v}_{ij}^0$. Note also that we have explicitly

---

[2] We utilize the neural network convention in defining links. In GLIM theory, the convention is that the link function relates η to μ; thus, $\eta = h(\mu)$, where h is equivalent to our f^{-1}.

[3] Not all exponential family densities have a dispersion parameter; in particular, the Bernoulli density discussed below has no dispersion parameter.

indicated the dependence of the probabilities g_i and $g_{j|i}$ on the input $\mathbf{x}$ and on the parameters. In the remainder of the paper we drop the explicit reference to the input and the parameters to simplify the notation:

$$P(\mathbf{y}|\mathbf{x}, \theta^0) = \sum_i g_i^0 \sum_j g_{j|i}^0 P_{ij}^0(\mathbf{y}) \tag{2.9}$$

We also utilize equation 2.9 without the superscripts to refer to the probability model defined by a particular HME architecture, irrespective of any reference to a "true" model.

2.2.1 Example (Regression). In the case of regression the probabilistic component of the model is generally assumed to be gaussian. Assuming identical covariance matrices of the form $\sigma^2 I$ for each of the experts yields the following hierarchical probability model:

$$P(\mathbf{y}|\mathbf{x}, \theta) = \frac{1}{(2\pi)^{n/2}\sigma^n} \sum_i g_i \sum_j g_{j|i} e^{-(1/2\sigma^2)(\mathbf{y}-\mu_{ij})^T(\mathbf{y}-\mu_{ij})}$$

2.2.2 Example (Binary Classification). In binary classification problems the output y is a discrete random variable having possible outcomes of "failure" and "success." The probabilistic component of the model is generally assumed to be the Bernoulli distribution (Cox 1970). In this case, the mean μ_{ij} is the conditional probability of classifying the input as "success." The resulting hierarchical probability model is a mixture of Bernoulli densities:

$$P(y|\mathbf{x}, \theta) = \sum_i g_i \sum_j g_{j|i} \mu_{ij}^y (1 - \mu_{ij})^{1-y}$$

2.3 Posterior Probabilities. In developing the learning algorithms to be presented in the remainder of the paper, it will prove useful to define posterior probabilities associated with the nodes of the tree. The terms "posterior" and "prior" have meaning in this context during the training of the system. We refer to the probabilities g_i and $g_{j|i}$ as *prior* probabilities, because they are computed based only on the input $\mathbf{x}$, without knowledge of the corresponding target output $\mathbf{y}$. A *posterior* probability is defined once both the input and the target output are known. Using Bayes' rule, we define the posterior probabilities at the nodes of the tree as follows:

$$h_i = \frac{g_i \sum_j g_{j|i} P_{ij}(\mathbf{y})}{\sum_i g_i \sum_j g_{j|i} P_{ij}(\mathbf{y})} \tag{2.10}$$

and

$$h_{j|i} = \frac{g_{j|i} P_{ij}(\mathbf{y})}{\sum_j g_{j|i} P_{ij}(\mathbf{y})} \tag{2.11}$$

We will also find it useful to define the joint posterior probability h_{ij}, the product of h_i and $h_{j|i}$:

$$h_{ij} = \frac{g_i g_{j|i} P_{ij}(\mathbf{y})}{\sum_i g_i \sum_j g_{j|i} P_{ij}(\mathbf{y})} \tag{2.12}$$

This quantity is the probability that expert network (i, j) can be considered to have generated the data, based on knowledge of both the input and the output. Once again, we emphasize that all of these quantities are conditional on the input $\mathbf{x}$.

In deeper trees, the posterior probability associated with an expert network is simply the product of the conditional posterior probabilities along the path from the root of the tree to that expert.

2.4 The Likelihood and a Gradient Ascent Learning Algorithm. Jordan and Jacobs (1992) presented a gradient ascent learning algorithm for the hierarchical architecture. The algorithm was based on earlier work by Jacobs *et al.* (1991), who treated the problem of learning in mixture-of-experts architectures as a maximum likelihood estimation problem. The log likelihood of a data set $\mathcal{X} = \{(\mathbf{x}^{(t)}, \mathbf{y}^{(t)})\}_1^N$ is obtained by taking the log of the product of N densities of the form of equation 2.9, which yields the following log likelihood:

$$l(\boldsymbol{\theta}; \mathcal{X}) = \sum_t \ln \sum_i g_i^{(t)} \sum_j g_{j|i}^{(t)} P_{ij}(\mathbf{y}^{(t)}) \tag{2.13}$$

Let us assume that the probability density P is gaussian with an identity covariance matrix and that the link function is the identity. In this case, by differentiating $l(\boldsymbol{\theta}; \mathcal{X})$ with respect to the parameters, we obtain the following gradient ascent learning rule for the weight matrix U_{ij}:

$$\Delta U_{ij} = \rho \sum_t h_i^{(t)} h_{j|i}^{(t)} (\mathbf{y}^{(t)} - \boldsymbol{\mu}^{(t)}) \mathbf{x}^{(t)T} \tag{2.14}$$

where ρ is a learning rate. The gradient ascent learning rule for the ith weight vector in the top-level gating network is given by

$$\Delta \mathbf{v}_i = \rho \sum_t (h_i^{(t)} - g_i^{(t)}) \mathbf{x}^{(t)} \tag{2.15}$$

and the gradient ascent rule for the jth weight vector in the ith lower-level gating network is given by

$$\Delta \mathbf{v}_{ij} = \rho \sum_t h_i^{(t)} (h_{j|i}^{(t)} - g_{j|i}^{(t)}) \mathbf{x}^{(t)} \tag{2.16}$$

Updates can also be obtained for covariance matrices (Jordan and Jacobs 1992).

The algorithm given by equations 2.14, 2.15, and 2.16 is a batch learning algorithm. The corresponding on-line algorithm is obtained by simply dropping the summation sign and updating the parameters after each stimulus presentation. Thus, for example,

$$U_{ij}^{(t+1)} = U_{ij}^{(t)} + \rho h_i^{(t)} h_{j|i}^{(t)} (\mathbf{y}^{(t)} - \boldsymbol{\mu}^{(t)}) \mathbf{x}^{(t)T} \qquad (2.17)$$

is the stochastic update rule for the weights in the (i,j)th expert network based on the tth stimulus pattern.

2.5 The EM Algorithm. In the following sections we develop a learning algorithm for the HME architecture based on the Expectation–Maximization (EM) framework of Dempster *et al.* (1977). We derive an EM algorithm for the architecture that consists of the iterative solution of a coupled set of iteratively-reweighted least-squares problems.

The EM algorithm is a general technique for maximum likelihood estimation. In practice EM has been applied almost exclusively to unsupervised learning problems. This is true of the neural network literature and machine learning literature, in which EM has appeared in the context of clustering (Cheeseman *et al.* 1988; Nowlan 1991) and density estimation (Specht 1991), as well as the statistics literature, in which applications include missing data problems (Little and Rubin 1987), mixture density estimation (Redner and Walker 1984), and factor analysis (Dempster *et al.* 1977). Another unsupervised learning application is the learning problem for Hidden Markov Models, for which the Baum–Welch reestimation formulas are a special case of EM. There is nothing in the EM framework that precludes its application to regression or classification problems; however, such applications have been few.[4]

EM is an iterative approach to maximum likelihood estimation. Each iteration of an EM algorithm is composed of two steps: an Estimation (E) step and a Maximization (M) step. The M step involves the maximization of a likelihood function that is redefined in each iteration by the E step. If the algorithm simply increases the function during the M step, rather than maximizing the function, then the algorithm is referred to as a Generalized EM (GEM) algorithm. The Boltzmann learning algorithm (Hinton and Sejnowski 1986) is a neural network example of a GEM algorithm. GEM algorithms are often significantly slower to converge than EM algorithms.

An application of EM generally begins with the observation that the optimization of the likelihood function $l(\boldsymbol{\theta}; \mathcal{X})$ would be simplified if only a set of additional variables, called "missing" or "hidden" variables, were known. In this context, we refer to the observable data $\mathcal{X}$ as the "incomplete data" and posit a "complete data" set $\mathcal{Y}$ that includes the missing variables $\mathcal{Z}$. We specify a probability model that links the fictive missing variables to the actual data: $P(\mathbf{y}, \mathbf{z} | \mathbf{x}, \boldsymbol{\theta})$. The logarithm of the density P defines the "complete-data likelihood," $l_c(\boldsymbol{\theta}; \mathcal{Y})$. The original likelihood,

---

[4]An exception is the "switching regression" model of Quandt and Ramsey (1972). For further discussion of switching regression, see Jordan and Xu (1993).

$l(\boldsymbol{\theta}; \mathcal{X})$, is referred to in this context as the "incomplete-data likelihood." It is the relationship between these two likelihood functions that motivates the EM algorithm. Note that the complete-data likelihood is a random variable, because the missing variables $\mathcal{Z}$ are in fact unknown. An EM algorithm first finds the expected value of the complete-data likelihood, given the observed data and the current model. This is the E step:

$$Q(\boldsymbol{\theta}, \boldsymbol{\theta}^{(p)}) = E[l_c(\boldsymbol{\theta}; \mathcal{Y}) | \mathcal{X}]$$

where $\boldsymbol{\theta}^{(p)}$ is the value of the parameters at the pth iteration and the expectation is taken with respect to $\boldsymbol{\theta}^{(p)}$. This step yields a deterministic function Q. The M step maximizes this function with respect to $\boldsymbol{\theta}$ to find the new parameter estimates $\boldsymbol{\theta}^{(p+1)}$:

$$\boldsymbol{\theta}^{(p+1)} = \arg\max_{\boldsymbol{\theta}} Q(\boldsymbol{\theta}, \boldsymbol{\theta}^{(p)})$$

The E step is then repeated to yield an improved estimate of the complete likelihood and the process iterates.

An iterative step of EM chooses a parameter value that increases the value of Q, the expectation of the complete likelihood. What is the effect of such a step on the incomplete likelihood? Dempster *et al.* proved that an increase in Q implies an increase in the incomplete likelihood:

$$l(\boldsymbol{\theta}^{(p+1)}; \mathcal{X}) \geq l(\boldsymbol{\theta}^{(p)}; \mathcal{X})$$

Equality obtains only at the stationary points of l (Wu 1983). Thus the likelihood l increases monotonically along the sequence of parameter estimates generated by an EM algorithm. In practice this implies convergence to a local maximum.

2.6 Applying EM to the HME Architecture.
To develop an EM algorithm for the HME architecture, we must define appropriate "missing data" so as to simplify the likelihood function. We define indicator variables z_i and $z_{j|i}$, such that one and only one of the z_i is equal to one, and one and only one of the $z_{j|i}$ is equal to one. These indicator variables have an interpretation as the labels that correspond to the decisions in the probability model. We also define the indicator variable z_{ij}, which is the product of z_i and $z_{j|i}$. This variable has an interpretation as the label that specifies the expert (the regressive process) in the probability model. If the labels z_i, $z_{j|i}$, and z_{ij} were known, then the maximum likelihood problem would decouple into a separate set of regression problems for each expert network and a separate set of multiway classification problems for the gating networks. These problems would be solved independently of each other, yielding a rapid one-pass learning algorithm. Of course, the missing variables are not known, but we can specify a probability model

that links them to the observable data. This probability model can be
written in terms of the z_{ij} as follows:

$$P(\mathbf{y}^{(t)}, z_{ij}^{(t)} | \mathbf{x}^{(t)}, \boldsymbol{\theta}) = g_i^{(t)} g_{j|i}^{(t)} P_{ij}(\mathbf{y}^{(t)}) \tag{2.18}$$

$$= \prod_i \prod_j \{ g_i^{(t)} g_{j|i}^{(t)} P_{ij}(\mathbf{y}^{(t)}) \}^{z_{ij}^{(t)}} \tag{2.19}$$

using the fact that $z_{ij}^{(t)}$ is an indicator variable. Taking the logarithm of
this probability model yields the following complete-data likelihood:

$$l_c(\boldsymbol{\theta}; \mathcal{Y}) = \sum_t \sum_i \sum_j z_{ij}^{(t)} \ln\{ g_i^{(t)} g_{j|i}^{(t)} P_{ij}(\mathbf{y}^{(t)}) \} \tag{2.20}$$

$$= \sum_t \sum_i \sum_j z_{ij}^{(t)} \{ \ln g_i^{(t)} + \ln g_{j|i}^{(t)} + \ln P_{ij}(\mathbf{y}^{(t)}) \} \tag{2.21}$$

Note the relationship of the complete-data likelihood in equation 2.21
to the incomplete-data likelihood in equation 2.13. The use of the indicator variables z_{ij} has allowed the logarithm to be brought inside the
summation signs, substantially simplifying the maximization problem.
We now define the E step of the EM algorithm by taking the expectation
of the complete-data likelihood:

$$Q(\boldsymbol{\theta}, \boldsymbol{\theta}^{(p)}) = \sum_t \sum_i \sum_j h_{ij}^{(t)} \{ \ln g_i^{(t)} + \ln g_{j|i}^{(t)} + \ln P_{ij}(\mathbf{y}^{(t)}) \} \tag{2.22}$$

where we have used the fact that

$$E[z_{ij}^{(t)} | \mathcal{X}] = P(z_{ij}^{(t)} = 1 | \mathbf{y}^{(t)}, \mathbf{x}^{(t)}, \boldsymbol{\theta}^{(p)}) \tag{2.23}$$

$$= \frac{P(\mathbf{y}^{(t)} | z_{ij}^{(t)} = 1, \mathbf{x}^{(t)}, \boldsymbol{\theta}^{(p)}) P(z_{ij}^{(t)} = 1 | \mathbf{x}^{(t)}, \boldsymbol{\theta}^{(p)})}{P(\mathbf{y}^{(t)} | \mathbf{x}^{(t)}, \boldsymbol{\theta}^{(p)})} \tag{2.24}$$

$$= \frac{P(\mathbf{y}^{(t)} | \mathbf{x}^{(t)}, \boldsymbol{\theta}_{ij}^{(p)}) g_i^{(t)} g_{j|i}^{(t)}}{\sum_i g_i^{(t)} \sum_j g_{j|i}^{(t)} P(\mathbf{y}^{(t)} | \mathbf{x}^{(t)}, \boldsymbol{\theta}_{ij}^{(p)})} \tag{2.25}$$

$$= h_{ij}^{(t)} \tag{2.26}$$

(Note also that $E[z_i^{(t)} | \mathcal{X}] = h_i^{(t)}$ and $E[z_{j|i}^{(t)} | \mathcal{X}] = h_{j|i}^{(t)}$.)

The M step requires maximizing $Q(\boldsymbol{\theta}, \boldsymbol{\theta}^{(p)})$ with respect to the expert network parameters and the gating network parameters. Examining
equation 2.22, we see that the expert network parameters influence the
Q function only through the terms $h_{ij}^{(t)} \ln P_{ij}(\mathbf{y}^{(t)})$, and the gating network
parameters influence the Q function only through the terms $h_{ij}^{(t)} \ln g_i^{(t)}$ and
$h_{ij}^{(t)} \ln g_{j|i}^{(t)}$. Thus the M step reduces to the following separate maximization problems:

$$\boldsymbol{\theta}_{ij}^{(p+1)} = \arg\max_{\boldsymbol{\theta}_{ij}} \sum_t h_{ij}^{(t)} \ln P_{ij}(\mathbf{y}^{(t)}) \tag{2.27}$$

$$\mathbf{v}_i^{(p+1)} = \arg\max_{\mathbf{v}_i} \sum_t \sum_k h_k^{(t)} \ln g_k^{(t)} \tag{2.28}$$

and

$$\mathbf{v}_{ij}^{(p+1)} = \arg\max_{\mathbf{v}_{ij}} \sum_t \sum_k h_k^{(t)} \sum_l h_{l|k}^{(t)} \ln g_{l|k}^{(t)} \qquad (2.29)$$

Each of these maximization problems is itself a maximum likelihood problem. This is clearly true in the case of equation 2.27, which is simply a weighted maximum likelihood problem in the probability density P_{ij}. Given our parameterization of P_{ij}, the log likelihood in equation 2.27 is a weighted log likelihood for a GLIM. An efficient algorithm known as iteratively reweighted least-squares (IRLS) is available to solve the maximum likelihood problem for such models (McCullagh and Nelder 1983). We discuss IRLS in Appendix A.

Equation 2.28 involves maximizing the cross-entropy between the posterior probabilities $h_k^{(t)}$ and the prior probabilities $g_k^{(t)}$. This cross-entropy is the log likelihood associated with a multinomial logit probability model in which the $h_k^{(t)}$ act as the output observations (see Appendix B). Thus the maximization in equation 2.28 is also a maximum likelihood problem for a GLIM and can be solved using IRLS. The same is true of equation 2.29, which is a weighted maximum likelihood problem with output observations $h_{l|k}^{(t)}$ and observation weights $h_k^{(t)}$.

In summary, the EM algorithm that we have obtained involves a calculation of posterior probabilities in the outer loop (the E step), and the solution of a set of IRLS problems in the inner loop (the M step). We summarize the algorithm as follows:

Algorithm 1

1. For each data pair $(\mathbf{x}^{(t)}, \mathbf{y}^{(t)})$, compute the posterior probabilities $h_i^{(t)}$ and $h_{j|i}^{(t)}$ using the current values of the parameters.

2. For each expert (i, j), solve an IRLS problem with observations $\{(\mathbf{x}^{(t)}, \mathbf{y}^{(t)})\}_1^N$ and observation weights $\{h_{ij}^{(t)}\}_1^N$.

3. For each top-level gating network, solve an IRLS problem with observations $\{(\mathbf{x}^{(t)}, h_k^{(t)})\}_1^N$.

4. For each lower-level gating network, solve a weighted IRLS problem with observations $\{(\mathbf{x}^{(t)}, h_{l|k}^{(t)})\}_1^N$ and observation weights $\{h_k^{(t)}\}_1^N$.

5. Iterate using the updated parameter values.

2.7 A Least-Squares Algorithm. In the case of regression, in which a gaussian probability model and an identity link function are used, the IRLS loop for the expert networks reduces to weighted least squares, which can be solved (in one pass) by any of the standard least-squares algorithms (Golub and van Loan 1989). The gating networks still require iterative processing. Suppose, however, that we fit the parameters of the gating networks using least squares rather than maximum likelihood. In this case, we might hope to obtain an algorithm in which the gating network parameters are fit by a one-pass algorithm. To motivate this approach, note that we can express the IRLS problem for the gating networks as follows. Differentiating the cross-entropy (equation 2.28) with respect to the parameters $\mathbf{v}_i$ (using the fact that $\partial g_i/\partial \xi_j = g_i(\delta_{ij} - g_j)$, where δ_{ij} is the Kronecker delta) and setting the derivatives to zero yields the following equations:

$$\sum_t (h_i^{(t)} - g_i(\mathbf{x}^{(t)}, \mathbf{v}_i))\mathbf{x}^{(t)} = 0 \qquad (2.30)$$

which are a coupled set of equations that must be solved for each i. Similarly, for each gating network at the second level of the tree, we obtain the following equations:

$$\sum_t h_i^{(t)} (h_{j|i}^{(t)} - g_{j|i}(\mathbf{x}^{(t)}, \mathbf{v}_{ij}))\mathbf{x}^{(t)} = 0 \qquad (2.31)$$

which must be solved for each i and j. There is one aspect of these equations that renders them unusual. Recall that if the labels $z_i^{(t)}$ and $z_{j|i}^{(t)}$ were known, then the gating networks would be essentially solving a set of multiway classification problems. The supervised errors $(z_i^{(t)} - g_i^{(t)})$ and $(z_{j|i}^{(t)} - g_{j|i}^{(t)})$ would appear in the algorithm for solving these problems. Note that these errors are differences between indicator variables and probabilities. In equations 2.30 and 2.31, on the other hand, the errors that drive the algorithm are the differences $(h_i^{(t)} - g_i^{(t)})$ and $(h_{j|i}^{(t)} - g_{j|i}^{(t)})$, which are differences between probabilities. The EM algorithm effectively "fills in" the missing labels with estimated probabilities h_i and $h_{j|i}$. These estimated probabilities can be thought of as targets for the g_i and the $g_{j|i}$. This suggests that we can compute "virtual targets" for the underlying linear predictors ξ_i and $\xi_{j|i}$, by inverting the softmax function. (Note that this option would not be available for the z_i and $z_{j|i}$, even if they were known, because zero and one are not in the range of the softmax function.) Thus the targets for the ξ_i are the values:

$$\ln h_i^{(t)} - \ln C$$

where $C = \sum_k e^{\xi_k}$ is the normalization constant in the softmax function. Note, however, that constants that are common to all of the ξ_i can be omitted, because such constants disappear when ξ_i are converted to g_i (cf. equation 2.3). Thus the values $\ln h^{(t)}_i$ can be used as targets for the ξ_i. A similar argument shows that the values $\ln h^{(t)}_{l|k}$ can be used as targets for the ξ_{ij}, with observation weights $h^{(t)}_k$.

The utility of this approach is that once targets are available for the linear predictors ξ_i and ξ_{ij}, the problem of finding the parameters $\mathbf{v}_i$ and $\mathbf{v}_{ij}$ reduces to a coupled set of weighted least-squares problems. Thus we obtain an algorithm in which all of the parameters in the hierarchy, both in the expert networks and the gating networks, can be obtained by solving least-squares problems. This yields the following learning algorithm:

Algorithm 2

1. For each data pair $(\mathbf{x}^{(t)}, \mathbf{y}^{(t)})$, compute the posterior probabilities $h_i^{(t)}$ and $h_{j|i}^{(t)}$ using the current values of the parameters.

2. For each expert (i, j), solve a weighted least-squares problem with observations $\{(\mathbf{x}^{(t)}, \mathbf{y}^{(t)})\}_1^N$ and observation weights $\{h_{ij}^{(t)}\}_1^N$.

3. For each top-level gating network, solve a least-squares problem with observations $\{(\mathbf{x}^{(t)}, \ln h_k^{(t)})\}_1^N$.

4. For each lower-level gating network, solve a weighted least-squares problem with observations $\{(\mathbf{x}^{(t)}, \ln h_{l|k}^{(t)})\}_1^N$ and observation weights $\{h_k^{(t)}\}_1^N$.

5. Iterate using the updated parameter values.

It is important to note that this algorithm does not yield the same parameter estimates as Algorithm 1; the gating network residuals $(h_i^{(t)} - g_i^{(t)})$ are being fit by least squares rather than maximum likelihood. The algorithm can be thought of as an approximation to Algorithm 1, an approximation based on the assumption that the differences between $h_i^{(t)}$ and $g_i^{(t)}$ are small. This assumption is equivalent to the assumption that the architecture can fit the underlying regression surface (a consistency condition) and the assumption that the noise is small. In practice we have found that the least-squares algorithm works reasonably well, even in the early stages of fitting when the residuals can be large. The ability to use least squares is certainly appealing from a computational point of view. One possible hybrid algorithm involves using the least-squares algorithm to converge quickly to the neighborhood of a solution and then using IRLS to refine the solution.

2.8 Simulation Results. We tested Algorithm 1 and Algorithm 2 on a nonlinear system identification problem. The data were obtained from a simulation of a four-joint robot arm moving in three-dimensional space (Fun and Jordan 1993). The network must learn the *forward dynamics* of the arm; a state-dependent mapping from joint torques to joint accelerations. The state of the arm is encoded by eight real-valued variables: four positions (rad) and four angular velocities (rad/sec). The torque was encoded as four real-valued variables (N · m). Thus there were 12 inputs to the learning system. Given these 12 input variables, the network must predict the four accelerations at the joints (rad/sec^2). This mapping is highly nonlinear due to the rotating coordinate systems and the interaction torques between the links of the arm.

We generated 15,000 data points for training and 5,000 points for testing. For each epoch (i.e., each pass through the training set), we computed the relative error on the test set. Relative error is computed as a ratio between the mean squared error and the mean squared error that would be obtained if the learner were to output the mean value of the accelerations for all data points.

We compared the performance of a binary hierarchy to that of a backpropagation network. The hierarchy was a four-level hierarchy with 16 expert networks and 15 gating networks. Each expert network had 4 output units and each gating network had 1 output unit. The backpropagation network had 60 hidden units, which yields approximately the same number of parameters in the network as in the hierarchy.

The HME architecture was trained by Algorithms 1 and 2, utilizing Cholesky decomposition to solve the weighted least-squares problems (Golub and van Loan 1989). Note that the HME algorithms have no free parameters. The free parameters for the backpropagation network (the learning rate and the momentum term) were chosen based on a coarse search of the parameter space. (Values of 0.00001 and 0.15 were chosen for these parameters.) There were difficulties with local minima (or plateaus) using the backpropagation algorithm: Five of 10 runs failed to converge to "reasonable" error values. (As we report in the next section, no such difficulties were encountered in the case of *on-line* backpropagation.) We report average convergence times and average relative errors only for those runs that converged to "reasonable" error values. All 10 runs for both of the HME algorithms converged to "reasonable" error values.

Figure 2 shows the performance of the hierarchy and the backpropagation network. The horizontal axis of the graph gives the training time in epochs. The vertical axis gives generalization performance as measured by the average relative error on the test set.

Table 1 reports the average relative errors for both architectures measured at the minima of the relative error curves. (Minima were defined by a sequence of three successive increases in the relative error.) We also report values of relative error for the best linear approximation, the CART algorithm, and the MARS algorithm. Both CART and MARS were run four times, once for each of the output variables. We combined the results from these four computations to compute the total relative error. Two versions of CART were run; one in which the splits were restricted to be parallel to the axes and one in which linear combinations of the input variables were allowed.

The MARS algorithm requires choices to be made for the values of two structural parameters: the maximum number of basis functions and the maximum number of interaction terms. Each basis function in MARS yields a linear surface defined over a rectangular region of the input

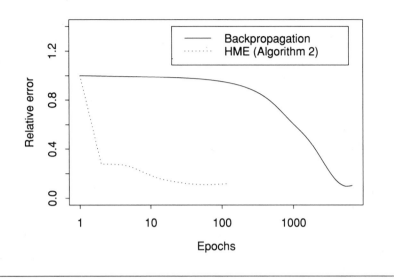

Figure 2: Relative error on the test set for a backpropagation network and a four-level HME architecture trained with batch algorithms. The standard errors at the minima of the curves are 0.013 for backpropagation and 0.002 for HME.

Table 1: Average Values of Relative Error and Number of Epochs Required for Convergence for the Batch Algorithms.

Architecture	Relative Error	# Epochs
Linear	0.31	1
Backpropagation	0.09	5,500
HME (Algorithm 1)	0.10	35
HME (Algorithm 2)	0.12	39
CART	0.17	NA
CART (linear)	0.13	NA
MARS	0.16	NA

space, corresponding roughly to the function implemented by a single expert in the HME architecture. Therefore we chose a maximum of 16 basis functions to correspond to the 16 experts in the four-level hierarchy. To choose the maximum number of interactions (mi), we compared the performance of MARS for $mi = 1, 2, 3, 6$, and 12, and chose the value that yielded the best performance ($mi = 3$).

For the iterative algorithms, we also report the number of epochs required for convergence. Because the learning curves for these algorithms generally have lengthy tails, we defined convergence as the first epoch at which the relative error drops within 5% of the minimum.

All of the architectures that we studied performed significantly better than the best linear approximation. As expected, the CART architecture with linear combinations performed better than CART with axis-parallel splits.[5] The HME architecture yielded a modest improvement over MARS and CART. Backpropagation produced the lowest relative error of the algorithms tested (ignoring the difficulties with convergence).

These differences in relative error should be treated with some caution. The need to set free parameters for some of the architectures (e.g., backpropagation) and the need to make structural choices (e.g., number of hidden units, number of basis functions, number of experts) make it difficult to match architectures. The HME architecture, for example, involves parameter dependencies that are not present in a backpropagation network. A gating network at a high level in the tree can "pinch off" a branch of the tree, rendering useless the parameters in that branch of the tree. Raw parameter count is therefore only a very rough guide to architecture capacity; more precise measures are needed (e.g., VC dimension) before definitive quantitative comparisons can be made.

The differences between backpropagation and HME in terms of convergence time are more definitive. Both HME algorithms reliably converge more than two orders of magnitude faster than backpropagation.

As shown in Figure 3, the HME architecture lends itself well to graphic investigation. This figure displays the time sequence of the distributions of posterior probabilities across the training set at each node of the tree. At Epoch 0, before any learning has taken place, most of the posterior probabilities at each node are approximately 0.5 across the training set. As the training proceeds, the histograms flatten out, eventually approaching bimodal distributions in which the posterior probabilities are either one or zero for most of the training patterns. This evolution is indicative of increasingly sharp splits being fit by the gating networks. Note that there is a tendency for the splits to be formed more rapidly at higher levels in the tree than at lower levels.

Figure 4 shows another graphic device that can be useful for understanding the way in which an HME architecture fits a data set. This figure, which we refer to as a "deviance tree," shows the deviance (mean squared error) that would be obtained at each level of the tree if the tree were clipped at that level. We construct a clipped tree at a given level by replacing each nonterminal at that level with a matrix that is a weighted average of the experts below that nonterminal. The weights are the total prior probabilities associated with each expert across the training set. The error for each output unit is then calculated by passing the test set through the clipped tree. As can be seen in the figure, the deviance is

---

[5]It should be noted that CART is at an advantage relative to the other algorithms in this comparison, because no structural parameters were fixed for CART. That is, CART is allowed to find the best tree of any size to fit the data.

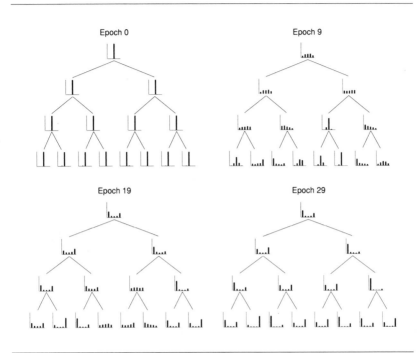

Figure 3: A sequence of histogram trees for the HME architecture. Each histogram displays the distribution of posterior probabilities across the training set at each node in the tree.

substantially smaller for deeper trees (note that the ordinate of the plots is on a log scale). The deviance in the right branch of the tree is larger than in the left branch of the tree. Information such as this can be useful for purposes of exploratory data analysis and for model selection.

2.9 An On-Line Algorithm. The batch least-squares algorithm that we have described (Algorithm 2) can be converted into an on-line algorithm by noting that linear least squares and weighted linear least squares problems can be solved by recursive procedures that update the parameter estimates with each successive data point (Ljung and Söderström 1986). Our application of these recursive algorithms is straightforward; however, care must be taken to handle the observation weights (the posterior probabilities) correctly. These weights change as a function of the changing parameter values. This implies that the recursive least squares algorithm must include a decay parameter that allows the system to "forget" older values of the posterior probabilities.

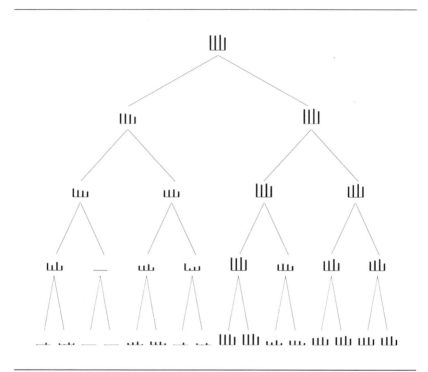

Figure 4: A deviance tree for the HME architecture. Each plot displays the mean squared error (MSE) for the four output units of the clipped tree. The plots are on a log scale covering approximately three orders of magnitude.

In this section we present the equations for the on-line algorithm. These equations involve an update not only of the parameters in each of the networks,[6] but also the storage and updating of an inverse covariance matrix for each network. Each matrix has dimensionality $m \times m$, where m is the dimensionality of the input vector. (Note that the size of these matrices depends on the square of the number of *input* variables, not the square of the number of *parameters*. Note also that the update equation for the inverse covariance matrix updates the inverse matrix directly; there is never a need to invert matrices.)

The on-line update rule for the parameters of the expert networks is given by the following recursive equation:

$$U_{ij}^{(t+1)} = U_{ij}^{(t)} + h_i^{(t)} h_{j|i}^{(t)} (\mathbf{y}^{(t)} - \boldsymbol{\mu}_{ij}^{(t)}) \mathbf{x}^{(t)T} R_{ij}^{(t)} \tag{2.32}$$

---

[6]Note that in this section we use the term "parameters" for the variables that are traditionally called "weights" in the neural network literature. We reserve the term "weights" for the observation weights.

where R_{ij} is the inverse covariance matrix for expert network (i, j). This matrix is updated via the equation:

$$R_{ij}^{(t)} = \lambda^{-1}R_{ij}^{(t-1)} - \lambda^{-1}\frac{R_{ij}^{(t-1)}\mathbf{x}^{(t)}\mathbf{x}^{(t)T}R_{ij}^{(t-1)}}{\lambda[h_{ij}^{(t)}]^{-1} + \mathbf{x}^{(t)T}R_{ij}^{(t-1)}\mathbf{x}^{(t)}} \tag{2.33}$$

where λ is the decay parameter.

It is interesting to note the similarity between the parameter update rule in equation 2.32 and the gradient rule presented earlier (cf. equation 2.14). These updates are essentially the same, except that the scalar ρ is replaced by the matrix $R_{ij}^{(t)}$. It can be shown, however, that $R_{ij}^{(t)}$ is an estimate of the inverse Hessian of the least-squares cost function (Ljung and Söderström 1986), thus equation 2.32 is in fact a stochastic approximation to a Newton–Raphson method rather than a gradient method.[7]

Similar equations apply for the updates of the gating networks. The update rule for the parameters of the top-level gating network is given by the following equation (for the ith output of the gating network):

$$\mathbf{v}_i^{(t+1)} = \mathbf{v}_i^{(t)} + S_i^{(t)}(\ln h_i^{(t)} - \xi_i^{(t)})\mathbf{x}^{(t)} \tag{2.34}$$

where the inverse covariance matrix S_i is updated by

$$S_i^{(t)} = \lambda^{-1}S_i^{(t-1)} - \lambda^{-1}\frac{S_i^{(t-1)}\mathbf{x}^{(t)}\mathbf{x}^{(t)T}S_i^{(t-1)}}{\lambda + \mathbf{x}^{(t)T}S_i^{(t-1)}\mathbf{x}^{(t)}} \tag{2.35}$$

Finally, the update rule for the parameters of the lower-level gating network is as follows:

$$\mathbf{v}_{ij}^{(t+1)} = \mathbf{v}_{ij}^{(t)} + S_{ij}^{(t)}h_i^{(t)}(\ln h_{j|i}^{(t)} - \xi_{ij}^{(t)})\mathbf{x}^{(t)} \tag{2.36}$$

where the inverse covariance matrix S_i is updated by

$$S_{ij}^{(t)} = \lambda^{-1}S_{ij}^{(t-1)} - \lambda^{-1}\frac{S_{ij}^{(t-1)}\mathbf{x}^{(t)}\mathbf{x}^{(t)T}S_{ij}^{(t-1)}}{\lambda[h_i^{(t)}]^{-1} + \mathbf{x}^{(t)T}S_{ij}^{(t-1)}\mathbf{x}^{(t)}} \tag{2.37}$$

2.10 Simulation Results. The on-line algorithm was tested on the robot dynamics problem described in the previous section. Preliminary simulations convinced us of the necessity of the decay parameter (λ). We also found that this parameter should be slowly increased as training proceeds—on the early trials the posterior probabilities are changing rapidly so that the covariances should be decayed rapidly, whereas on later trials the posterior probabilities have stabilized and the covariances should be decayed less rapidly. We used a simple fixed schedule: λ was

---

[7]This is true for fixed values of the posterior probabilities. These posterior probabilities are also changing over time, however, as required by the EM algorithm. The overall convergence rate of the algorithm is determined by the convergence rate of EM, not the convergence rate of Newton–Raphson.

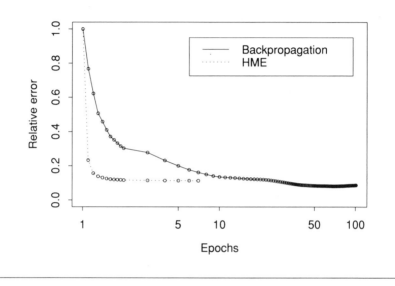

Figure 5: Relative error on the test set for a backpropagation network and a four-level hierarchy trained with on-line algorithms. The standard errors at the minima of the curves are 0.008 for backpropagation and 0.009 for HME.

initialized to 0.99 and increased a fixed fraction (0.6) of the remaining distance to 1.0 every 1000 time steps.

The performance of the on-line algorithm was compared to an on-line backpropagation network. Parameter settings for the backpropagation network were obtained by a coarse search through the parameter space, yielding a value of 0.15 for the learning rate and 0.20 for the momentum. The results for both architectures are shown in Figure 5. As can be seen, the on-line algorithm for backpropagation is significantly faster than the corresponding batch algorithm (cf. Fig. 2). This is also true of the on-line HME algorithm, which has nearly converged within the first epoch.

The minimum values of relative error and the convergence times for both architectures are provided in Table 2. We also provide the corresponding values for a simulation of the on-line gradient algorithm for the HME architecture (equation 2.17).

We also performed a set of simulations which tested a variety of different HME architectures. We compared a one-level hierarchy with 32 experts to hierarchies with five levels (32 experts), and six levels (64 experts). We also simulated two three-level hierarchies, one with branching factors of 4, 4, and 2 (proceeding from the top of the tree to the bottom), and one with branching factors of 2, 4, and 4. (Each three-level hierarchy contained 32 experts.) The results are shown in Figure 6. As can be

Table 2: Average Values of Relative Error and Number of Epochs Required for Convergence for the On-Line Algorithms.

Architecture	Relative Error	Number of Epochs
Linear	0.32	1
Backpropagation (on-line)	0.08	63
HME (on-line)	0.12	2
HME (gradient)	0.15	104

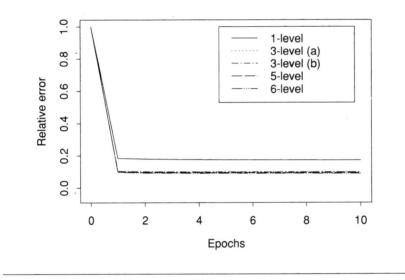

Figure 6: Relative error on the test set for HME hierarchies with different structures. "3-level (a)" refers to a 3-level hierarchy with branching factors of 4, 4, and 2, and "3-level (b)" refers to a 3-level hierarchy with branching factors of 2, 4, and 4. The standard errors for all curves at their respective minima were approximately 0.009.

seen, there was a significant difference between the one-level hierarchy and the other architectures. There were smaller differences among the multilevel hierarchies. No significant difference was observed between the two different 3-level architectures.

3 Model Selection

Utilizing the HME approach requires that choices be made regarding the structural parameters of the model, in particular the number of levels and the branching factor of the tree. As with other flexible estimation techniques, it is desirable to allow these structural parameters to be chosen based at least partly on the data. This model selection problem can be addressed in a variety of ways. In this paper we have utilized a test set approach to model selection, stopping the training when the error on the test set reaches a minimum. As is the case with other neural network algorithms, this procedure can be justified as a complexity control measure. As we have noted, when the parameters in the gating networks of an HME architecture are small, the entire system reduces to a single "averaged" GLIM at the root of the tree. As the training proceeds, the parameters in the gating networks begin to grow in magnitude and splits are formed. When a split is formed the parameters in the branches of the tree on either side of the split are decoupled and the effective number of degrees of freedom in the system increases. This increase in complexity takes place gradually as the values of the parameters increase and the splits sharpen. By stopping the training of the system based on the performance on a test set, we obtain control over the effective number of degrees of freedom in the architecture.

Other approaches to model selection can also be considered. One natural approach is to use ridge regression in each of the expert networks and the gating networks. This approach extends naturally to the on-line setting in the form of a "weight decay." It is also worth considering Bayesian techniques of the kind considered in the decision tree literature by Buntine (1991), as well as the MDL methods of Quinlan and Rivest (1989).

4 Related work

There are a variety of ties that can be made between the HME architecture and related work in statistics, machine learning, and neural networks. In this section we briefly mention some of these ties and make some comparative remarks.

Our architecture is not the only nonlinear approximator to make substantial use of GLIMs and the IRLS algorithm. IRLS also figures prominently in a branch of nonparametric statistics known as generalized additive models (GAMs; Hastie and Tibshirani 1990). It is interesting to note the complementary roles of IRLS in these two architectures. In the GAM model, the IRLS algorithm appears in the outer loop, providing an adjusted dependent variable that is fit by a backfitting procedure in the inner loop. In the HME approach, on the other hand, the outer loop is the E step of EM and IRLS is in the inner loop. This complementarity suggests that it might be of interest to consider hybrid models in which a HME is nested inside a GAM or vice versa.

We have already mentioned the close ties between the HME approach and other tree-structured estimators such as CART and MARS. Our approach differs from MARS and related architectures—such as the basis-function trees of Sanger (1991)—by allowing splits that are oblique with respect to the axes. We also differ from these architectures by using a statistical model—the multinomial logit model—for the splits. We believe that both of these features can play a role in increasing predictive ability—the use of oblique splits should tend to decrease bias, and the use of smooth multinomial logit splits should generally decrease variance. Oblique splits also render the HME architecture insensitive to the particular choice of coordinates used to encode the data. Finally, it is worth emphasizing the difference in philosophy behind these architectures. Whereas CART and MARS are entirely nonparametric, the HME approach has a strong flavor of parametric statistics, via its use of generalized linear models, mixture models, and maximum likelihood.

Similar comments can be made with respect to the decision tree methodology in the machine learning literature. Algorithms such as ID3 build trees that have axis-parallel splits and use heuristic splitting algorithms (Quinlan 1986). More recent research has studied decision trees with oblique splits (Murthy *et al.* 1993; Utgoff and Brodley 1990). None of these papers, however, has treated the problem of splitting data as a statistical problem, nor have they provided a global goodness-of-fit measure for their trees.

There are a variety of neural network architectures that are related to the HME architecture. The multiresolution aspect of HME is reminiscent of Moody's (1989) multiresolution CMAC hierarchy, differing in that Moody's levels of resolution are handled explicitly by separate networks. The "neural tree" algorithm (Strömberg *et al.* 1991) is a decision tree with multilayer perceptions (MLPs) at the nonterminals. This architecture can form oblique (or curvilinear) splits, however, the MLPs are trained by a heuristic that has no clear relationship to overall classification performance. Finally, Hinton and Nowlan (see Nowlan 1991) have independently proposed extending the Jacobs *et al.* (1991) modular architecture to a tree-structured system. They did not develop a likelihood approach to the problem, however, proposing instead a heuristic splitting scheme.

5 Conclusions

We have presented a tree-structured architecture for supervised learning. We have developed the learning algorithm for this architecture within the framework of maximum likelihood estimation, utilizing ideas from mixture model estimation and generalized linear model theory. The maximum likelihood framework allows standard tools from statistical theory to be brought to bear in developing inference procedures and measures of uncertainty for the architecture (Cox and Hinkley 1974). It also opens the door to the Bayesian approaches that have been found to be useful in the context of unsupervised mixture model estimation (Cheeseman *et al.* 1988).

Although we have not emphasized theoretical issues in this paper, there are a number of points that are worth mentioning. First, the set of exponentially smoothed piecewise linear functions that we have utilized is clearly dense in the set of piecewise linear functions on compact sets in $\Re^m$, thus it is straightforward to show that the hierarchical architecture is dense in the set of continuous functions on compact sets in $\Re^m$. That is, the architecture is "universal" in the sense of Hornik *et al.* (1989). From this result it would seem straightforward to develop consistency results for the architecture (cf. Geman *et al.* 1992; Stone 1977). We are currently developing this line of argument and are studying the asymptotic distributional properties of fixed hierarchies. Second, convergence results are available for the architecture. We have shown that the convergence rate of the algorithm is linear in the condition number of a matrix that is the product of an inverse covariance matrix and the Hessian of the log likelihood for the architecture (Jordan and Xu 1993).

Finally, it is worth noting a number of possible extensions of the work reported here. Our earlier work on hierarchical mixtures of experts utilized the multilayer perceptron as the primitive function for the expert networks and gating networks (Jordan and Jacobs 1992). That option is still available, although we lose the EM proof of convergence (cf. Jordan and Xu 1993) and we lose the ability to fit the subnetworks efficiently with IRLS. One interesting example of such an application is the case where the experts are autoassociators (Bourlard and Kamp 1988), in which case the architecture fits hierarchically nested local principal component decompositions. Another area in unsupervised learning worth exploring is the nonassociative version of the hierarchical architecture. Such a model would be a recursive version of classical mixture-likelihood clustering and may have interesting ties to hierarchical clustering models. Finally, it is also of interest to note that the recursive least squares algorithm that we utilized in obtaining an on-line variant of Algorithm 2 is not the only possible on-line approach. Any of the fast filter algorithms (Haykin 1991) could also be utilized, giving rise to a family of on-line algorithms. Also, it is worth studying the application of the recursive algorithms to PRESS-like cross-validation calculations to efficiently compute the changes in likelihood that arise from adding or deleting parameters or data points.

Appendix A: Iteratively Reweighted Least Squares

The iteratively reweighted least squares (IRLS) algorithm is the inner loop of the algorithm that we have proposed for the HME architecture. In this section, we describe the IRLS algorithm, deriving it as a special case of the Fisher scoring method for generalized linear models. Our presentation derives from McCullagh and Nelder (1983).

IRLS is an iterative algorithm for computing the maximum likelihood estimates of the parameters of a generalized linear model. It is a special case of a general algorithm for maximum likelihood estimation known as the Fisher scoring method (Finney 1973). Let $l(\beta; \mathcal{X})$ be a log likelihood function—a function of the parameter vector β—and let $(\partial l / \partial \beta \partial \beta^T)$ denote the Hessian of the log likelihood. The Fisher scoring method updates the parameter estimates β as follows:

$$\beta_{r+1} = \beta_r - \left\{ E \left[\frac{\partial l}{\partial \beta \partial \beta^T} \right] \right\}^{-1} \frac{\partial l}{\partial \beta} \tag{5.1}$$

where β_r denotes the parameter estimate at the rth iteration and $\partial l / \partial \beta$ is the gradient vector. Note that the Fisher scoring method is essentially the same as the Newton–Raphson algorithm, except that the expected value of the Hessian replaces the Hessian. There are statistical reasons for preferring the expected value of the Hessian—and the expected value of the Hessian is often easier to compute—but Newton–Raphson can also be used in many cases.

The likelihood in generalized linear model theory is a product of densities from the exponential family of distributions. This family is an important class in statistics and includes many useful densities, such as the normal, the Poisson, the binomial, and the gamma. The general form of a density in the exponential family is the following:

$$P(y, \eta, \phi) = \exp\{(\eta y - b(\eta))/\phi + c(y, \phi)\} \tag{5.2}$$

where η is known as the "natural parameter" and ϕ is the dispersion parameter.[8]

Example (Bernoulli Density). The Bernoulli density with mean π has the following form:

$$
\begin{aligned}
P(y, \pi) &= \pi^y (1 - \pi)^{1-y} \\
&= \exp\{\ln(\frac{\pi}{1 - \pi})y + \ln(1 - \pi)\} \\
&= \exp\{\eta y - \ln(1 + e^\eta)\}
\end{aligned}
\tag{5.3}
$$

where $\eta = \ln(\pi/1 - \pi)$ is the natural parameter of the Bernoulli density. This parameter has the interpretation as the log odds of "success" in a random Bernoulli experiment.

In a generalized linear model, the parameter η is modeled as a linear function of the input $\mathbf{x}$:

$$\eta = \beta^T \mathbf{x}$$

---

[8]We restrict ourselves to scalar-valued random variables to simplify the presentation, and describe the (straightforward) extension to vector-valued random variables at the end of the section.

where β is a parameter vector. Substituting this expression into equation 5.2 and taking the product of N such densities yields the following log likelihood for a data set $\mathcal{X} = \{(\mathbf{x}^{(t)}, y^{(t)})\}_1^N$:

$$l(\beta, \mathcal{X}) = \sum_t \{((\beta^T \mathbf{x}^{(t)} y^{(t)} - b(\beta^T \mathbf{x}^{(t)}))/\phi + c(y^{(t)}, \phi)\}$$

The observations $y^{(t)}$ are assumed to be sampled independently from densities $P(y, \eta^{(t)}, \phi)$, where $\eta^{(t)} = \beta^T \mathbf{x}^{(t)}$.

We now compute the gradient of the log likelihood:

$$\frac{\partial l}{\partial \beta} = \sum_t (y^{(t)} - b'(\beta^T \mathbf{x}^{(t)})) \mathbf{x}^{(t)}/\phi \tag{5.4}$$

and the Hessian of the log likelihood:

$$\frac{\partial l}{\partial \beta \partial \beta^T} = -\sum_t b''(\beta^T \mathbf{x}^{(t)}) \mathbf{x}^{(t)} \mathbf{x}^{(t)T}/\phi \tag{5.5}$$

These quantities could be substituted directly into equation 5.1, however, there is additional mathematical structure that can be exploited. First note the following identity, which is true of any log likelihood:

$$E\left[\frac{\partial l}{\partial \beta}\right] = 0$$

(This fact can be proved by differentiating both sides of the identity $\int P(y, \beta, \phi) dy = 1$ with respect to β.) Because this identity is true for any set of observed data, including all subsets of $\mathcal{X}$, we have the following:

$$E[y^{(t)}] = b'(\beta^T \mathbf{x}^{(t)})$$

for all t. This equation implies that the mean of $y^{(t)}$, which we denote as $\mu^{(t)}$, is a function of $\eta^{(t)}$. We therefore include in the generalized linear model the *link function*, which models μ as a function of η:

$$\mu^{(t)} = f(\eta^{(t)})$$

Example (Bernoulli Density). Equation 5.3 shows that $b(\eta) = \ln(1 + e^\eta)$ for the Bernoulli density. Thus

$$\mu = b'(\eta) = \frac{e^\eta}{1 + e^\eta}$$

which is the logistic function. Inverting the logistic function yields $\eta = \ln(\mu/1 - \mu)$; thus, μ equals π, as it must.

The link function $f(\eta) = b'(\eta)$ is known in generalized linear model theory as the *canonical link*. By parameterizing the exponential family density in terms of η (cf. equation 5.2), we have forced the choice of the canonical link. It is also possible to use other links, in which case η

no longer has the interpretation as the natural parameter of the density. There are statistical reasons, however, to prefer the canonical link (McCullagh and Nelder 1983). Moreover, by choosing the canonical link, the Hessian of the likelihood turns out to be constant (cf. equation 5.5), and the Fisher scoring method therefore reduces to Newton–Raphson.[9]

To continue the development, we need an additional fact about log likelihoods. By differentiating the identity $\int P(y, \beta) dy = 1$ twice with respect to β, the following identity can be established:

$$E\left[\frac{\partial l}{\partial \beta \partial \beta^T}\right] = -E\left[\frac{\partial l}{\partial \beta}\right]\left[\frac{\partial l}{\partial \beta}\right]^T$$

This identity can be used to obtain a relationship between the variance of η and the function $b(\eta)$ in the exponential family density. Beginning with equation 5.5, we have

$$-E\left[\sum_t b''(\beta^T \mathbf{x}^{(t)})\mathbf{x}^{(t)}\mathbf{x}^{(t)T}/\phi\right]$$

$$= E\left[\frac{\partial l}{\partial \beta \partial \beta^T}\right]$$

$$= -E\left[\frac{\partial l}{\partial \beta}\right]\left[\frac{\partial l}{\partial \beta}\right]^T$$

$$= -\frac{1}{\phi^2}E\left[\sum_t (y^{(t)} - b'(\beta^T \mathbf{x}^{(t)}))\mathbf{x}^{(t)} \sum_s (y^{(s)} - b'(\beta^T \mathbf{x}^{(s)}))\mathbf{x}^{(s)T}\right]$$

$$= -\frac{1}{\phi^2}E\left[\sum_t (y^{(t)} - b'(\beta^T \mathbf{x}^{(t)}))^2 \mathbf{x}^{(t)}\mathbf{x}^{(t)T}\right]$$

$$= -\frac{1}{\phi^2}\sum_t \text{Var}[y^{(t)}]\mathbf{x}^{(t)}\mathbf{x}^{(t)T}$$

where we have used the independence assumption in the fourth step. Comparing equation 5.5 with the last equation, we obtain the following relationship:

$$\text{Var}[y^{(t)}] = \phi b''(\beta^T \mathbf{x}^{(t)})$$

Moreover, because $f(\eta) = b'(\eta)$, we have

$$\text{Var}[y^{(t)}] = \phi f'(\beta^T \mathbf{x}^{(t)}) \tag{5.6}$$

We now assemble the various pieces. First note that equation 5.6 can be utilized to express the Hessian (equation 5.5) in the following form:

$$\frac{\partial l}{\partial \beta \partial \beta^T} = -\sum_t \mathbf{x}^{(t)}\mathbf{x}^{(t)T}w^{(t)}$$

---

[9]Whether or not the canonical link is used, the results presented in the remainder of this section are correct for the Fisher scoring method. If noncanonical links are used, then Newton–Raphson will include additional terms (terms that vanish under the expectation operator).

where the weight $w^{(t)}$ is defined as follows:

$$w^{(t)} = \frac{f'(\eta^{(t)})^2}{\text{Var}[y^{(t)}]}$$

In matrix notation we have

$$\frac{\partial l}{\partial \beta \partial \beta^T} = -X^T W X \tag{5.7}$$

where X is the matrix whose rows are the input vectors $\mathbf{x}^{(t)}$ and W is a diagonal matrix whose diagonal elements are $w^{(t)}$. Note also that the Hessian is a constant, thus the expected value of the Hessian is also $X^T W X$.

Similarly, equation 5.6 can be used to remove the dependence of the gradient (equation 5.4) on ϕ:

$$\frac{\partial l}{\partial \beta} = \sum_t (y^{(t)} - \mu^{(t)}) \mathbf{x}^{(t)} w^{(t)} / f'(\eta^{(t)})$$

This equation can be written in matrix notation as follows:

$$\frac{\partial l}{\partial \beta} = X^T W \mathbf{e} \tag{5.8}$$

where $\mathbf{e}$ is the vector whose components are

$$e^{(t)} = (y^{(t)} - \mu^{(t)}) / f'(\eta^{(t)})$$

Finally, substitute equation 5.7 and equation 5.8 into equation 5.1 to obtain

$$\begin{aligned} \beta_{r+1} &= \beta_r + (X^T W X)^{-1} X^T W \mathbf{e} \tag{5.9} \\ &= (X^T W X)^{-1} X^T W \mathbf{z} \tag{5.10} \end{aligned}$$

where $\mathbf{z} = X\beta_r + \mathbf{e}$.[10] These equations are the normal equations for a weighted least squares problem with observations $\{(\mathbf{x}^{(t)}, z^{(t)})\}_1^N$ and observation weights $w^{(t)}$. The weights change from iteration to iteration, because they are a function of the parameters β_r. The resulting iterative algorithm is known as iteratively reweighted least squares (IRLS).

It is easy to generalize the derivation to allow additional fixed observation weights to be associated with the data pairs. Such weights simply multiply the iteratively varying weights $w^{(t)}$, leading to an iteratively reweighted *weighted* least squares algorithm. Such a generalization is in fact necessary in our application of IRLS: the EM algorithm defines observation weights in the outer loop that IRLS must treat as fixed during the inner loop.

Finally, it is also straightforward to generalize the derivation in this section to the case of vector outputs. In the case of vector outputs, each row of the weight matrix (e.g., U for the expert networks) is a separate parameter vector corresponding to the vector β of this section. These row vectors are updated independently and in parallel.

---

[10]As McCullagh and Nelder (1983) note, $\mathbf{z}$ has the interpretation as the linearization of the link function around the current value of the mean.

Appendix B: Multinomial Logit Models

The multinomial logit model is a special case of the generalized linear model in which the probabilistic component is the multinomial density or the Poisson density. It is of particular interest to us because the gating networks in the HME architecture are multinomial logit models.

Consider a multiway classification problem on n variables $y_1, y_2, \ldots, y_n$. A natural probability model for multiway classification is the multinomial density:

$$P(y_1, y_2, \ldots, y_n) = \frac{m!}{(y_1!)(y_2!) \cdots (y_n!)} p_1^{y_1} p_2^{y_2} \cdots p_n^{y_n}$$

where the p_i are the multinomial probabilities associated with the different classes and $m = \sum_{i=1}^{n} y_i$ is generally taken to equal one for classification problems. The multinomial density is an member of the exponential family and can be written in the following form:

$$P(y_1, y_2, \ldots, y_n) = \exp \left\{ \ln \frac{m!}{(y_1!)(y_2!) \cdots (y_n!)} + \sum_{i=1}^{n} y_i \ln p_i \right\} \quad (6.1)$$

Taking the logarithm of both sides, and dropping the terms that do not depend on the parameters p_i, we see that the log likelihood for the multinomial logit model is the cross-entropy between the observations y_i and the parameters p_i.

Implicit in equation 6.1 is the constraint that the p_i sum to one. This constraint can be made explicit by defining p_n as follows: $p_n = 1 - \sum_{i}^{n-1} p_i$, and rewriting equation 6.1:

$$P(y_1, y_2, \ldots, y_n) = \exp \left\{ \ln \frac{m!}{(y_1!)(y_2!) \cdots (y_n!)} + \sum_{i=1}^{n-1} y_i \ln \frac{p_i}{p_n} + n \ln p_n \right\} \quad (6.2)$$

The natural parameters in an exponential family density are those quantities that appear linearly in the y_i (cf. equation 5.2), thus we define

$$\eta_i = \ln \frac{p_i}{p_n} \quad (6.3)$$

Using $p_n = 1 - \sum_{i}^{n-1} p_i$ implies

$$p_n = \frac{1}{1 + \sum_{i=1}^{n-1} e^{\eta_i}}$$

and therefore equation 6.3 can be inverted to yield

$$p_i = \frac{e^{\eta_i}}{1 + \sum_{j=1}^{n-1} e^{\eta_j}}$$

$$= \frac{e^{\eta_i}}{\sum_{j=1}^{n} e^{\eta_j}} \quad (6.4)$$

using $\eta_n = 0$ from equation 6.3. This latter expression is the "softmax" function (Bridle 1989).

Finally, note that equation 6.2 implies that $b(\eta)$ must be defined as follows (cf. equation 5.2):

$$b(\eta) = n \ln \left(\sum_{i=1}^{n} e^{\eta_i} \right)$$

which implies

$$\mu_i = \frac{\partial b(\eta)}{\partial \eta_i} = \frac{n e^{\eta_i}}{\sum_{j=1}^{n} e^{\eta_j}} = n p_i \tag{6.5}$$

The fitting of a multinomial logit model proceeds by IRLS as described in Appendix A, using equations 6.4 and 6.5 for the link function and the mean, respectively.

Acknowledgments

We want to thank Geoffrey Hinton, Tony Robinson, Mitsuo Kawato, Carlotta Domeniconi, and Daniel Wolpert for helpful comments on the manuscript. This project was supported in part by a grant from the McDonnell-Pew Foundation, by a grant from ATR Human Information Processing Research Laboratories, by a grant from Siemens Corporation, by Grant IRI-9013991 from the National Science Foundation, and by Grant N00014-90-J-1942 from the Office of Naval Research. The project was also supported by NSF Grant ASC-9217041 in support of the Center for Biological and Computational Learning at MIT, including funds provided by DARPA under the HPCC program, and NSF Grant ECS-9216531 to support an Initiative in Intelligent Control at MIT. Michael I. Jordan is an NSF Presidential Young Investigator.

References

Bourlard, H., and Kamp, Y. 1988. Auto-association by multilayer perceptrons and singular value decomposition. *Biol. Cybern.* **59**, 291–294.

Breiman, L., Friedman, J. H., Olshen, R. A., and Stone, C. J. 1984. *Classification and Regression Trees.* Wadsworth International Group, Belmont, CA.

Bridle, J. 1989. Probabilistic interpretation of feedforward classification network outputs, with relationships to statistical pattern recognition. In *Neurocomputing: Algorithms, Architectures, and Applications*, F. Fogelman-Soulie and J. Hérault, eds. Springer-Verlag, New York.

Buntine, W. 1991. *Learning classification trees.* NASA Ames Tech. Rep. FIA-90-12-19-01, Moffett Field, CA.

Cheeseman, P., Kelly, J., Self, M., Stutz, J., Taylor, W., and Freeman, D. 1988. Autoclass: A Bayesian classification system. In *Proceedings of the Fifth International Conference on Machine Learning*, Ann Arbor, MI.

Cox, D. R. 1970. *The Analysis of Binary Data.* Chapman-Hall, London.

Cox, D. R., and Hinkley, D. V. 1974. *Theoretical Statistics*. Chapman-Hall, London.

Dempster, A. P., Laird, N. M., and Rubin, D. B. 1977. Maximum likelihood from incomplete data via the EM algorithm. *J. R. Statist. Soc. B* **39**, 1–38.

Duda, R. O., and Hart, P. E. 1973. *Pattern Classification and Scene Analysis*. John Wiley, New York.

Finney, D. J. 1973. *Statistical Methods in Biological Assay*. Hafner, New York.

Friedman, J. H. 1991. Multivariate adaptive regression splines. *Ann. Statist.* **19**, 1–141.

Fun, W., and Jordan, M. I. 1993. *The Moving Basin: Effective Action Search in Forward Models*. MIT Computational Cognitive Science Tech. Report 9205, Cambridge, MA.

Geman, S., Bienenstock, E., and Doursat, R. 1992. Neural networks and the bias/variance dilemma. *Neural Comp.* **4**, 1–52.

Golub, G. H., and Van Loan, G. F. 1989. *Matrix Computations*. The Johns Hopkins University Press, Baltimore, MD.

Hastie, T. J., and Tibshirani, R. J. 1990. *Generalized Additive Models*. Chapman and Hall, London.

Haykin, S. 1991. *Adaptive Filter Theory*. Prentice-Hall, Englewood Cliffs, NJ.

Hinton, G. E., and Sejnowski, T. J. 1986. Learning and relearning in Boltzmann machines. In *Parallel Distributed Processing*, D. E. Rumelhart and J. L. McClelland, eds., Vol. 1, pp. 282–317. MIT Press, Cambridge, MA.

Hornik, K., Stinchcombe, M., and White, H. 1989. Multilayer feedforward networks are universal approximators. *Neural Networks* **2**, 359–366.

Jacobs, R. A., Jordan, M. I., Nowlan, S. J., and Hinton, G. E. 1991. Adaptive mixtures of local experts. *Neural Comp.* **3**, 79–87.

Jordan, M. I., and Jacobs, R. A. 1992. Hierarchies of adaptive experts. In *Advances in Neural Information Processing Systems 4*, J. Moody, S. Hanson, and R. Lippmann, eds., pp. 985–993. Morgan Kaufmann, San Mateo, CA.

Jordan, M. I., and Xu, L. 1993. *Convergence Properties of the EM Approach to Learning in Mixture-of-Experts Architectures*. Computational Cognitive Science Tech. Rep. 9301, MIT, Cambridge, MA.

Little, R. J. A., and Rubin, D. B. 1987. *Statistical Analysis with Missing Data*. John Wiley, New York.

Ljung, L., and Söderström, T. 1986. *Theory and Practice of Recursive Identification*. MIT Press, Cambridge.

McCullagh, P., and Nelder, J. A. 1983. *Generalized Linear Models*. Chapman and Hall, London.

Moody, J. 1989. Fast learning in multi-resolution hierarchies. In *Advances in Neural Information Processing Systems*, D. S. Touretzky, ed. Morgan Kaufmann, San Mateo, CA.

Murthy, S. K., Kasif, S., and Salzberg, S. 1993. *OC1: A Randomized Algorithm for Building Oblique Decision Trees*. Tech. Rep., Department of Computer Science, The Johns Hopkins University.

Nowlan, S. J. 1990. Maximum likelihood competitive learning. In *Advances in Neural Information Processing Systems 2*, D. S. Touretzky, ed. Morgan Kaufmann, San Mateo, CA.

Nowlan, S. J. 1991. *Soft Competitive Adaptation: Neural Network Learning Algorithms Based on Fitting Statistical Mixtures.* Tech. Rep. CMU-CS-91-126, CMU, Pittsburgh, PA.

Quandt, R. E., and Ramsey, J. B. 1972. A new approach to estimating switching regressions. *J. Am. Statist. Soc.* **67**, 306–310.

Quinlan, J. R. 1986. Induction of decision trees. *Machine Learn.* **1**, 81–106.

Quinlan, J. R., and Rivest, R. L. 1989. Inferring decision trees using the Minimum Description Length Principle. *Information and Computation* **80**, 227–248.

Redner, R. A., and Walker, H. F. 1984. Mixture densities, maximum likelihood and the EM algorithm. *SIAM Rev.* **26**, 195–239.

Sanger, T. D. 1991. A tree-structured adaptive network for function approximation in high dimensional spaces. *IEEE Transact. Neural Networks* **2**, 285–293.

Scott, D. W. 1992. *Multivariate Density Estimation.* John Wiley, New York.

Specht, D. F. 1991. A general regression neural network. *IEEE Transact. Neural Networks* **2**, 568–576.

Stone, C. J. 1977. Consistent nonparametric regression. *Ann. Statist.* **5**, 595–645.

Strömberg, J. E., Zrida, J., and Isaksson, A. 1991. Neural trees—using neural nets in a tree classifier structure. *IEEE International Conference on Acoustics, Speech and Signal Processing,* 137–140.

Titterington, D. M., Smith, A. F. M., and Makov, U. E. 1985. *Statistical Analysis of Finite Mixture Distributions.* John Wiley, New York.

Utgoff, P. E., and Brodley, C. E. 1990. An incremental method for finding multivariate splits for decision trees. In *Proceedings of the Seventh International Conference on Machine Learning,* Los Altos, CA.

Wahba, G., Gu, C., Wang, Y., and Chappell, R. 1993. *Soft Classification, a.k.a. Risk Estimation, via Penalized Log Likelihood and Smoothing Spline Analysis of Variance.* Tech. Rep. 899, Department of Statistics, University of Wisconsin, Madison.

Wu, C. F. J. 1983. On the convergence properties of the EM algorithm. *Ann. Statist.* **11**, 95–103.

12

Hidden Neural Networks

Anders Krogh
Center for Biological Sequence Analysis, Building 208, Technical University of Denmark,
2800 Lyngby, Denmark

Søren Kamaric Riis
Department of Mathematical Modeling, Section for Digital Signal Processing, Technical University of Denmark, Building 321, 2800 Lyngby, Denmark

A general framework for hybrids of hidden Markov models (HMMs) and neural networks (NNs) called hidden neural networks (HNNs) is described. The article begins by reviewing standard HMMs and estimation by conditional maximum likelihood, which is used by the HNN. In the HNN, the usual HMM probability parameters are replaced by the outputs of state-specific neural networks. As opposed to many other hybrids, the HNN is normalized globally and therefore has a valid probabilistic interpretation. All parameters in the HNN are estimated simultaneously according to the discriminative conditional maximum likelihood criterion. The HNN can be viewed as an undirected probabilistic independence network (a graphical model), where the neural networks provide a compact representation of the clique functions. An evaluation of the HNN on the task of recognizing broad phoneme classes in the TIMIT database shows clear performance gains compared to standard HMMs tested on the same task.

1 Introduction

Hidden Markov models (HMMs) is one of the most successful modeling approaches for acoustic events in speech recognition (Rabiner, 1989; Juang & Rabiner, 1991), and more recently they have proved useful for several problems in biological sequence analysis like protein modeling and gene finding (see, e.g., Durbin, Eddy, Krogh, & Mitchison, 1998; Eddy, 1996; Krogh, Brown, Mian, Sjölander, & Haussler, 1994). Although the HMM is good at capturing the temporal nature of processes such as speech, it has a very limited capacity for recognizing complex patterns involving more than first-order dependencies in the observed data. This is due to the first-order state process and the assumption of state-conditional independence of observations. Multilayer perceptrons are almost the opposite: they cannot model temporal phenomena very well but are good at recognizing complex patterns. Combining the two frameworks in a sensible way can therefore lead to a more powerful model with better classification abilities.

The starting point for this work is the so-called class HMM (CHMM), which is basically a standard HMM with a distribution over classes assigned to each state (Krogh, 1994). The CHMM incorporates conditional maximum likelihood (CML) estimation (Juang & Rabiner, 1991; Nádas, 1983; Nádas, Nahamoo, & Picheny, 1988). In contrast to the widely used maximum likelihood (ML) estimation, CML estimation is a discriminative training algorithm that aims at maximizing the ability of the model to discriminate between different classes. The CHMM can be normalized globally, which allows for nonnormalizing parameters in the individual states, and this enables us to generalize the CHMM to incorporate neural networks in a valid probabilistic way.

In the CHMM/NN hybrid, which we call a hidden neural network (HNN), some or all CHMM probability parameters are replaced by the outputs of state-specific neural networks that take the observations as input. The model can be trained as a whole from observation sequences with labels by a gradient-descent algorithm. It turns out that in this algorithm, the neural networks are updated by standard backpropagation, where the errors are calculated by a slightly modified forward-backward algorithm.

In this article, we first give a short introduction to standard HMMs. The CHMM and conditional ML are then introduced, and a gradient descent algorithm is derived for estimation. Based on this, the HNN is described next along with training issues for this model, and finally we give a comparison to other hybrid models. The article concludes with an evaluation of the HNN on the recognition of five broad phoneme classes in the TIMIT database (Garofolo et al., 1993). Results on this task clearly show a better performance of the HNN compared to a standard HMM.

2 Hidden Markov Models

To establish notation and set the stage for describing CHMMs and HNNs, we start with a brief overview of standard hidden Markov models. (For a more comprehensive introduction, see Rabiner, 1989; Juang & Rabiner, 1991.) In this description we consider discrete first-order HMMs, where the observations are symbols from a finite alphabet $\mathcal{A}$. The treatment of continuous observations is very similar (see, e.g., Rabiner, 1989).

The standard HMM is characterized by a set of N states and two concurrent stochastic processes: a first-order Markov process between states modeling the temporal structure of the data and an emission process for each state modeling the locally stationary part of the data. The state process is given by a set of transition probabilities, θ_{ij}, giving the probability of making a transition from state i to state j, and the emission process in state i is described by the probabilities, $\phi_i(a)$, of emitting symbol $a \in \mathcal{A}$ in state i. The ϕ's are usually called emission probabilities, but we use the term *match probabilities* here. We observe only the sequence of outputs from the model, and not the underlying (hidden) state sequence, hence the name *hidden* Markov model. The set Θ of all transition and emission probabilities completely specifies the model.

Given an HMM, the probability of an observation sequence, $x = x_1, \ldots, x_L$, of L symbols from the alphabet $\mathcal{A}$ is defined by

$$P(x|\Theta) = \sum_\pi P(x, \pi|\Theta) = \sum_\pi \prod_{l=1}^{L} \theta_{\pi_{l-1}\pi_l} \phi_{\pi_l}(x_l). \tag{2.1}$$

Here $\pi = \pi_1, \ldots, \pi_L$ is a state sequence; π_i is the number of the ith state in the sequence. Such a state sequence is called a *path* through the model. An auxiliary start state, $\pi_0 = 0$, has been introduced such that θ_{0i} denotes the probability of starting a path in state i. In the following we assume that state N is an end state: a nonmatching state with no outgoing transitions.

The probability 2.1 can be calculated efficiently by a dynamic programming-like algorithm known as the forward algorithm. Let $\alpha_i(l) = P(x_1, \ldots, x_l, \pi_l = i \mid \Theta)$, that is, the probability of having matched observations $x_1, \ldots, x_l$ and being in state i at time l. Then the following recursion holds for $1 \leq i \leq N$ and $1 < l \leq L$,

$$\alpha_i(l) = \phi_i(x_l) \sum_j \alpha_j(l-1)\theta_{ji}, \tag{2.2}$$

and $P(x|\Theta) = \alpha_N(L)$. The recursion is initialized by $\alpha_i(1) = \theta_{0i}\phi_i(x_1)$ for $1 \leq i \leq N$.

The parameters of the model can be estimated from data by an ML method. If multiple sequences of observations are available for training, they are assumed independent, and the total likelihood of the model is just a product of probabilities of the form 2.1 for each of the sequences. The generalization from one to many observation sequences is therefore trivial, and we will consider only one training sequence in the following. The likelihood of the model, $P(x|\Theta)$, given in equation 2.1, is commonly maximized by the Baum-Welch algorithm, which is an expectation-maximization (EM) algorithm (Dempster, Laird, & Rubin, 1977) guaranteed to converge to a local maximum of the likelihood. The Baum-Welch algorithm iteratively reestimates the model parameters until convergence, and for the transition probabilities the reestimation formulas are given by

$$\theta_{ij} \leftarrow \frac{\sum_l n_{ij}(l)}{\sum_{j'l'} n_{ij'}(l')} = \frac{n_{ij}}{\sum_{j'} n_{ij'}}, \tag{2.3}$$

where $n_{ij}(l) = P(\pi_{l-1} = i, \pi_l = j \mid x, \Theta)$ is the expected number of times a transition from state i to state j is used at time l. The reestimation equations for the match probabilities can be expressed in a similar way by defining $n_i(l) = P(\pi_l = i \,|\, x, \Theta)$ as the expected number of times we are in state i at time l. Then the reestimation equations for the match probabilities are given by

$$\phi_i(a) \leftarrow \frac{\sum_l n_i(l)\delta_{x_l,a}}{\sum_{l a'} n_i(l)\delta_{x_l,a'}} = \frac{n_i(a)}{\sum_{a'} n_i(a')}. \tag{2.4}$$

The expected counts can be computed efficiently by the forward-backward algorithm. In addition to the forward recursion, a similar recursion for the backward variable $\beta_i(l)$ is introduced. Let $\beta_i(l) = P(x_{l+1}, \ldots, x_L \,|\, \pi_l = i, \Theta)$, that is, the probability of matching the rest of the sequence $x_{l+1}, \ldots, x_L$ given that we are in state i at time l. After initializing by $\beta_N(L) = 1$, the recursion runs from $l = L - 1$ to $l = 1$ as

$$\beta_i(l) = \sum_{j=1}^{N} \theta_{ij}\beta_j(l+1)\phi_j(x_{l+1}), \tag{2.5}$$

for all states $1 \le i \le N$. Using the forward and backward variables, $n_{ij}(l)$ and $n_i(l)$ can easily be computed:

$$n_{ij}(l) = P(\pi_{l-1}=i, \pi_l=j \,|\, x, \Theta) = \frac{\alpha_i(l-1)\theta_{ij}\phi_j(x_l)\beta_j(l)}{P(x|\Theta)} \tag{2.6}$$

$$n_i(l) = P(\pi_l=i \,|\, x, \Theta) = \frac{\alpha_i(l)\beta_i(l)}{P(x|\Theta)}. \tag{2.7}$$

2.1 Discriminative Training. In many problems, the aim is to predict what class an input belongs to or what sequence of classes it represents. In continuous speech recognition, for instance, the object is to predict the sequence of words or phonemes for a speech signal. To achieve this, a (sub)model for each class is usually estimated by ML independent of all other models and using only the data belonging to this class. This procedure maximizes the ability of the model to reproduce the observations in each class and can be expressed as

$$\hat{\Theta}^{ML} = \operatorname*{argmax}_{\Theta} P(x, y|\Theta) = \operatorname*{argmax}_{\Theta}[P(x|\Theta_y)P(y|\Theta)], \tag{2.8}$$

where y is the class or sequence of class labels corresponding to the observation sequence x and Θ_y is the model for class y or a concatenation of submodels corresponding to the observed labels. In speech recognition, $P(x|\Theta_y)$ is often denoted the acoustic model probability, and the language model probability $P(y|\Theta)$ is usually assumed constant during training of the acoustic models. If the true source producing the data is contained in the model space, ML estimation based on an infinite training set can give the optimal parameters for classification (Nádas et al., 1988; Nádas, 1983), provided that the global maximum of the likelihood can be reached. However, in any real-world application, it is highly unlikely that the true source is contained in the space of HMMs, and the training data are indeed limited. This is the motivation for using discriminative training.

To accommodate discriminative training, we use one big model and assign a label to each state; all the states that are supposed to describe a certain class C are assigned label C. A state can also have a probability distribution $\psi_i(c)$ over labels, so that several labels are possible with different probabilities. This is discussed in Krogh (1994) and Riis (1998a), and it is somewhat similar to the input/output HMM (IOHMM) (Bengio & Frasconi, 1996). For brevity, however, we here limit ourselves to consider only one label for each state, which we believe is the most interesting for many applications. Because each state has a class label or a distribution over class labels, this sort of model was called a class HMM (CHMM) in Krogh (1994).

In the CHMM, the objective is to predict the labels associated with x, and instead of ML estimation, we therefore choose to maximize the probability of the correct labeling,

$$\hat{\Theta}^{CML} = \operatorname*{argmax}_{\Theta} P(y|x, \Theta) = \operatorname*{argmax}_{\Theta} \frac{P(x, y|\Theta)}{P(x|\Theta)}, \qquad (2.9)$$

which is also called conditional maximum likelihood (CML) estimation (Nádas, 1983). If the language model is assumed constant during training, CML estimation is equivalent to maximum mutual information estimation (Bahl, Brown, de Souza, & Mercer, 1986).

From equation 2.9, we observe that computing the probability of the labeling requires computation of (1) the probability $P(x, y|\Theta)$ in the clamped phase and (2) the probability $P(x|\Theta)$ in the free-running phase. The term *free running* means that the labels are not taken into account, so this phase is similar to the decoding phase, where we wish to find the labels for an observation sequence. The constraint by the labels during training gives rise to the name *clamped phase*; this terminology is borrowed from the Boltzmann machine literature (Ackley, Hinton, & Sejnowski, 1985; Bridle, 1990). Thus, CML estimation adjusts the model parameters so as to make the free-running recognition model as close as possible to the clamped model. The probability in the free-running phase is computed using the forward algorithm described for standard HMMs, whereas the probability in the clamped phase is computed by considering only paths $C(y)$ that are consistent with the observed labeling,

$$P(x, y|\Theta) = \sum_{\pi \in C(y)} P(x, \pi|\Theta). \qquad (2.10)$$

This quantity can be calculated by a variant of the forward algorithm to be discussed below.

Unfortunately the Baum-Welch algorithm is not applicable to CML estimation (see, e.g., Gopalakrishnan, Kanevsky, Nádas, & Nahamoo, 1991). Instead, one can use a gradient-descent-based approach, which is also applicable to the HNNs discussed later. To calculate the gradients, we switch to the negative log-likelihood, and define

$$\mathcal{L} = -\log P(y|x, \Theta) = \mathcal{L}_c - \mathcal{L}_f \tag{2.11}$$
$$\mathcal{L}_c = -\log P(x, y|\Theta) \tag{2.12}$$
$$\mathcal{L}_f = -\log P(x|\Theta). \tag{2.13}$$

The derivative of $\mathcal{L}_f$ for the free-running model with regard to a generic parameter $\omega \in \Theta$ can be expressed as,

$$
\begin{aligned}
\frac{\partial \mathcal{L}_f}{\partial \omega} &= -\frac{1}{P(x|\Theta)} \frac{\partial P(x|\Theta)}{\partial \omega} \\
&= -\sum_{\pi} \frac{1}{P(x|\Theta)} \frac{\partial P(x, \pi|\Theta)}{\partial \omega} \\
&= -\sum_{\pi} \frac{P(x, \pi|\Theta)}{P(x|\Theta)} \frac{\partial \log P(x, \pi|\Theta)}{\partial \omega} \\
&= -\sum_{\pi} P(\pi|x, \Theta) \frac{\partial \log P(x, \pi|\Theta)}{\partial \omega}.
\end{aligned}
\tag{2.14}
$$

This gradient is an expectation over all paths of the derivative of the complete data log-likelihood $\log P(x, \pi|\Theta)$. Using equation 2.1, this becomes

$$\frac{\partial \mathcal{L}_f}{\partial \omega} = -\sum_{l,i} \frac{n_i(l)}{\phi_i(x_l)} \frac{\partial \phi_i(x_l)}{\partial \omega} - \sum_{l,i,j} \frac{n_{ij}(l)}{\theta_{ij}} \frac{\partial \theta_{ij}}{\partial \omega}. \tag{2.15}$$

The gradient of the negative log-likelihood $\mathcal{L}_c$ in the clamped phase is computed similarly, but the expectation is taken only for the allowed paths $\mathcal{C}(y)$,

$$\frac{\partial \mathcal{L}_c}{\partial \omega} = -\sum_{l,i} \frac{m_i(l)}{\phi_i(x_l)} \frac{\partial \phi_i(x_l)}{\partial \omega} - \sum_{l,i,j} \frac{m_{ij}(l)}{\theta_{ij}} \frac{\partial \theta_{ij}}{\partial \omega}, \tag{2.16}$$

where $m_{ij}(l) = P(\pi_{l-1} = i, \pi_l = j | x, y, \Theta)$ is the expected number of times a transition from state i to state j is used at time l for the allowed paths. Similarly, $m_i(l) = P(\pi_l = i | x, y, \Theta)$ is the expected number of times we are in state i at time l for the allowed paths. These counts can be computed using the modified forward-backward algorithm, discussed below.

For a standard model, the derivatives in equations 2.15 and 2.16 are simple. When ω is a transition probability, we obtain

$$\frac{\partial \mathcal{L}}{\partial \theta_{ij}} = -\frac{m_{ij} - n_{ij}}{\theta_{ij}}. \tag{2.17}$$

The derivative $\frac{\partial \mathcal{L}}{\partial \phi_i(a)}$ is of exactly the same form, except that m_{ij} and n_{ij} are replaced by $m_i(a)$ and $n_i(a)$, and θ_{ij} by $\phi_i(a)$.

When minimizing $\mathcal{L}$ by gradient descent, it must be ensured that the probability parameters remain positive and properly normalized. Here we use the same method as Bridle (1990) and Baldi and Chauvin (1994) and do gradient descent in another set of unconstrained variables. For the transition probabilities, we define

$$\theta_{ij} = \frac{e^{z_{ij}}}{\sum_{j'} e^{z_{ij'}}}, \tag{2.18}$$

where z_{ij} are the new unconstrained auxiliary variables, and θ_{ij} always sum to one by construction. Gradient descent in the z's by $z_{ij} \leftarrow z_{ij} - \eta \frac{\partial \mathcal{L}}{\partial z_{ij}}$ yields a change in θ given by

$$\theta_{ij} \leftarrow \frac{\theta_{ij} \exp(-\eta \frac{\partial \mathcal{L}}{\partial z_{ij}})}{\sum_{j'} \theta_{ij'} \exp(-\eta \frac{\partial \mathcal{L}}{\partial z_{ij'}})}. \tag{2.19}$$

The gradients with respect to z_{ij} can be expressed entirely in terms of θ_{ij} and $m_{ij} - n_{ij}$,

$$\frac{\partial \mathcal{L}}{\partial z_{ij}} = -[m_{ij} - n_{ij} - \theta_{ij} \sum_{j'} (m_{ij'} - n_{ij'})], \tag{2.20}$$

and inserting equation 2.20 into 2.19 yields an expression entirely in θs. Equations for the emission probabilities are obtained in exactly the same way. This approach is slightly more straightforward than the one proposed in Baldi and Chauvin (1994), where the auxiliary variables are retained and the parameters of the model calculated explicitly from equation 2.18 after updating the auxiliary variables. This type of gradient descent is very similar to the exponentiated gradient descent proposed and investigated in Kivinen and Warmuth (1997) and Helmbold, Schapire, Singer, and Warmuth (1997).

2.2 The CHMM as a Probabilistic Independence Network.

A large variety of probabilistic models can be represented as graphical models (Lauritzen, 1996), including the HMM and its variants. The relation between HMMs and probabilistic independence networks is thoroughly described

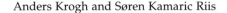

Figure 1: The DPIN (left) and UPIN (right) for an HMM.

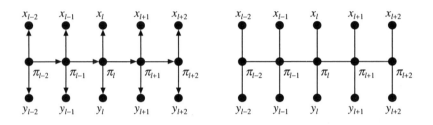

Figure 2: The DPIN (left) and UPIN (right) for a CHMM.

in Smyth, Heckerman, and Jordan (1997), and here we follow their terminology and refer the reader to that paper for more details.

An HMM can be represented as both a directed probabilistic independence network (DPIN) and an undirected one (UPIN) (see Figure 1). The DPIN shows the conditional dependencies of the variables in the HMM—both the observable ones (x) and the unobservable ones (π). For instance, the DPIN in Figure 1 shows that conditioned on π_l, x_l is independent of $x_1, \ldots, x_{l-1}$ and $\pi_1, \ldots, \pi_{l-1}$, that is, $P(x_l|x_1, \ldots, x_{l-1}, \pi_1, \ldots, \pi_l) = P(x_l|\pi_l)$. Similarly, $P(\pi_l|x_1, \ldots, x_{l-1}, \pi_1, \ldots, \pi_{l-1}) = P(\pi_l|\pi_{l-1})$. When "marrying" unconnected parents of all nodes in a DPIN and removing the directions, the moral graph is obtained. This is a UPIN for the model. For the HMM, the UPIN has the same topology as shown in Figure 1.

In the CHMM there is one more set of variables (the y's), and the PIN structures are shown in Figure 2. In a way, the CHMM can be seen as an HMM with two streams of observables, x and y, but they are usually not treated symmetrically. Again the moral graph is of the same topology, because no node has more than one parent.

It turns out that the graphical representation is the best way to see the difference between the CHMM and the IOHMM. In the IOHMM, the output y_l is conditioned on both the input x_l and the state π_l, but more important, the state is conditioned on the input. This is shown in the DPIN of Figure 3 (Bengio & Frasconi, 1996). In this case the moral graph is different, because π_l has two unconnected parents in the DPIN.

It is straightforward to extend the CHMM to have the label y conditioned on x, meaning that there would be arrows from x_l to y_l in the DPIN for the

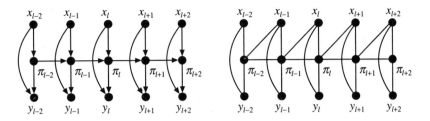

Figure 3: The DPIN for an IOHMM (left) is adapted from Bengio and Frasconi (1996). The moral graph to the right is a UPIN for an IOHMM.

CHMM. Then the only difference between the DPINs for the CHMM and the IOHMM would be the direction of the arrow between x_l and π_l. However, the DPIN for the CHMM would still not contain any "unmarried parents" and thus their moral graphs would be different.

2.3 Calculation of Quantities Consistent with the Labels. Generally there are two different types of labeling: incomplete and complete labeling (Juang & Rabiner, 1991). We describe the modified forward-backward algorithm for both types of labeling below.

2.3.1 Complete Labels. In this case, each observation has a label, so the sequence of labels denoted $y = y_1, \ldots, y_L$ is as long as the sequence of observations. Typically the labels come in groups, that is, several consecutive observations have the same label. In speech recognition, the complete labeling corresponds to knowing which word or phoneme each particular observation x_l is associated with.

For complete labeling, the expectations in the clamped phase are averages over "allowed" paths through the model—paths in which the labels of the states agree with the labeling of the observations. Such averages can be calculated by limiting the sum in the forward and backward recursions to states with the correct label. The new forward and backward variables, $\tilde{\alpha}_i(l)$ and $\tilde{\beta}_i(l)$, are defined as $\alpha_i(l)$ (see equation 2.2) and $\beta_i(l)$ (see equation 2.5), but with $\phi_i(x_l)$ replaced by $\phi_i(x_l)\delta_{y_l,c_i}$. The expected counts $m_{ij}(l)$ and $m_i(l)$ for the allowed paths are calculated exactly as $n_{ij}(l)$ and $n_i(l)$, but using the new forward and backward variables.

If we think of $\alpha_i(l)$ (or $\beta_i(l)$) as a matrix, the new algorithm corresponds to masking this matrix such that only allowed regions are calculated (see Figure 4). Therefore the calculation is faster than the standard forward (or backward) calculation of the whole matrix.

2.3.2 Incomplete Labels. When dealing with incomplete labeling, the whole sequence of observations is associated with a shorter sequence of

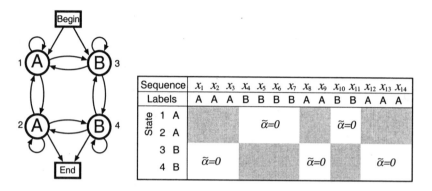

Figure 4: (Left) A very simple model with four states, two labeled A and two labeled B. (Right) The $\tilde{\alpha}$ matrix for an example of observations $x_1, \ldots, x_{14}$ with complete labels. The gray areas of the matrix are calculated as in the standard forward algorithm, whereas $\tilde{\alpha}$ is set to zero in the white areas. The $\tilde{\beta}$ matrix is calculated in the same way, but from right to left.

labels $y = y_1, \ldots, y_S$, where $S < L$. The label of each individual observation is unknown; only the order of labels is available. In continuous speech recognition, the correct string of phonemes is known (because the spoken words are known in the training set), but the time boundaries between them are unknown. In such a case, the sequence of observations may be considerably longer than the label sequence. The case $S = 1$ corresponds to classifying the whole sequence into one of the possible classes (e.g., isolated word recognition).

To compute the expected counts for incomplete labeling, one has to ensure that the sequence of labels matches the sequence of *groups of states with the same label*.[1] This is less restrictive than the complete label case. An easy way to ensure this is by rearranging the (big) model temporarily for each observation sequence and collecting the statistics (the m's) by running the standard forward-backward algorithm on this model. This is very similar to techniques already used in several speech applications (see, e.g., Lee, 1990), where phoneme (sub)models corresponding to the spoken word or sentence are concatenated. Note, however, that for the CHMM, the transitions between states with different labels retain their original value in the temporary model (see Figure 5).

---

[1] If multiple labels are allowed in each state, an algorithm similar to the forward-backward algorithm for asynchronous IOHMMs (Bengio & Bengio, 1996) can be used; see Riis (1998a).

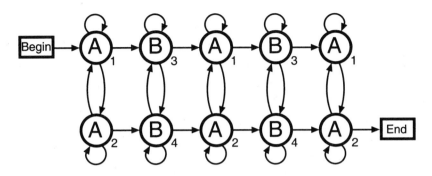

Figure 5: For the same model as in Figure 4, this example shows how the model is temporarily rearranged for gathering statistics (i.e., calculation of m values) for a sequence with incomplete labels *ABABA*.

3 Hidden Neural Networks

HMMs are based on a number of assumptions that limit their classification abilities. Combining the CHMM framework with neural networks can lead to a more flexible and powerful model for classification. The basic idea of the HNN presented here is to replace the probability parameters of the CHMM by state-specific multilayer perceptrons that take the observations as input. Thus, in the HNN, it is possible to assign up to three networks to each state: (1) a *match network* outputting the "probability" that the current observation matches a given state, (2) a *transition network* that outputs transition "probabilities" dependent on observations, and (3) a *label network* that outputs the probability of the different labels in this state. We have put "probabilities" in quotes because the output of the match and transition networks need not be properly normalized probabilities, since global normalization is used. For brevity we limit ourselves here to one label per state; the label networks are not present. The case of multiple labels in each state is treated in more detail in Riis (1998a).

The CHMM match probability $\phi_i(x_l)$ of observation x_l in state i is replaced by the output of a match network, $\phi_i(s_l; w^i)$, assigned to state i. The match network in state i is parameterized by a weight vector w^i and takes the vector s_l as input. Similarly, the probability θ_{ij} of a transition from state i to j is replaced by the output of a transition network $\theta_{ij}(s_l; u^i)$, which is parameterized by weights u^i. The transition network assigned to state i has $\mathcal{J}_i$ outputs, where $\mathcal{J}_i$ is the number of (nonzero) transitions *from* state i. Since we consider only states with one possible label, the label networks are just delta functions, as in the CHMM described earlier.

The network input s_l corresponding to x_l will usually be a window of context around x_l, such as a symmetrical context window of $2K + 1$

observations,[2] $x_{l-K}, x_{l-K+1}, \ldots, x_{l+K}$; however, it can be any sort of information related to x_l or the observation sequence in general. We will call s_l the *context* of observation x_l, but it can contain all sorts of other information and can differ from state to state. The only limitation is that it cannot depend on the path through the model, because then the state process is no longer first-order Markovian.

Each of the three types of networks in an HNN state can be omitted or replaced by standard CHMM probabilities. In fact, all sorts of combinations with standard CHMM states are possible. If an HNN contains only transition networks (that is, $\phi_i(s_l; w^i) = 1$ for all i, l) the model can be normalized locally by using a softmax output function as in the IOHMM. However, if it contains match networks, it is usually impossible to make $\sum_{x \in \mathcal{X}} P(x|\Theta) = 1$ by normalizing locally even if the transition networks are normalized. A probabilistic interpretation of the HNN is instead ensured by global normalization. We define the joint probability

$$
\begin{aligned}
P(x, y, \pi|\Theta) &= \frac{1}{Z(\Theta)} R(x, y, \pi|\Theta) \\
&= \frac{1}{Z(\Theta)} \prod_l \theta_{\pi_{l-1}\pi_l}(s_l; u^{\pi_{l-1}}) \phi_{\pi_l}(s_l; w^{\pi_l}) \delta_{y_l, c^{\pi_l}},
\end{aligned}
\tag{3.1}
$$

where the normalizing constant is $Z(\Theta) = \sum_{x,y,\pi} R(x, y, \pi|\Theta)$. From this,

$$
\begin{aligned}
P(x, y|\Theta) &= \frac{1}{Z(\Theta)} R(x, y|\Theta) = \frac{1}{Z(\Theta)} \sum_{\pi} R(x, y, \pi|\Theta) \\
&= \frac{1}{Z(\Theta)} \sum_{\pi \in \mathcal{C}(y)} R(x, \pi|\Theta),
\end{aligned}
\tag{3.2}
$$

where

$$
R(x, \pi|\Theta) = \prod_l \theta_{\pi_{l-1}\pi_l}(s_l; u^{\pi_{l-1}}) \phi_{\pi_l}(s_l; w^{\pi_l}).
\tag{3.3}
$$

Similarly,

$$
\begin{aligned}
P(x|\Theta) &= \frac{1}{Z(\Theta)} R(x|\Theta) = \frac{1}{Z(\Theta)} \sum_{y,\pi} R(x, y, \pi|\Theta) \\
&= \frac{1}{Z(\Theta)} \sum_{\pi} R(x, \pi|\Theta).
\end{aligned}
\tag{3.4}
$$

---

[2] If the observations are inherently discrete (as in protein modeling), they can be encoded in binary vectors and then used in the same manner as continuous observation vectors.

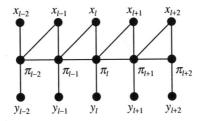

Figure 6: The UPIN for an HNN using transition networks that take only the current observation as input ($s_l = x_l$).

It is sometimes possible to compute the normalization factor Z, but not in all cases. However, for CML estimation, the normalization factor cancels out,

$$P(y|x, \Theta) = \frac{R(x, y|\Theta)}{R(x|\Theta)}. \qquad (3.5)$$

The calculation of $R(x|\Theta)$ and $R(x, y|\Theta)$ can be done exactly as the calculation of $P(x|\Theta)$ and $P(x, y|\Theta)$ in the CHMM, because the forward and backward algorithms are not dependent on the normalization of probabilities.

Because one cannot usually normalize the HNN locally, there exists no directed graph (DPIN) for the general HNN. For UPINs, however, local normalization is not required. For instance, the Boltzmann machine can be drawn as a UPIN, and the Boltzmann chain (Saul & Jordan, 1995) can actually be described by a UPIN identical to the one for a globally normalized discrete HMM in Figure 1. A model with a UPIN is characterized by its clique functions, and the joint probability is the product of all the clique functions (Smyth et al., 1997). The three different clique functions are clearly seen in equation 3.1. In Figure 6 the UPIN for an HNN with transition networks and $s_l = x_l$ is shown; this is identical to Figure 3 for the IOHMM, except that it does not have edges from x to y. Note that the UPIN remains the same if match networks (with $s_l = x_l$) are used as well. The graphical representation as a UPIN for an HNN with no transition networks and match networks having a context of one to each side is shown in Figure 7 along with the three types of cliques.

A number of authors have investigated compact representations of conditional probability tables in DPINs (see Boutilier, Friedman, Goldszmidt, & Koller, 1996, and references therein). The HNN provides a similar compact representation of clique functions in UPINs, and this holds also for models that are more general than the HMM-type graphs discussed in this article.

The fact that the individual neural network outputs do not have to normalize gives us a great deal of freedom in selecting the output activation

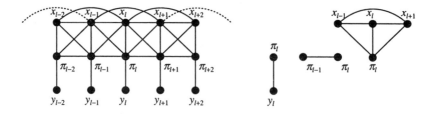

Figure 7: (Left) The UPIN of an HNN with no transition networks and match networks having a context of one to each side. (Right) The three different clique types contained in the graph.

function. A natural choice is a standard (asymmetric) sigmoid or an exponential output activation function, $g(h) = \exp(h)$, where h is the input to the output unit in question.

Although the HNN is a very intuitive and simple extension of the standard CHMM, it is a much more powerful model. First, neural networks can implement complex functions using far fewer parameters than, say, a mixture of gaussians. Furthermore, the HNN can directly use observation context as input to the neural networks and thereby exploit higher-order correlations between consecutive observations, which is difficult in standard HMMs. This property can be particularly useful in problems like speech recognition, where the pronunciation of one phoneme is highly influenced by the acoustic context in which it is uttered. Finally, the observation context dependency on the transitions allows the HNN to model the data as successive steady-state segments connected by "nonstationary" transitional regions. For speech recognition this is believed to be very important (see, e.g., Bourlard, Konig, & Morgan, 1994; Morgan, Bourlard, Greenberg, and Hermansky, 1994).

3.1 Training an HNN. As for the CHMM, it is not possible to train the HNN using an EM algorithm; instead, we suggest training the model using gradient descent. From equations 2.15 and 2.16, we find the following gradients of $\mathcal{L} = -\log P(y|x, \Theta)$ with regard to a generic weight ω^i in the match or transition network assigned to state i,

$$\frac{\partial \mathcal{L}}{\partial \omega^i} = -\sum_l \frac{m_i(l) - n_i(l)}{\phi_i(s_l; w^i)} \frac{\partial \phi_i(s_l; w^i)}{\partial \omega^i} - \sum_{lj} \frac{m_{ij}(l) - n_{ij}(l)}{\theta_{ij}(s_l; u^i)} \frac{\partial \theta_{ij}(s_l; u^i)}{\partial \omega^i}, \quad (3.6)$$

where it is assumed that networks are not shared between states. In the backpropagation algorithm for neural networks (Rumelhart, Hinton, & Williams, 1986) the squared error of the network is minimized by gradient descent. For an activation function g, this gives rise to a weight update of the form $\Delta w \propto -\mathcal{E} \times \frac{\partial g}{\partial w}$. We therefore see from equation 3.6 that the neural networks are trained using the standard backpropagation algorithm where the quantity to backpropagate is $\mathcal{E} = [m_i(l) - n_i(l)]/\phi_i(s_l; w^i)$ for the match networks and $\mathcal{E} = [m_{ij}(l) - n_{ij}(l)]/\theta_{ij}(s_l; u^i)$ for the transition networks. The m and n counts are calculated as before by running two forward-backward passes: once in the clamped phase (the m's) and once in the free-running phase (the n's).

The training can be done in either batch mode, where all the networks are updated after the entire training set has been presented to the model, or sequence on-line mode, where the update is performed after the presentation of each sequence. There are many other variations possible. Because of the l dependence of $m_{ij}(l)$, $m_i(l)$ and the similar n's, the training algorithm is not as simple as for standard HMMs; we have to do a backpropagation pass for each l. Because the expected counts are not available before the forward-backward passes have been completed, we must either store or recalculate all the neural network unit activations for each input s_l before running backpropagation. Storing all activations can require large amounts of memory even for small networks if the observation sequences are very long (which they typically are in continuous speech). For such tasks, it is necessary to recalculate the network unit activations before each backpropagation pass. Many of the standard modifications of the backpropagation algorithm can be incorporated, such as momentum and weight decay (Hertz, Krogh, & Palmer, 1991). It is also possible to use conjugate gradient descent or approximative second-order methods like pseudo-Gauss-Newton. However, in a set of initial experiments for the speech recognition task reported in section 4, on-line gradient methods consistently gave the fastest convergence.

4 Comparison to Other Work

Recently several HMM/NN hybrids have been proposed in the literature. The hybrids can roughly be divided into those estimating the parameters of the HMM and the NN separately (see, e.g., Renals, Morgan, Bourlard, Cohen, & Franco, 1994; Robinson, 1994; Le Cerf, Ma, & Compernolle, 1994; McDermott & Katagiri, 1991) and those applying simultaneous or joint estimation of all parameters as in the HNN (see, e.g., Baldi & Chauvin, 1996; Konig, Bourlard, & Morgan, 1996; Bengio, De Mori, Flammia, & Kompe, 1992; Johansen, 1994; Valtchev, Kapadia, & Young, 1993; Bengio & Frasconi, 1996; Hennebert, Ris, Bourlard, Renals, & Morgan, 1997; Bengio, LeCun, Nohl, & Burges, 1995).

In Renals et al. (1994) a multilayer perceptron is trained separately to estimate phoneme posterior probabilities, which are scaled with the observed phoneme frequencies and then used instead of the usual emission densities in a continuous HMM. A similar approach is taken in Robinson (1994), but here a recurrent NN is used. A slightly different method is used in McDermott and Katagiri (1991) and Le Cerf et al. (1994), where the vector quantizer front end in a discrete HMM is replaced by a multilayer perceptron or a learning vector quantization network (Kohonen, Barna, & Chrisley, 1988). In contrast, our approach uses only one output for each match network whereby continuous and discrete observations are treated the same.

Several authors have proposed methods in which all parameters are estimated simultaneously as in the HNN. In some hybrids, a big multilayer perceptron (Bengio et al., 1992; Johansen & Johnsen, 1994) or recurrent network (Valtchev et al., 1993) performs an adaptive input transformation of the observation vectors. Thus, the network outputs are used as new observation vectors in a continuous density HMM, and simultaneous estimation of all parameters is performed by backpropagating errors calculated by the HMM into the neural network in a way similar to the HNN training. Our approach is somewhat similar to the idea of adaptive input transformations, but instead of retaining the computationally expensive mixture densities, we replace these by match networks. This is also done in Bengio et al. (1995), where a large network with the same number of outputs as there are states in the HMM is trained by backpropagating errors calculated by the HMM. Instead of backpropagating errors from the HMM into the neural network, Hennebert et al. (1997) and Senior and Robinson (1996) use a two-step iterative procedure to train the networks. In the first step, the current model is used for estimating a set of "soft" targets for the neural networks, and then the network is trained on these targets. This method extends the scaled likelihood approach by Renals et al. (1994) to use global estimation where training is performed by a generalized EM (GEM) algorithm (Hennebert et al., 1997).

The IOHMM (Bengio and Frasconi, 1996) and the CHMM/HNN have different graphical representations, as seen in Figures 2, 3, and 7. However, the IOHMM is very similar to a locally normalized HNN with a label and transition network in each state, but no match network. An important difference between the two is in the decoding, where the IOHMM uses only a forward pass, which makes it insensitive to future events but makes the decoding "real time." (See Riis, 1998a, for more details.)

5 Experiments

In this section we give an evaluation of the HNN on the task introduced in Johansen (1994) of recognizing five broad phoneme classes in continuous read speech from the TIMIT database (Garofolo et al., 1993): vowels (V), consonants (C), nasals (N), liquids (L) and silence (S) (see Table 1).

We use one sentence from each of the 462 speakers in the TIMIT training set for training, and the results are reported for the recommended TIMIT core test set containing 192 sentences. An additional validation set of 144 sentences has been used to monitor performance during training. The raw speech signal is preprocessed using a standard mel cepstral preprocessor, which outputs a 26-dimensional feature vector each 10 ms (13 mel cepstral features and 13 delta features). These vectors are normalized to zero mean

Table 1: Definition of Broad Phoneme Classes.

Broad Class	TIMIT Phoneme Label
Vowel (V)	iy ih eh ae ix ax ah ax-h uw uh ao aa ey ay oy aw ow ux
Consonant (C)	ch jh dh b d dx g p t k z zh v f th s sh hh hv
Nasal (N)	m n en ng em nx eng
Liquid (L)	l el r y w er axr
Silence (S)	h# pau

and unit variance. Each of the five classes is modeled by a simple left-to-right three-state model. The last state in any submodel is fully connected to the first state of all other submodels. (Further details are given in Riis & Krogh, 1997.)

5.1 Baseline Results. In Table 2, the results for complete label training are shown for the baseline system, which is a discrete CHMM using a codebook of 256 codebook vectors. The results are reported in the standard measure of percentage accuracy, $\%Acc = 100\% - \%Ins - \%Del - \%Sub$, where $\%Ins$, $\%Del$ and $\%Sub$ denote the percentage of insertions, deletions and substitutions used for aligning the observed and the predicted transcription.[3] In agreement with results reported in Johansen (1994), we have observed an increased performance for CML estimated models when using a forward or all-paths decoder instead of the best-path Viterbi decoder. In this work we use an N-best decoder (Schwarz & Chow, 1990) with 10 active hypotheses during decoding. Only the top-scoring hypothesis is used at the end of decoding. The N-best decoder finds (approximatively) the most probable labels, which depends on many different paths, whereas the Viterbi algorithm finds only the most probable path. For ML-trained models, the N-best and Viterbi decoder yield approximately the same accuracy (see Table 2). As shown by an example in Figure 8, several paths contribute to the optimal labeling in the CML estimated models, whereas only a few paths contribute significantly for the ML estimated models.

Table 2 shows that additional incomplete label training of a complete label trained model does not improve performance for the ML estimated model. However, for the CML estimation, there is a significant gain in accuracy by incomplete label training. The reason is that the CML criterion is very sensitive to mislabelings, because it is dominated by training sequences with an unlikely labeling. Although the phoneme segmentation (complete labeling) in TIMIT is done by hand, it is imperfect. Furthermore, it is often impossible—or even meaningless—to assign exact boundaries between phonemes.

---

[3] The NIST standard scoring package "sclite" version 1.1 is used in all experiments.

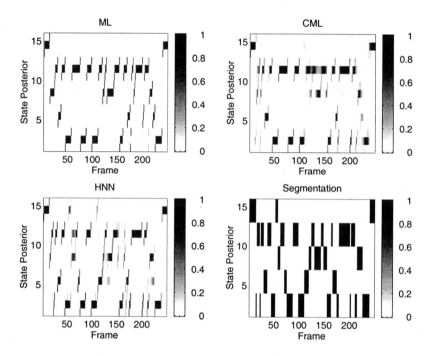

Figure 8: State posterior plots ($P(\pi_l = i \mid x, \Theta)$) for baseline and HNN for the test sentence "But in this one section we welcomed auditors" (TIMIT id: si1361). States 1–3 belong to the consonant model, 4–6 to the nasal model, 7–9 to the liquid model, 10–12 to the vowel model, and 13–15 to the silence model. (Top left) ML-trained baseline, which yield %Acc = 62.5 for this sentence. (Top right) CML-trained baseline (%Acc = 78.1). (Bottom left) HNN using both match and transition networks with 10 hidden units and context $K = 1$ (%Acc = 93.7). (Bottom right) The observed segmentation.

Table 2: Baseline Recognition Accuracies.

	Viterbi	N-Best
Complete labels		
ML	75.9	76.1
CML	76.6	79.0
Incomplete labels		
ML	75.8	75.2
CML	78.4	81.3

Note: The baseline system contains 3856 free parameters.

CML gives a big improvement from an accuracy of around 76% for the ML estimated models to around 81%. Statistical significance is hard to assess, because of the computational requirements for this task, but in a set of 10 CML training sessions of random initial models, we observed a deviation of no more than ±0.2% in accuracy. For comparison, a MMI-trained model with a single diagonal covariance gaussian per state achieved a result of 72.4% accuracy in Johansen and Johnsen (1994).

5.2 HNN Results. For the HNN, two series of experiments were conducted. In the first set of experiments, only a match network is used in each state, and the transitions are standard HMM transitions. In the second set of experiments, we also use match networks, but the match distribution *and* the standard transitions in the last state of each submodel are replaced by a transition network. All networks use the same input s_l, have the same number of hidden units, are fully connected, and have sigmoid output functions. This also applies for the transition networks; that is, a softmax output function is *not* used for the transition networks.

Although the HNN with match networks and no hidden units has far fewer parameters than the baseline system, it achieves a comparable performance of 80.8% accuracy using only the current observation x_l as input ($K = 0$) and 81.7% accuracy for a context of one left and right observation ($K = 1$) (see Table 3). No further improvement was observed for larger contexts. Note that the match networks without hidden units just implement linear weighted sums of input features (passed through a sigmoid output function). For approximately the same number of parameters as used in the baseline system, the HNN with 10 hidden units and no context ($K = 0$) yields 84.0% recognition accuracy. Increasing the context or number of hidden units for this model yields a slightly lower accuracy due to overfitting.

In Johansen (1994) a multilayer perceptron was used as a global adaptive input transformation to a continuous density HMM with a single diagonal covariance gaussian per state. Using N-best decoding and CML estimation, a result of 81.3% accuracy was achieved on the broad phoneme class task.

When using a transition network in the last state of each submodel, the accuracy increases, as shown in Table 3. Thus, for the model with context $K = 1$ and no hidden units, an accuracy of 82.3% is obtained compared to 81.7% for the same model with only match networks. The best result on the five broad class task is an accuracy of 84.4% obtained by the HNN with context $K = 1$, match and transition networks and 10 hidden units in all networks (see Table 3).

6 Conclusion

In this article we described the HNN, which in a very natural way replaces the probability parameters of an HMM with the output of state-specific

Table 3: Recognition Accuracies for HNNs.

	Context K	Number of Parameters	Accuracy
No hidden units			
HNN, match networks	0	436	80.8
HNN, match networks	1	1,216	81.7
HNN, match and transition networks	1	2411	82.3
Ten hidden units			
HNN, match networks	0	4,246	84.0
HNN, match networks	1	12,046	83.8
HNN, match and transition networks	1	12,191	84.4

Note: "HNN, match networks" are models using only match networks and standard CHMM transitions, whereas "HNN, match and transition networks" use both match and transition networks. Decoding is done by N-best.

neural networks. The model is normalized at a global level, which ensures a proper probabilistic interpretation of the HNN. All the parameters in the model are trained simultaneously from labeled data using gradient-descent-based CML estimation. The architecture is very flexible in that all combinations with standard CHMM probability parameters are possible. The relation to graphical models was discussed, and it was shown that the HNN can be viewed as an undirected probabilistic independence network, where the neural networks provide a compact representation of the clique functions.

Finally, it was shown that the HNN improves on the results of a speech recognition problem with a reduced set of phoneme classes. The HNN has also been applied to the recognition of task-independent isolated words from the PHONEBOOK database (Riis, 1998b) and preliminary results on the 39 phoneme TIMIT problem are presented in Riis (1998a).

Acknowledgments

We thank Steve Renals and Finn T. Johansen for valuable comments and suggestions to this work. We also thank the anonymous referees for pointing our attention to graphical models. This work was supported by the Danish National Research Foundation.

References

Ackley, D. H., Hinton, G. E., & Sejnowski, T. J. (1985). A learning algorithm for Boltzmann machines. *Cognitive Science, 9,* 147–169.
Bahl, L. R., Brown, P. F., de Souza, P. V., & Mercer, R. L. (1986). Maximum mu-

tual information estimation of hidden Markov model parameters for speech recognition. In *Proceedings of ICASSP'86* (pp. 49–52).

Baldi, P., & Chauvin, Y. (1994). Smooth on-line learning algorithms for hidden Markov models. *Neural Computation, 6*(2), 307–318.

Baldi, P., & Chauvin, Y. (1996). Hybrid modeling, HMM/NN architectures, and protein applications. *Neural Computation, 8*, 1541–1565.

Bengio, S., & Bengio, Y. (1996). An EM algorithm for asynchronous input/output hidden Markov models. In *Proceedings of the ICONIP'96*.

Bengio, Y., De Mori, R., Flammia, G., & Kompe, R. (1992). Global optimization of a neural network–hidden Markov model hybrid. *IEEE Transactions on Neural Networks, 3*(2), 252–259.

Bengio, Y., & Frasconi, P. (1996). Input/output HMMs for sequence processing. *IEEE Transactions on Neural Networks, 7*(5), 1231–1249.

Bengio, Y., LeCun, Y., Nohl, C., & Burges, C. (1995). Lerec: A NN/HMM hybrid for on-line handwritting recognition. *Neural Computation, 7*(5).

Bourlard, H., Konig, Y., & Morgan, N. (1994). *REMAP: Recursive estimation and maximization of a posteriori probabilities* (Tech. Rep. TR-94-064). Berkeley, CA: International Computer Science Institute.

Boutilier, C., Friedman, N., Goldszmidt, M., & Koller, D. (1996). Context-specific independence in Bayesian networks. In E. Horvitz & F. V. Jensen (Eds.), *Proceedings of the Twelfth Conference on Uncertainty in Artificial Intelligence* (pp. 115–123). San Francisco: Morgan Kaufmann.

Bridle, J. S. (1990). Alphanets: A recurrent "neural" network architecture with a hidden Markov model interpretation. *Speech Communication, 9*, 83–92.

Dempster, A. P., Laird, N. M., & Rubin, D. B. (1977). Maximum likelihood from incomplete data via the EM algorithm. *Royal Statistical Society B, 39*, 1–38.

Durbin, R. M., Eddy, S. R., Krogh, A., & Mitchison, G. (1998). *Biological sequence analysis.* Cambridge: Cambridge University Press.

Eddy, S. R. (1996). Hidden Markov models. *Current Opinion in Structural Biology, 6*, 361–365.

Garofolo, J. S., Lamel, L. F., Fisher, W. M., Fiscus, J. G., Pallet, D. S., & Dahlgren, N. L. (1993). *DARPA TIMIT Acoustic-Phonetic Continuous Speech Corpus CD-ROM.* Gaithersburg, MD: National Institute of Standards.

Gopalakrishnan, P. S., Kanevsky, D., Nádas, A., & Nahamoo, D. (1991). An inequality for rational functions with applications to some statistical estimation problems. *IEEE Transactions on Information Theory, 37*(1), 107–113.

Helmbold, D. P., Schapire, R. E., Singer, Y., & Warmuth, M. K. (1997). A comparison of new and old algorithms for a mixture estimation problem. *Machine Learning, 27*(1), 97–119.

Hennebert, J., Ris, C., Bourlard, H., Renals, S., & Morgan, N. (1997). Estimation of global posteriors and forward-backward training of hybrid HMM/ANN systems. In *Proceedings of EUROSPEECH'97*.

Hertz, J. A., Krogh, A., & Palmer, R. (1991). *Introduction to the theory of neural computation.* Redwood City, CA: Addison-Wesley.

Johansen, F. T. (1994). Global optimisation of HMM input transformations. In *Proceedings of ICSLP'94* (Vol. 1, pp. 239–242).

Johansen, F. T., & Johnsen, M. H. (1994). Non-linear input transformations for discriminative HMMs. In *Proceedings of ICASSP'94* (Vol. 1, pp. 225–228).

Juang, B. H., & Rabiner, L. R. (1991). Hidden Markov models for speech recognition. *Technometrics, 33*(3), 251–272.

Kivinen, J., & Warmuth, M. K. (1997). Exponentiated gradient versus gradient descent for linear predictors. *Information and Computation, 132*(1), 1–63.

Kohonen, T., Barna, G., & Chrisley, R. (1988). Statistical pattern recognition with neural networks: Benchmarking studies. In *Proceedings of ICNN'88* (Vol. 1, pp. 61–68).

Konig, Y., Bourlard, H., & Morgan, N. (1996). REMAP: Recursive estimation and maximization of a posteriori probabilities—application to transition-based connectionist speech recognition. In D. S. Touretzky, M. C. Mozer, & M. E. Hasselmo (Eds.), *Advances in neural information processing systems, 8* (pp. 388–394). Cambridge, MA: MIT Press.

Krogh, A. (1994). Hidden Markov models for labeled sequences. In *Proceedings of the 12th IAPR ICPR'94* (pp. 140–144).

Krogh, A., Brown, M., Mian, I. S., Sjölander, K., & Haussler, D. (1994). Hidden Markov models in computational biology: Applications to protein modeling. *Journal of Molecular Biology, 235*, 1501–1531.

Lauritzen, S. L. (1996). *Graphical models*. New York: Oxford University Press.

Le Cerf, P., Ma, W., & Compernolle, D. V. (1994). Multilayer perceptrons as labelers for hidden Markov models. *IEEE Transactions on Speech and Audio Processing, 2*(1), 185–193.

Lee, K.-F. (1990). Context-dependent phonetic hidden Markov models for speaker-independent continuous speech recognition. *IEEE Transactions on Acoustics, Speech and Signal Processing, 38*(4), 599–609.

McDermott, E., & Katagiri, S. (1991). LVQ-based shift-tolerant phoneme recognition. *IEEE Transactions on Acoustics, Speech and Signal Processing, 39*, 1398–1411.

Morgan, N., Bourlard, H., Greenberg, S., & Hermansky, H. (1994). Stochastic perceptual auditory-event-based models for speech recognition. In *Proceedings of Interternational Conference on Spoken Language Processing* (pp. 1943–1946).

Nádas, A. (1983). A decision-theoretic formulation of a training problem in speech recognition and a comparison of training by unconditional versus conditional maximum likelihood. *IEEE Transactions on Acoustics, Speech and Signal Processing, 31*(4), 814–817.

Nádas, A., Nahamoo, D., & Picheny, M. A. (1988). On a model-robust training method for speech recognition. *IEEE Transactions on Acoustics, Speech and Signal Processing, 36*(9), 814–817.

Rabiner, L. R. (1989). A tutorial on hidden Markov models and selected applications in speech recognition. *Proceedings of IEEE, 77*(2), 257–286.

Renals, S., Morgan, N., Bourlard, H., Cohen, M., & Franco, H. (1994). Connectionist probability estimators in HMM speech recognition. *IEEE Transactions on Speech and Audio Processing, 2*(1), 161–174.

Riis, S. K. (1998a). *Hidden Markov models and neural networks for speech recognition.* Doctoral dissertation, IMM-PHD-1998-46, Technical University of Denmark.

Riis, S. K. (1998b). Hidden neural networks: Application to speech recognition. In *In Proceedings of ICASSP'98* (Vol. 2, pp. 1117–1121).

Riis, S. K., & Krogh, A. (1997). Hidden neural networks: A framework for HMM/NN hybrids. In *Proceedings of ICASSP'97* (pp. 3233–3236).

Robinson, A. J. (1994). An application of recurrent nets to phone probability estimation. *IEEE Transactions on Neural Networks, 5,* 298–305.

Rumelhart, D. E., Hinton, G. E., & Williams, R. J. (1986). Learning representations by back-propagating errors. *Nature, 323,* 533–536.

Saul, L. K., & Jordan, M. I. (1995). Boltzman chains and hidden Markov models. In G. Tesauro, D. Touretzky, & T. Leen (Eds.), *Advances in neural information processing systems, 7* (pp. 435–442). San Mateo, CA: Morgan Kaufmann.

Schwarz, R., & Chow, Y.-L. (1990). The N-best algorithm: An efficient and exact procedure for finding the N most likely hypotheses. In *Proceedings of ICASSP'90* (pp. 81–84).

Senior, A., & Robinson, T. (1996). Forward-backward retraining of recurrent neural networks. In D. Touretzky, M. Mozer, & M. Hasselmo (Eds.), *Advances in neural information processing dystems, 8* (pp. 743–749). San Mateo, CA: Morgan Kaufmann.

Smyth, P., Heckerman, D., & Jordan, M. I. (1997). Probabilistic independence networks for hidden Markov probability models. *Neural Computation, 9,* 227–269.

Valtchev, V., Kapadia, S., & Young, S. (1993). Recurrent input transformations for hidden Markov models. In *Proceedings of ICASSP'93* (pp. 287–290).

13

Variational Learning for Switching State-Space Models

Zoubin Ghahramani
Geoffrey E. Hinton
Gatsby Computational Neuroscience Unit, University College London, London WC1N 3AR, U.K.

We introduce a new statistical model for time series that iteratively segments data into regimes with approximately linear dynamics and learns the parameters of each of these linear regimes. This model combines and generalizes two of the most widely used stochastic time-series models—hidden Markov models and linear dynamical systems—and is closely related to models that are widely used in the control and econometrics literatures. It can also be derived by extending the mixture of experts neural network (Jacobs, Jordan, Nowlan, & Hinton, 1991) to its fully dynamical version, in which both expert and gating networks are recurrent. Inferring the posterior probabilities of the hidden states of this model is computationally intractable, and therefore the exact expectation maximization (EM) algorithm cannot be applied. However, we present a variational approximation that maximizes a lower bound on the log-likelihood and makes use of both the forward and backward recursions for hidden Markov models and the Kalman filter recursions for linear dynamical systems. We tested the algorithm on artificial data sets and a natural data set of respiration force from a patient with sleep apnea. The results suggest that variational approximations are a viable method for inference and learning in switching state-space models.

1 Introduction

Most commonly used probabilistic models of time series are descendants of either hidden Markov models (HMM) or stochastic linear dynamical systems, also known as state-space models (SSM). HMMs represent information about the past of a sequence through a single discrete random variable—the hidden state. The prior probability distribution of this state is derived from the previous hidden state using a stochastic transition matrix. Knowing the state at any time makes the past, present, and future observations statistically independent. This is the Markov independence property that gives the model its name.

SSMs represent information about the past through a real-valued hidden state vector. Again, conditioned on this state vector, the past, present, and future observations are statistically independent. The dependency between the present state vector and the previous state vector is specified through the dynamic equations of the system and the noise model. When these equations are linear and the noise model is gaussian, the SSM is also known as a linear dynamical system or Kalman filter model.

Unfortunately, most real-world processes cannot be characterized by either purely discrete or purely linear-gaussian dynamics. For example, an industrial plant may have multiple discrete modes of behavior, each with approximately linear dynamics. Similarly, the pixel intensities in an image of a translating object vary according to approximately linear dynamics for subpixel translations, but as the image moves over a larger range, the dynamics change significantly and nonlinearly.

This article addresses models of dynamical phenomena that are characterized by a combination of discrete and continuous dynamics. We introduce a probabilistic model called the switching SSM inspired by the divide-and-conquer principle underlying the mixture-of-experts neural network (Jacobs, Jordan, Nowlan, & Hinton, 1991). Switching SSMs are a natural generalization of HMMs and SSMs in which the dynamics can transition in a discrete manner from one linear operating regime to another. There is a large literature on models of this kind in econometrics, signal processing, and other fields (Harrison & Stevens, 1976; Chang & Athans, 1978; Hamilton, 1989; Shumway & Stoffer, 1991; Bar-Shalom & Li, 1993). Here we extend these models to allow for multiple real-valued state vectors, draw connections between these fields and the relevant literature on neural computation and probabilistic graphical models, and derive a learning algorithm for all the parameters of the model based on a structured variational approximation that rigorously maximizes a lower bound on the log-likelihood.

In the following section we review the background material on SSMs, HMMs, and hybrids of the two. In section 3, we describe the generative model—the probability distribution defined over the observation sequences—for switching SSMs. In section 4, we describe a learning algorithm for switching state-space models that is based on a structured variational approximation to the expectation-maximization algorithm. In section 5 we present simulation results in both an artificial domain, to assess the quality of the approximate inference method, and a natural domain. We conclude with section 6.

2 Background

2.1 State-Space Models. An SSM defines a probability density over time series of real-valued observation vectors $\{Y_t\}$ by assuming that the observations were generated from a sequence of hidden state vectors $\{X_t\}$. (Appendix A describes the variables and notation used throughout this article.) In particular, the SSM specifies that given the hidden state vector at one time step, the observation vector at that time step is statistically independent from all other observation vectors, and that the hidden state vectors

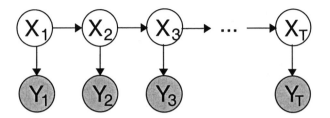

Figure 1: A directed acyclic graph (DAG) specifying conditional independence relations for a state-space model. Each node is conditionally independent from its nondescendants given its parents. The output Y_t is conditionally independent from all other variables given the state X_t; and X_t is conditionally independent from $X_1, \ldots, X_{t-2}$ given X_{t-1}. In this and the following figures, shaded nodes represent observed variables, and unshaded nodes represent hidden variables.

obey the Markov independence property. The joint probability for the sequences of states X_t and observations Y_t can therefore be factored as:

$$P(\{X_t, Y_t\}) = P(X_1)P(Y_1|X_1) \prod_{t=2}^{T} P(X_t|X_{t-1})P(Y_t|X_t). \tag{2.1}$$

The conditional independencies specified by equation 2.1 can be expressed graphically in the form of Figure 1. The simplest and most commonly used models of this kind assume that the transition and output functions are linear and time invariant and the distributions of the state and observation variables are multivariate gaussian. We use the term *state-space model* to refer to this simple form of the model. For such models, the state transition function is

$$X_t = AX_{t-1} + w_t, \tag{2.2}$$

where A is the state transition matrix and w_t is zero-mean gaussian noise in the dynamics, with covariance matrix Q. $P(X_1)$ is assumed to be gaussian. Equation 2.2 ensures that if $P(X_{t-1})$ is gaussian, so is $P(X_t)$. The output function is

$$Y_t = CX_t + v_t, \tag{2.3}$$

where C is the output matrix and v_t is zero-mean gaussian output noise with covariance matrix R; $P(Y_t|X_t)$ is therefore also gaussian:

$$P(Y_t|X_t) = (2\pi)^{-D/2}|R|^{-1/2} \exp\left\{-\frac{1}{2}(Y_t - CX_t)' R^{-1}(Y_t - CX_t)\right\}, \tag{2.4}$$

where D is the dimensionality of the Y vectors.

Often the observation vector can be divided into input (or predictor) variables and output (or response) variables. To model the input-output behavior of such a system—the conditional probability of output sequences given input sequences—the linear gaussian SSM can be modified to have a state-transition function,

$$X_t = AX_{t-1} + BU_t + w_t, \qquad (2.5)$$

where U_t is the input observation vector and B is the (fixed) input matrix.[1]

The problem of *inference* or *state estimation* for an SSM with known parameters consists of estimating the posterior probabilities of the hidden variables given a sequence of observed variables. Since the local likelihood functions for the observations are gaussian and the priors for the hidden states are gaussian, the resulting posterior is also gaussian. Three special cases of the inference problem are often considered: filtering, smoothing, and prediction (Anderson & Moore, 1979; Goodwin & Sin, 1984). The goal of filtering is to compute the probability of the current hidden state X_t given the sequence of inputs and outputs up to time t—$P(X_t|\{Y\}_1^t, \{U\}_1^t)$.[2] The recursive algorithm used to perform this computation is known as the *Kalman filter* (Kalman & Bucy, 1961). The goal of *smoothing* is to compute the probability of X_t given the sequence of inputs and outputs up to time T, where $T > t$. The Kalman filter is used in the forward direction to compute the probability of X_t given $\{Y\}_1^t$ and $\{U\}_1^t$. A similar set of *backward* recursions from T to t completes the computation by accounting for the observations after time t (Rauch, 1963). We will refer to the combined forward and backward recursions for smoothing as the Kalman smoothing recursions (also known as the RTS, or Rauch-Tung-Striebel smoother). Finally, the goal of *prediction* is to compute the probability of future states and observations given observations up to time t. Given $P(X_t|\{Y\}_1^t, \{U\}_1^t)$ computed as before, the model is simulated in the forward direction using equations 2.2 (or 2.5 if there are inputs) and 2.3 to compute the probability density of the state or output at future time $t + \tau$.

The problem of learning the parameters of an SSM is known in engineering as the *system identification* problem; in its most general form it assumes access only to sequences of input and output observations. We focus on maximum likelihood learning in which a single (locally optimal) value of the parameters is estimated, rather than Bayesian approaches that treat the parameters as random variables and compute or approximate the posterior distribution of the parameters given the data. One can also distinguish between on-line and off-line approaches to learning. On-line recursive algorithms, favored in real-time adaptive control applications, can be obtained by computing the gradient or the second derivatives of the log-likelihood (Ljung

---

[1] One can also define the state such that $X_{t+1} = AX_t + BU_t + w_t$.

[2] The notation $\{Y\}_1^t$ is shorthand for the sequence $Y_1, \ldots, Y_t$.

& Söderström, 1983). Similar gradient-based methods can be obtained for off-line methods. An alternative method for off-line learning makes use of the expectation maximization (EM) algorithm (Dempster, Laird, & Rubin, 1977). This procedure iterates between an E-step that fixes the current parameters and computes posterior probabilities over the hidden states given the observations, and an M-step that maximizes the expected log-likelihood of the parameters using the posterior distribution computed in the E-step. For linear gaussian state-space models, the E-step is exactly the Kalman smoothing problem as defined above, and the M-step simplifies to a linear regression problem (Shumway & Stoffer, 1982; Digalakis, Rohlicek, & Ostendorf, 1993). Details on the EM algorithm for SSMs can be found in Ghahramani and Hinton (1996a), as well as in the original Shumway and Stoffer (1982) article.

2.2 Hidden Markov Models. Hidden Markov models also define probability distributions over sequences of observations $\{Y_t\}$. The distribution over sequences is obtained by specifying a distribution over observations at each time step t given a *discrete* hidden state S_t, and the probability of transitioning from one hidden state to another. Using the Markov property, the joint probability for the sequences of states S_t and observations Y_t, can be factored in exactly the same manner as equation 2.1, with S_t taking the place of X_t:

$$P(\{S_t, Y_t\}) = P(S_1)P(Y_1|S_1) \prod_{t=2}^{T} P(S_t|S_{t-1})P(Y_t|S_t). \qquad (2.6)$$

Similarly, the conditional independencies in an HMM can be expressed graphically in the same form as Figure 1. The state is represented by a single multinomial variable that can take one of K discrete values, $S_t \in \{1, \ldots, K\}$. The state transition probabilities, $P(S_t|S_{t-1})$, are specified by a $K \times K$ transition matrix. If the observables are discrete symbols taking on one of L values, the observation probabilities $P(Y_t|S_t)$ can be fully specified as a $K \times L$ observation matrix. For a continuous observation vector, $P(Y_t|S_t)$ can be modeled in many different forms, such as a gaussian, mixture of gaussians, or neural network. HMMs have been applied extensively to problems in speech recognition (Juang & Rabiner, 1991), computational biology (Baldi, Chauvin, Hunkapiller, & McClure, 1994), and fault detection (Smyth, 1994).

Given an HMM with known parameters and a sequence of observations, two algorithms are commonly used to solve two different forms of the inference problem (Rabiner & Juang, 1986). The first computes the posterior probabilities of the hidden states using a recursive algorithm known as the *forward-backward* algorithm. The computations in the forward pass are exactly analogous to the Kalman filter for SSMs, and the computations in the backward pass are analogous to the backward pass of the Kalman smoothing equations. As noted by Bridle (pers. comm., 1985) and Smyth, Heckerman, and Jordan (1997), the forward-backward algorithm is a special case of exact inference algorithms for more general graphical probabilistic models (Lauritzen & Spiegelhalter, 1988; Pearl, 1988). The same observation holds true for the Kalman smoothing recursions. The other inference problem commonly posed for HMMs is to compute the single most likely sequence of hidden states. The solution to this problem is given by the Viterbi algorithm, which also consists of a forward and backward pass through the model.

To learn maximum likelihood parameters for an HMM given sequences of observations, one can use the well-known Baum-Welch algorithm (Baum, Petrie, Soules, & Weiss, 1970). This algorithm is a special case of EM that uses the forward-backward algorithm to infer the posterior probabilities of the hidden states in the E-step. The M-step uses expected counts of transitions and observations to reestimate the transition and output matrices (or linear regression equations in the case where the observations are gaussian distributed). Like SSMs, HMMs can be augmented to allow for input variables, such that they model the conditional distribution of sequences of output observations given sequences of inputs (Cacciatore & Nowlan, 1994; Bengio & Frasconi, 1995; Meila & Jordan, 1996).

2.3 Hybrids. A burgeoning literature on models that combine the discrete transition structure of HMMs with the linear dynamics of SSMs has developed in fields ranging from econometrics to control engineering (Harrison & Stevens, 1976; Chang & Athans, 1978; Hamilton, 1989; Shumway & Stoffer, 1991; Bar-Shalom & Li, 1993; Deng, 1993; Kadirkamanathan & Kadirkamanathan, 1996; Chaer, Bishop, & Ghosh, 1997). These models are known alternately as hybrid models, SSMs with switching, and jump-linear systems. We briefly review some of this literature, including some related neural network models.[3]

Shortly after Kalman and Bucy solved the problem of state estimation for linear gaussian SSMs, attention turned to the analogous problem for switching models (Ackerson & Fu, 1970). Chang and Athans (1978) derive the equations for computing the conditional mean and variance of the state when the parameters of a linear SSM switch according to arbitrary and Markovian dynamics. The prior and transition probabilities of the switching process are assumed to be known. They note that for M models (sets of parameters) and an observation length T, the exact conditional distribution of the state is a gaussian mixture with M^T components. The conditional mean and variance, which require far less computation, are therefore only summary statistics.

---

[3] A review of how SSMs and HMMs are related to simpler statistical models such as principal components analysis, factor analysis, mixture of gaussians, vector quantization, and independent components analysis (ICA) can be found in Roweis and Ghahramani (1999).

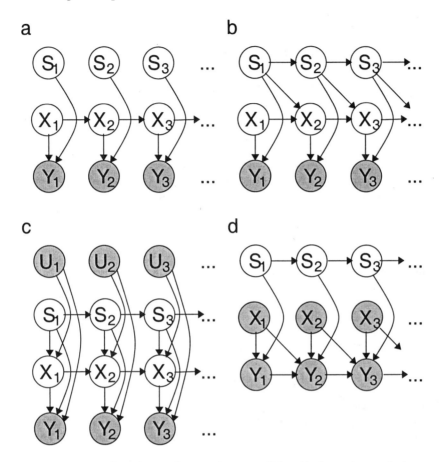

Figure 2: Directed acyclic graphs specifying conditional independence relations for various switching state-space models. (a) Shumway and Stoffer (1991): the output matrix (C in equation 2.3) switches independently between a fixed number of choices at each time step. Its setting is represented by the discrete hidden variable S_t; (b) Bar-Shalom and Li (1993): both the output equation and the dynamic equation can switch, and the switches are Markov; (c) Kim (1994); (d) Fraser and Dimitriadis (1993): outputs and states are observed. Here we have shown a simple case where the output depends directly on the current state, previous state, and previous output.

Shumway and Stoffer (1991) consider the problem of learning the parameters of SSMs with a single real-valued hidden state vector and switching output matrices. The probability of choosing a particular output matrix is a prespecified time-varying function, independent of previous choices (see Figure 2a). A pseudo-EM algorithm is derived in which the E-step, which in its exact form would require computing a gaussian mixture with M^T components, is approximated by a single gaussian at each time step.

Bar-Shalom and Li (1993; sec. 11.6) review models in which both the state dynamics and the output matrices switch, and where the switching follows Markovian dynamics (see Figure 2b). They present several methods for approximately solving the state-estimation problem in switching models (they do not discuss parameter estimation for such models). These methods, referred to as generalized pseudo-Bayesian (GPB) and interacting multiple models (IMM), are all based on the idea of collapsing into one gaussian the mixture of M gaussians that results from considering all the settings of the switch state at a given time step. This avoids the exponential growth of mixture components at the cost of providing an approximate solution. More sophisticated but computationally expensive methods that collapse M^2 gaussians into M gaussians are also derived. Kim (1994) derives a similar approximation for a closely related model, which also includes observed input variables (see Figure 2c). Furthermore, Kim discusses parameter estimation for this model, although without making reference to the EM algorithm. Other authors have used Markov chain Monte Carlo methods for state and parameter estimation in switching models (Carter & Kohn, 1994; Athaide, 1995) and in other related dynamic probabilistic networks (Dean & Kanazawa, 1989; Kanazawa, Koller, & Russell, 1995).

Hamilton (1989, 1994, sec. 22.4) describes a class of switching models in which the real-valued observation at time t, Y_t, depends on both the observations at times $t-1$ to $t-r$ and the discrete states at time t to $t-r$. More precisely, Y_t is gaussian with mean that is a linear function of $Y_{t-1}, \ldots, Y_{t-r}$ and of binary indicator variables for the discrete states, $S_t, \ldots, S_{t-r}$. The system can therefore be seen as an $(r+1)$th order HMM driving an rth order autoregressive process, and is tractable for small r and number of discrete states in S.

Hamilton's models are closely related to hidden filter HMM (HFHMM; Fraser & Dimitriadis, 1993). HFHMMs have both discrete and real-valued states. However, the real-valued states are assumed to be either observed or a known, deterministic function of the past observations (i.e., an embedding). The outputs depend on the states and previous outputs, and the form of this dependence can switch randomly (see Figure 2d). Because at any time step the only hidden variable is the switch state, S_t, exact inference in this model can be carried out tractably. The resulting algorithm is a variant of the forward-backward procedure for HMMs. Kehagias and Petridis (1997) and Pawelzik, Kohlmorgen, and Müller (1996) present other variants of this model.

Elliott, Aggoun, and Moore (1995; sec. 12.5) present an inference algorithm for hybrid (Markov switching) systems for which there is a separate observable from which the switch state can be estimated. The true switch states, S_t, are represented as unit vectors in $\Re^M$, and the estimated switch state is a vector in the unit square with elements corresponding to the estimated probability of being in each switch state. The real-valued state, X_t, is approximated as a gaussian given the estimated switch state by forming a linear combination of the transition and observation matrices for the different SSMs weighted by the estimated switch state. Eliott et al. also derive control equations for such hybrid systems and discuss applications of the change-of-measures whitening procedure to a large family of models.

With regard to the literature on neural computation, the model presented in this article is a generalization of both the mixture-of-experts neural network (Jacobs et al., 1991; Jordan & Jacobs, 1994) and the related mixture of factor analyzers (Hinton, Dayan, & Revow, 1997; Ghahramani & Hinton, 1996b). Previous dynamical generalizations of the mixture-of-experts architecture consider the case in which the gating network has Markovian dynamics (Cacciatore & Nowlan, 1994; Kadirkamanathan & Kadirkamanathan, 1996; Meila & Jordan, 1996). One limitation of this generalization is that the entire past sequence is summarized in the value of a single discrete variable (the gating activation), which for a system with M experts can convey on average at most $\log M$ bits of information about the past. In the models we consider here, both the experts and the gating network have Markovian dynamics. The past is therefore summarized by a state composed of the cross-product of the discrete variable and the combined real-valued state-space of all the experts. This provides a much wider information channel from the past. One advantage of this representation is that the real-valued state can contain componential structure. Thus, attributes such as the position, orientation, and scale of an object in an image, which are most naturally encoded as independent real-valued variables, can be accommodated in the state without the exponential growth required of a discretized HMM-like representation.

It is important to place the work in this article in the context of the literature we have just reviewed. The hybrid models, state-space models with switching, and jump-linear systems we have described all assume a single real-valued state vector. The model considered in this article generalizes this to multiple real-valued state vectors.[4] Unlike the models described in Hamilton (1994), Fraser and Dimitradis (1993), and the current dynamical extensions of mixtures of experts, in the model we present, the real-valued state vectors are hidden. The inference algorithm we derive, which is based on making a structured variational approximation, is entirely novel in the context of switching SSMs. Specifically, our method is unlike all the approximate methods we have reviewed in that it is not based on fitting a single gaussian to a mixture of gaussians by computing the mean and covariance of the mixture.[5] We derive a learning algorithm for all of the parameters

---

[4] Note that the state vectors could be concatenated into one large state vector with factorized (block-diagonal) transition matrices (cf. factorial hidden Markov model; Ghahramani & Jordan, 1997). However, this obscures the decoupled structure of the model.

[5] Both classes of methods can be seen as minimizing Kullback-Liebler (KL) diver-

of the model, including the Markov switching parameters. This algorithm maximizes a lower bound on the log-likelihood of the data rather than a heuristically motivated approximation to the likelihood. The algorithm has a simple and intuitive flavor: It decouples into forward-backward recursions on a HMM, and Kalman smoothing recursions on each SSM. The states of the HMM determine the soft assignment of each observation to an SSM; the prediction errors of the SSMs determine the observation probabilities for the HMM.

3 The Generative Model

In switching SSMs, the sequence of observations $\{Y_t\}$ is modeled by specifying a probabilistic relation between the observations and a hidden state-space comprising M real-valued state vectors, $X_t^{(m)}$, and one discrete state vector S_t. The discrete state, S_t, is modeled as a multinomial variable that can take on M values: $S_t \in \{1, \ldots, M\}$; for reasons that will become obvious we refer to it as the *switch* variable. The joint probability of observations and hidden states can be factored as

$$
P\left(\left\{S_t, X_t^{(1)}, \ldots, X_t^{(M)}, Y_t\right\}\right)
$$
$$
= P(S_1) \prod_{t=2}^{T} P(S_t|S_{t-1}) \cdot \prod_{m=1}^{M} P\left(X_1^{(m)}\right) \prod_{t=2}^{T} P\left(X_t^{(m)}|X_{t-1}^{(m)}\right)
$$
$$
\cdot \prod_{t=1}^{T} P\left(Y_t|X_t^{(1)}, \ldots, X_t^{(M)}, S_t\right), \tag{3.1}
$$

which corresponds graphically to the conditional independencies represented by Figure 3. Conditioned on a setting of the switch state, $S_t = m$, the observable is multivariate gaussian with output equation given by state-space model m. Notice that m is used as both an index for the real-valued state variables and a value for the switch state. The probability of the observation vector Y_t is therefore

$$
P\left(Y_t|X_t^{(1)}, \ldots, X_t^{(M)}, S_t = m\right)
$$
$$
= |2\pi R|^{-\frac{1}{2}} \exp\left\{-\frac{1}{2}\left(Y_t - C^{(m)}X_t^{(m)}\right)' R^{-1}\left(Y_t - C^{(m)}X_t^{(m)}\right)\right\}, \tag{3.2}
$$

where R is the observation noise covariance matrix and $C^{(m)}$ is the output matrix for SSM m (cf. equation 2.4 for a single linear-gaussian SSM). Each

---

gences. However, the KL divergence is asymmetrical, and whereas the variational methods minimize it in one direction, the methods that merge gaussians minimize it in the other direction. We return to this point in section 4.2.

a   b

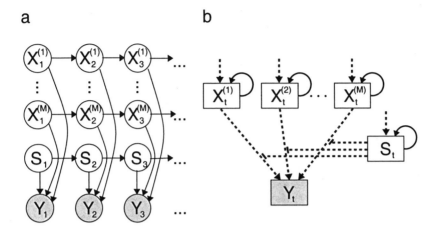

Figure 3: (a) Graphical model representation for switching state-space models. S_t is the discrete switch variable, and $X_t^{(m)}$ are the real-valued state vectors. (b) Switching state-space model depicted as a generalization of the mixture of experts. The dashed arrows correspond to the connections in a mixture of experts. In a switching state-space model, the states of the experts and the gating network also depend on their previous states (solid arrows).

real-valued state vector evolves according to the linear gaussian dynamics of an SSM with differing initial state, transition matrix, and state noise (see equation 2.2). For simplicity we assume that all state vectors have identical dimensionality; the generalization of the algorithms we present to models with different-sized state-spaces is immediate. The switch state itself evolves according to the discrete Markov transition structure specified by the initial state probabilities $P(S_1)$ and the $M \times M$ state transition matrix $P(S_t|S_{t-1})$.

An exact analogy can be made to the mixture-of-experts architecture for modular learning in neural networks (see Figure 3b; Jacobs et al., 1991). Each SSM is a linear expert with gaussian output noise model and linear-gaussian dynamics. The switch state "gates" the outputs of the M SSMs, and therefore plays the role of a gating network with Markovian dynamics.

There are many possible extensions of the model; we shall consider three obvious and straightforward ones:

(Ex1) Differing output covariances, $R^{(m)}$, for each SSM;

(Ex2) Differing output means, $\mu_Y^{(m)}$, for each SSM, such that each model is allowed to capture observations in a different operating range

(Ex3) Conditioning on a sequence of observed input vectors, $\{U_t\}$

4 Learning ───

An efficient learning algorithm for the parameters of a switching SSM can be derived by generalizing the EM algorithm (Baum et al., 1970; Dempster et al., 1977). EM alternates between optimizing a distribution over the hidden states (the E-step) and optimizing the parameters given the distribution over hidden states (the M-step). Any distribution over the hidden states, $Q(\{S_t, X_t\})$, where $X_t = [X_t^{(1)}, \dots X_t^{(M)}]$ is the combined state of the SSMs, can be used to define a lower bound, $\mathcal{B}$, on the log probability of the observed data:

$$\log P(\{Y_t\}|\theta) = \log \sum_{\{S_t\}} \int P(\{S_t, X_t, Y_t\}|\theta) \, d\{X_t\} \qquad (4.1)$$

$$= \log \sum_{\{S_t\}} \int Q(\{S_t, X_t\}) \left[\frac{P(\{S_t, X_t, Y_t\}|\theta)}{Q(\{S_t, X_t\})} \right] d\{X_t\} \qquad (4.2)$$

$$\geq \sum_{\{S_t\}} \int Q(\{S_t, X_t\}) \, \log \left[\frac{P(\{S_t, X_t, Y_t\}|\theta)}{Q(\{S_t, X_t\})} \right] d\{X_t\}$$

$$= \mathcal{B}(Q, \theta), \qquad (4.3)$$

where θ denotes the parameters of the model and we have made use of Jensen's inequality (Cover & Thomas, 1991) to establish equation 4.3. Both steps of EM increase the lower bound on the log probability of the observed data. The E-step holds the parameters fixed and sets Q to be the posterior distribution over the hidden states given the parameters,

$$Q(\{S_t, X_t\}) = P(\{S_t, X_t\}|\{Y_t\}, \theta). \qquad (4.4)$$

This maximizes $\mathcal{B}$ with respect to the distribution, turning the lower bound into an equality, which can be easily seen by substitution. The M-step holds the distribution fixed and computes the parameters that maximize $\mathcal{B}$ for that distribution. Since $\mathcal{B} = \log P(\{Y_t\}|\theta)$ at the start of the M-step and since the E-step does not affect $\log P$, the two steps combined can never decrease $\log P$. Given the change in the parameters produced by the M-step, the distribution produced by the previous E-step is typically no longer optimal, so the whole procedure must be iterated.

Unfortunately, the exact E-step for switching SSMs is intractable. Like the related hybrid models described in section 2.3, the posterior probability of the real-valued states is a gaussian mixture with M^T terms. This can be seen by using the semantics of directed graphs, in particular the d-separation criterion (Pearl, 1988), which implies that the hidden state variables in Figure 3, while marginally independent, become conditionally dependent given the observation sequence. This induced dependency effectively couples all of the real-valued hidden state variables to the discrete switch variable, as a consequence of which the exact posteriors become Gaussian mixtures with an exponential number of terms.[6]

In order to derive an efficient learning algorithm for this system, we relax the EM algorithm by approximating the posterior probability of the hidden states. The basic idea is that since expectations with respect to P are intractable, rather than setting $Q(\{S_t, X_t\}) = P(\{S_t, X_t\}|\{Y_t\})$ in the E-step, a tractable distribution Q is used to *approximate* P. This results in an EM learning algorithm that maximizes a lower bound on the log-likelihood. The difference between the bound $\mathcal{B}$ and the log-likelihood is given by the Kullback-Liebler (KL) divergence between Q and P:

$$ \text{KL}(Q\|P) = \sum_{\{S_t\}} \int Q(\{S_t, X_t\}) \log \left[\frac{Q(\{S_t, X_t\})}{P(\{S_t, X_t\}|\{Y_t\})} \right] d\{X_t\}. \qquad (4.5) $$

Since the complexity of exact inference in the approximation given by Q is determined by its conditional independence relations, not by its parameters, we can choose Q to have a tractable structure—a graphical representation that eliminates some of the dependencies in P. Given this structure, the parameters of Q are varied to obtain the tightest possible bound by minimizing equation 4.5. Therefore, the algorithm alternates between optimizing the parameters of the distribution Q to minimize equation 4.5 (the E-step) and optimizing the parameters of P given the distribution over the hidden states (the M-step). As in exact EM, both steps increase the lower bound $\mathcal{B}$ on the log-likelihood; however, equality is not reached in the E-step.

We will refer to the general strategy of using a parameterized approximating distribution as a *variational approximation* and refer to the free parameters of the distribution as *variational parameters*. A completely factorized approximation is often used in statistical physics, where it provides the basis for simple yet powerful mean-field approximations to statistical mechanical systems (Parisi, 1988). Theoretical arguments motivating approximate E-steps are presented in Neal and Hinton (1998; originally in a technical report in 1993). Saul and Jordan (1996) showed that approximate E-steps could be used to maximize a lower bound on the log-likelihood, and proposed the powerful technique of structured variational approximations to intractable probabilistic networks. The key insight of their work, which this article makes use of, is that by judicious use of an approximation Q, exact inference algorithms can be used on the tractable substructures in an intractable network. A general tutorial on variational approximations can be found in Jordan, Ghahramani, Jaakkola, and Saul (1998).

---

[6] The intractability of the E-step or smoothing problem in the simpler single-state switching model has been noted by Ackerson and Fu (1970), Chang and Athans (1978), Bar-Shalom and Li (1993), and others.

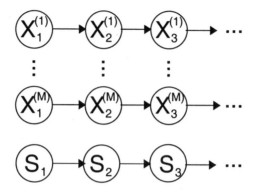

Figure 4: Graphical model representation for the structured variational approximation to the posterior distribution of the hidden states of a switching state-space model.

The parameters of the switching SSM are $\theta = \{A^{(m)}, C^{(m)}, Q^{(m)}, \mu_{X_1}^{(m)}, Q_1^{(m)}, R, \pi, \Phi\}$, where $A^{(m)}$ is the state dynamics matrix for model m, $C^{(m)}$ is its output matrix, $Q^{(m)}$ is its state noise covariance, $\mu_{X_1}^{(m)}$ is the mean of the initial state, $Q_1^{(m)}$ is the covariance of the initial state, R is the (tied) output noise covariance, $\pi = P(S_1)$ is the prior for the discrete Markov process, and $\Phi = P(S_t|S_{t-1})$ is the discrete transition matrix. Extensions (Ex1) through (Ex3) can be readily implemented by substituting $R^{(m)}$ for R, adding means $\mu_Y^{(m)}$ and input matrices $B^{(m)}$.

Although there are many possible approximations to the posterior distribution of the hidden variables that one could use for learning and inference in switching SSMs, we focus on the following:

$$Q(\{S_t, X_t\}) = \frac{1}{Z_Q} \left[\psi(S_1) \prod_{t=2}^{T} \psi(S_{t-1}, S_t) \right] \prod_{m=1}^{M} \psi\left(X_1^{(m)}\right)$$
$$\cdot \prod_{t=2}^{T} \psi\left(X_{t-1}^{(m)}, X_t^{(m)}\right), \qquad (4.6)$$

where the ψ are unnormalized probabilities, which we will call *potential functions* and define soon, and Z_Q is a normalization constant ensuring that Q integrates to one. Although Q has been written in terms of potential functions rather than conditional probabilities, it corresponds to the simple graphical model shown in Figure 4. The terms involving the switch variables S_t define a discrete Markov chain, and the terms involving the state vectors $X_t^{(m)}$ define M *uncoupled* SSMs. As in mean-field approximations, we have approximated the stochastically coupled system by removing some of the couplings of the original system. Specifically, we have removed the stochastic coupling between the chains that results from the fact that the observation at time t depends on all the hidden variables at time t. However, we retain the coupling between the hidden variables at successive time steps since these couplings can be handled exactly using the forward-backward and Kalman smoothing recursions. This approximation is therefore structured, in the sense that not all variables are uncoupled.

The discrete switching process is defined by

$$\psi(S_1 = m) = P(S_1 = m)\, q_1^{(m)} \tag{4.7}$$

$$\psi(S_{t-1}, S_t = m) = P(S_t = m | S_{t-1})\, q_t^{(m)}, \tag{4.8}$$

where the $q_t^{(m)}$ are variational parameters of the Q distribution. These parameters scale the probabilities of each of the states of the switch variable at each time step, so that $q_t^{(m)}$ plays exactly the same role that the observation probability $P(Y_t | S_t = m)$ would play in a regular HMM. We will soon see that minimizing KL$(Q\|P)$ results in an equation for $q_t^{(m)}$ that supports this intuition.

The uncoupled SSMs in the approximation Q are also defined by potential functions that are related to probabilities in the original system. These potentials are the prior and transition probabilities for $X^{(m)}$ multiplied by a factor that changes these potentials to try to account for the data:

$$\psi\left(X_1^{(m)}\right) = P\left(X_1^{(m)}\right) \left[P\left(Y_1 | X_1^{(m)}, S_1 = m\right)\right]^{h_1^{(m)}} \tag{4.9}$$

$$\psi\left(X_{t-1}^{(m)}, X_t^{(m)}\right) = P\left(X_t^{(m)} | X_{t-1}^{(m)}\right) \left[P\left(Y_t | X_t^{(m)}, S_t = m\right)\right]^{h_t^{(m)}}, \tag{4.10}$$

where the $h_t^{(m)}$ are variational parameters of Q. The vector h_t plays a role very similar to the switch variable S_t. Each component $h_t^{(m)}$ can range between 0 and 1. When $h_t^{(m)} = 0$, the posterior probability of $X_t^{(m)}$ under Q does not depend on the observation at time Y_t. When $h_t^{(m)} = 1$, the posterior probability of $X_t^{(m)}$ under Q includes a term that assumes that SSM m generated Y_t. We call $h_t^{(m)}$ the *responsibility* assigned to SSM m for the observation vector Y_t. The difference between $h_t^{(m)}$ and $S_t^{(m)}$ is that $h_t^{(m)}$ is a deterministic parameter, while $S_t^{(m)}$ is a stochastic random variable.

To maximize the lower bound on the log-likelihood, KL$(Q\|P)$ is minimized with respect to the variational parameters $h_t^{(m)}$ and $q_t^{(m)}$ separately for each sequence of observations. Using the definition of P for the switching state-space model (equations 3.1 and 3.2) and the approximating distribution Q, the minimum of KL satisfies the following fixed-point equations for the variational parameters (see appendix B):

$$h_t^{(m)} = Q(S_t = m) \tag{4.11}$$

$$q_t^{(m)} = \exp\left\{-\frac{1}{2}\left\langle\left(Y_t - C^{(m)}X_t^{(m)}\right)' R^{-1}\left(Y_t - C^{(m)}X_t^{(m)}\right)\right\rangle\right\}, \qquad (4.12)$$

where $\langle\cdot\rangle$ denotes expectation over the Q distribution. Intuitively, the responsibility, $h_t^{(m)}$ is equal to the probability under Q that SSM m generated observation vector Y_t, and $q_t^{(m)}$ is an unnormalized gaussian function of the expected squared error if SSM m generated Y_t.

To compute $h_t^{(m)}$ it is necessary to sum Q over all the S_τ variables not including S_t. This can be done efficiently using the forward-backward algorithm on the switch state variables, with $q_t^{(m)}$ playing exactly the same role as an observation probability associated with each setting of the switch variable. Since $q_t^{(m)}$ is related to the prediction error of model m on data Y_t, this has the intuitive interpretation that the switch state associated with models with smaller expected prediction error on a particular observation will be favored at that time step. However, the forward-backward algorithm ensures that the final responsibilities for the models are obtained after considering the entire sequence of observations.

To compute $q_t^{(m)}$, it is necessary to calculate the expectations of $X_t^{(m)}$ and $X_t^{(m)}X_t^{(m)'}$ under Q. We see this by expanding equation 4.12:

$$q_t^{(m)} = \exp\left\{-\frac{1}{2}Y_t'R^{-1}Y_t + Y_t'R^{-1}C^{(m)}\langle X_t^{(m)}\rangle\right.$$
$$\left.-\frac{1}{2}tr\left[C^{(m)'}R^{-1}C^{(m)}\left\langle X_t^{(m)}X_t^{(m)'}\right\rangle\right]\right\}, \qquad (4.13)$$

where tr is the matrix trace operator, and we have used $tr(AB) = tr(BA)$. The expectations of $X_t^{(m)}$ and $X_t^{(m)}X_t^{(m)'}$ can be computed efficiently using the Kalman smoothing algorithm on each SSM, where for model m at time t, the data are weighted by the responsibilities $h_t^{(m)}$.[7] Since the h parameters depend on the q parameters, and vice versa, the whole process has to be iterated, where each iteration involves calls to the forward-backward and Kalman smoothing algorithms. Once the iterations have converged, the E-step outputs the expected values of the hidden variables under the final Q.

The M-step computes the model parameters that optimize the expectation of the log-likelihood (see equation B.7), which is a function of the expectations of the hidden variables. For switching SSMs, all the parameter reestimates can be computed analytically. For example, taking derivatives of the expectation of equation B.7 with respect to $C^{(m)}$ and setting to zero,

---

[7] Weighting the data by $h_t^{(m)}$ is equivalent to running the Kalman smoother on the unweighted data using a time-varying observation noise covariance matrix $R_t^{(m)} = R/h_t^{(m)}$.

```
Initialize parameters of the model.

Repeat until bound on log likelihood has converged:
```

E step Repeat until convergence of $\text{KL}(Q\|P)$:

> E.1 Compute $q_t^{(m)}$ from the prediction error of state-space model m on observation Y_t
>
> E.2 Compute $h_t^{(m)}$ using the forward-backward algorithm on the HMM, with observation probabilities $q_t^{(m)}$
>
> E.3 For $m = 1$ to M
>
>> Run Kalman smoothing recursions, using the data weighted by $h_t^{(m)}$

M step

> M.1 Re-estimate parameters for each state-space model using the data weighted by $h_t^{(m)}$
>
> M.2 Re-estimate parameters for the switching process using Baum-Welch update equations.

Figure 5: Learning algorithm for switching state-space models.

we get

$$\hat{C}^{(m)} = \left(\sum_{t=1}^{T}\left\langle S_t^{(m)}\right\rangle Y_t\left\langle X_t^{(m)'}\right\rangle\right)\left(\sum_{t=1}^{T}\left\langle S_t^{(m)}\right\rangle\left\langle X_t^{(m)}X_t^{(m)'}\right\rangle\right)^{-1}, \qquad (4.14)$$

which is a weighted version of the reestimation equations for SSMs. Similarly, the reestimation equations for the switch process are analogous to the Baum-Welch update rules for HMMs. The learning algorithm for switching state-space models using the above structured variational approximation is summarized in Figure 5.

4.1 Deterministic Annealing. The KL divergence minimized in the E-step of the variational EM algorithm can have multiple minima in general. One way to visualize these minima is to consider the space of all possible segmentations of an observation sequence of length T, where by segmentation we mean a discrete partition of the sequence between the SSMs. If there are M SSMs, then there are M^T possible segmentations of the sequence. Given one such segmentation, inferring the optimal distribution for the real-valued states of the SSMs is a convex optimization problem, since these real-valued states are conditionally gaussian. So the difficulty in the KL minimization lies in trying to find the best (soft) partition of the data.

As in other combinatorial optimization problems, the possibility of getting trapped in local minima can be reduced by gradually annealing the cost function. We can employ a deterministic variant of the annealing idea by making the following simple modifications to the variational fixed-point equations 4.11 and 4.12:

$$h_t^{(m)} = \frac{1}{T} Q(S_t = m) \tag{4.15}$$

$$q_t^{(m)} = \exp \left\{ -\frac{1}{2T} \left\langle \left(Y_t - C^{(m)} X_t^{(m)} \right)' R^{-1} \left(Y_t - C^{(m)} X_t^{(m)} \right) \right\rangle \right\}. \tag{4.16}$$

Here T is a temperature parameter, which is initialized to a large value and gradually reduced to 1. The above equations maximize a modified form of the bound B in equation 4.3, where the entropy of Q has been multiplied by T (Ueda & Nakano, 1995).

4.2 Merging Gaussians. Almost all the approximate inference methods that are described in the literature for switching SSMs are based on the idea of merging, at each time step, a mixture of M gaussians into one gaussian. The merged gaussian is obtained by setting its mean and covariance equal to the mean and covariance of the mixture. Here we briefly describe, as an alternative to the variational approximation methods we have derived, how this more traditional gaussian merging procedure can be applied to the model we have defined.

In the switching state-space models described in section 3, there are M different SSMs, with possibly different state-space dimensionalities, so it would be inappropriate to merge their states into one gaussian. However, it is still possibly to apply a gaussian merging technique by considering each SSM separately. In each SSM, m, the hidden state density produces at each time step a mixture of two gaussians: one for the case $S_t = m$ and one for $S_t \neq m$. We merge these two gaussians, weighted the current estimates of $P(S_t = m|Y_1, \ldots Y_t)$ and $1 - P(S_t = m|Y_1, \ldots Y_t)$, respectively. This merged gaussian is used to obtain the gaussian prior for $X_{t+1}^{(m)}$ for the next time step. We implemented a forward-pass version of this approximate inference scheme, which is analogous to the IMM procedure described in Bar-Shalom and Li (1993).

This procedure finds at each time step the "best" gaussian fit to the current mixture of gaussians for each SSM. If we denote the approximating gaussian by Q and the mixture being approximated by P, "best" is defined here as minimizing KL($P\|Q$). Furthermore, gaussian merging techniques are greedy in that the "best" gaussian is computed at every time step and used immediately for the next time step. For a gaussian Q, KL($P\|Q$) has no local minima, and it is very easy to find the optimal Q by computing the first two moments of P. Inaccuracies in this greedy procedure arise because the estimates of $P(S_t|Y_1, \ldots, Y_t)$ are based on this single merged gaussian, not on the real mixture.

In contrast, variational methods seek to minimize $\text{KL}(Q\|P)$, which can have many local minima. Moreover, these methods are not greedy in the same sense: they iterate forward and backward in time until obtaining a locally optimal Q.

5 Simulations

5.1 Experiment 1: Variational Segmentation and Deterministic Annealing.
The goal of this experiment was to assess the quality of solutions found by the variational inference algorithm and the effect of using deterministic annealing on these solutions. We generated 200 sequences of length 200 from a simple model that switched between two SSMs. These SSMs and the switching process were defined by:

$$X_t^{(1)} = 0.99\, X_{t-1}^{(1)} + w_t^{(1)} \qquad w_t^{(1)} \sim \mathcal{N}(0,1) \tag{5.1}$$

$$X_t^{(2)} = 0.9\, X_{t-1}^{(2)} + w_t^{(2)} \qquad w_t^{(2)} \sim \mathcal{N}(0,10) \tag{5.2}$$

$$Y_t = X_t^{(m)} + v_t \qquad v_t \sim \mathcal{N}(0,0.1), \tag{5.3}$$

where the switch state m was chosen using priors $\pi^{(1)} = \pi^{(2)} = 1/2$ and transition probabilities $\Phi_{11} = \Phi_{22} = 0.95$; $\Phi_{12} = \Phi_{21} = 0.05$. Five sequences from this data set are shown in in Figure 6, along with the true state of the switch variable.

We compared three different inference algorithms: variational inference, variational inference with deterministic annealing (section 4.1), and inference by gaussian merging (section 4.2). For each sequence, we initialized the variational inference algorithms with equal responsibilities for the two SSMs and ran them for 12 iterations. The nonannealed inference algorithm ran at a fixed temperature of $T = 1$, while the annealed algorithm was initialized to a temperature of $T = 100$, which decayed down to 1 over the 12 iterations, using the decay function $T_{i+1} = \frac{1}{2}T_i + \frac{1}{2}$. To eliminate the effect of model inaccuracies we gave all three inference algorithms the true parameters of the generative model.

The segmentations found by the nonannealed variational inference algorithm showed little similarity to the true segmentations of the data (see Figure 7). Furthermore, the nonannealed algorithm generally underestimated the number of switches, often converging on solutions with no switches at all. Both the annealed variational algorithm and the gaussian merging method found segmentations that were more similar to the true segmentations of the data. Comparing percentage correct segmentations, we see that annealing substantially improves the variational inference method and that the gaussian merging and annealed variational methods perform comparably (see Figure 8). The average performance of the annealed variational method is only about 1.3% better than gaussian merging.

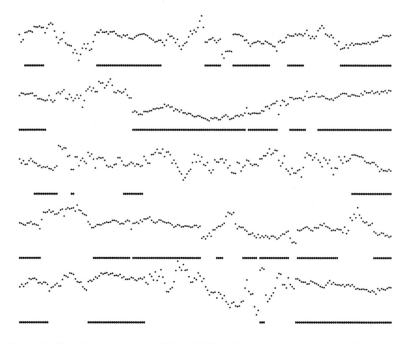

Figure 6: Five data sequences of length 200, with their true segmentations below them. In the segmentations, switch states 1 and 2 are represented with presence and absence of dots, respectively. Notice that it is difficult to segment the sequences correctly based only on knowing the dynamics of the two processes.

5.2 Experiment 2: Modeling Respiration in a Patient with Sleep Apnea.

Switching state-space models should prove useful in modeling time series that have dynamics characterized by several different regimes. To illustrate this point, we examined a physiological data set from a patient tentatively diagnosed with sleep apnea, a medical condition in which an individual intermittently stops breathing during sleep. The data were obtained from the repository of time-series data sets associated with the Santa Fe Time Series Analysis and Prediction Competition (Weigend & Gershenfeld, 1993) and is described in detail in Rigney et al. (1993).[8] The respiration pattern in sleep apnea is characterized by at least two regimes: no breathing and gasping breathing induced by a reflex arousal. Furthermore, in this patient there also seem to be periods of normal rhythmic breathing (see Figure 9).

---

[8] The data are available online at http://www.stern.nyu.edu/~aweigend/Time-Series/SantaFe.html#setB. We used samples 6201–7200 for training and 5201–6200 for testing.

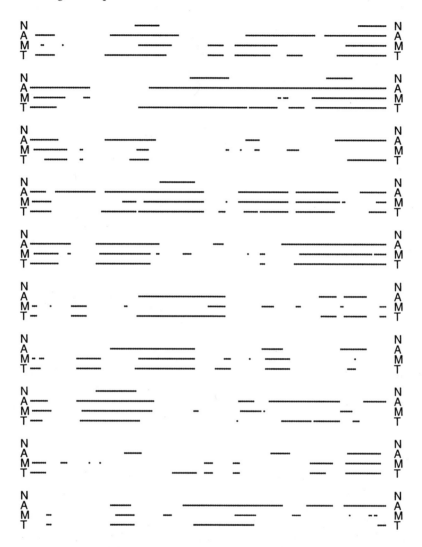

Figure 7: For 10 different sequences of length 200, segmentations are shown with presence and absence of dots corresponding to the two SSMs generating these data. The rows are the segmentations found using the variational method with no annealing (N), the variational method with deterministic annealing (A), the gaussian merging method (M), and the true segmentation (T). All three inference algorithms give real-valued $h_t^{(m)}$; hard segmentations were obtained by thresholding the final $h_t^{(m)}$ values at 0.5. The first five sequences are the ones shown in Figure 6.

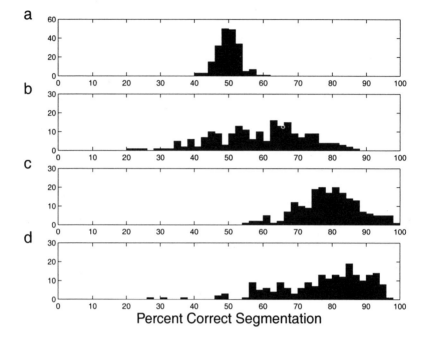

Figure 8: Histograms of percentage correct segmentations: (a) control, using random segmentation; (b) variational inference without annealing; (c) variational inference with annealing; (d) gaussian merging. Percentage correct segmentation was computed by counting the number of time steps for which the true and estimated segmentations agree.

We trained switching SSMs varying the random seed, the number of components in the mixture ($M = 2$ to 5), and the dimensionality of the state-space in each component ($K = 1$ to 10) on a data set consisting of 1000 consecutive measurements of the chest volume. As controls, we also trained simple SSMs (i.e., $M = 1$), varying the dimension of the state-space from $K = 1$ to 10, and simple HMMs (i.e., $K = 0$), varying the number of discrete hidden states from $M = 2$ to $M = 50$. Simulations were run until convergence or for 200 iterations, whichever came first; convergence was assessed by measuring the change in likelihood (or bound on the likelihood) over consecutive steps of EM.

The likelihood of the simple SSMs and the HMMs was calculated on a test set consisting of 1000 consecutive measurements of the chest volume. For the switching SSMs, the likelihood is intractable, so we calculated the lower bound on the likelihood, $\mathcal{B}$. The simple SSMs modeled the data very poorly for $K = 1$, and the performance was flat for values of $K = 2$ to 10 (see

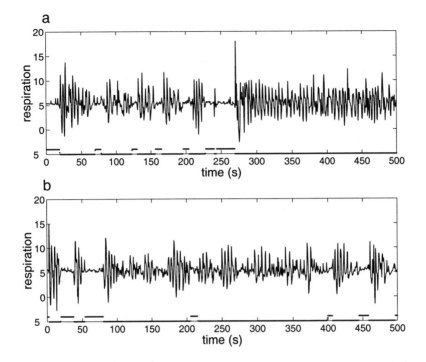

Figure 9: Chest volume (respiration force) of a patient with sleep apnea during two noncontinuous time segments of the same night (measurements sampled at 2 Hz). (a) Training data. Apnea is characterized by extended periods of small variability in chest volume, followed by bursts (gasping). Here we see such behavior around $t = 250$, followed by normal rhythmic breathing. (b) Test data. In this segment we find several instances of apnea and an approximately rhythmic region. (The thick lines at the bottom of each plot are explained in the main text.)

Figure 10a). The large majority of runs of the switching state-space model resulted in models with higher likelihood than those of the simple SMMs (see Figures 10b–10e). One consistent exception should be noted: for values of $M = 2$ and $K = 6$ to 10, the switching SSM performed almost identically to the simple SSM. Exploratory experiments suggest that in these cases, a single component takes responsibility for all the data, so the model has $M = 1$ effectively. This may be a local minimum problem or a result of poor initialization heuristics. Looking at the learning curves for simple and switching SSMs, it is easy to see that there are plateaus at the solutions found by the simple one-component SSMs that the switching SSM can get caught in (see Figure 11).

The likelihoods for HMMs with around $M = 15$ were comparable to those of the best switching SSMs (see Figure 10f). Purely in terms of cod-

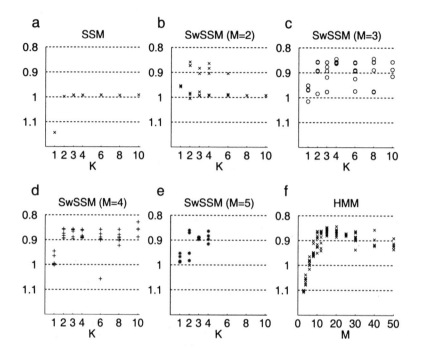

Figure 10: Log likelihood (nats per observation) on the test data from a total of almost 400 runs of simple state-space models (a), switching state-space models with differing numbers of components (b–e), and hidden Markov models (f).

ing efficiency, switching SSMs have little advantage over HMMs on this data.

However, it is useful to contrast the solutions learned by HMMs with the solutions learned by the switching SSMs. The thick dots at the bottom of the Figures 9a and 9b show the responsibility assigned to one of two components in a fairly typical switching SSM with $M = 2$ components of state size $K = 2$. This component has clearly specialized to modeling the data during periods of apnea, while the other component models the gasps and periods of rhythmic breathing. These two switching components provide a much more intuitive model of the data than the 10 to 20 discrete components needed in an HMM with comparable coding efficiency.[9]

---

[9] By using further assumptions to constrain the model, such as continuity of the real-valued hidden state at switch times, it should be possible to obtain even better performance on these data.

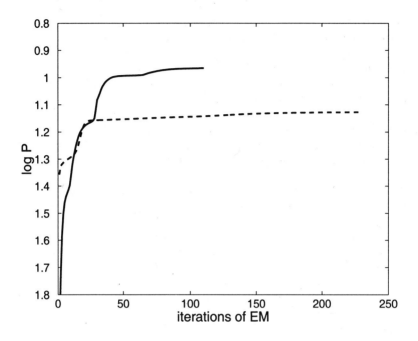

Figure 11: Learning curves for a state space model ($K = 4$) and a switching state-space model ($M = 2, K = 2$).

6 Discussion

The main conclusion we can draw from the first series of experiments is that even when given the correct model parameters, the problem of segmenting a switching time series into its components is difficult. There are combinatorially many alternatives to be considered, and the energy surface suffers from many local minima, so local optimization approaches like the variational method we used are limited by the quality of the initial conditions. Deterministic annealing can be thought of as a sophisticated initialization procedure for the hidden states: the final solution at each temperature provides the initial conditions at the next. We found that annealing substantially improved the quality of the segmentations found.

The first experiment also indicates that the much simpler gaussian merging method performs comparably to annealed variational inference. The gaussian merging methods have the advantage that at each time step, the cost function minimized has no local minima. This may account for how well they perform relative to the nonannealed variational method. On the other hand, the variational methods have the advantage that they iteratively improve their approximation to the posterior, and they define a lower bound on the likelihood. Our results suggest that it may be very fruitful to use the gaussian merging method to initialize the variational inference procedure. Furthermore, it is possible to derive variational approximations for other switching models described in the literature, and a combination of gaussian merging and variational approximation may provide a fast and robust method for learning and inference in those models.

The second series of experiments suggests that on a real data set believed to have switching dynamics, the switching SSM can indeed uncover multiple regimes. When it captures these regimes, it generalizes to the test set much better than the simple linear dynamical model. Similar coding efficiency can be obtained by using HMMs, which due to the discrete nature of the state-space, can model nonlinear dynamics. However, in doing so, the HMMs had to use 10 to 20 discrete states, which makes their solutions less interpretable.

Variational approximations provide a powerful tool for inference and learning in complex probabilistic models. We have seen that when applied to the switching SSM, they can incorporate within a single framework well-known exact inference methods like Kalman smoothing and the forward-backward algorithm. Variational methods can be applied to many of the other classes of intractable switching models described in section 2.3. However, training more complex models also makes apparent the importance of good methods for model selection and initialization.

To summarize, switching SSMs are a dynamical generalization of mixture-of-experts neural networks, are closely related to well-known models in econometrics and control, and combine the representations underlying HMMs and linear dynamical systems. For domains in which we have some a priori belief that there are multiple, approximately linear dynamical regimes, switching SSMs provide a natural modeling tool. Variational approximations provide a method to overcome the most difficult problem in learning switching SSMs: that the inference step is intractable. Deterministic annealing further improves on the solutions found by the variational method.

Appendix A: Notation

Symbol	Size	Description
Variables		
Y_t	$D \times 1$	observation vector at time t
$\{Y_t\}$	$D \times T$	sequence of observation vectors $[Y_1, Y_2, \ldots Y_T]$
$X_t^{(m)}$	$K \times 1$	state vector of state-space model (SSM) m at time t
X_t	$KM \times 1$	entire real-valued hidden state at time t: $X_t = [X_t^{(1)}, \ldots, X_t^{(M)}]$

S_t	$M \times 1$	switch state variable (represented either as discrete variable $S_t \in \{1, \ldots M\}$, or as an $M \times 1$ vector $S_t = [S_t^{(1)}, \ldots S_t^{(M)}]'$ where $S_t^{(m)} \in \{0, 1\}$)

Model parameters

$A^{(m)}$	$K \times K$	state dynamics matrix for SSM m
$C^{(m)}$	$D \times K$	output matrix for SSM m
$Q^{(m)}$	$K \times K$	state noise covariance matrix for SSM m
$\mu_{X_1}^{(m)}$	$K \times 1$	initial state mean for SSM m
$Q_1^{(m)}$	$K \times K$	initial state noise covariance matrix for SSM m
R	$D \times D$	output noise covariance matrix
π	$M \times 1$	initial state probabilities for switch state
Φ	$M \times M$	state transition matrix for switch state

Variational parameters

$h_t^{(m)}$	1×1	responsibility of SSM m for Y_t
$q_t^{(m)}$	1×1	related to expected squared error if SSM m generated Y_t

Miscellaneous

X'	matrix transpose of X
$\lvert X \rvert$	matrix determinant of X
$\langle X \rangle$	expected value of X under the Q distribution

Dimensions

D	size of observation vector
T	length of a sequence of observation vectors
M	number of state-space models
K	size of state vector in each state-space model

Appendix B: Derivation of the Variational Fixed-Point Equations _____

In this appendix we derive the variational fixed-point equations used in the learning algorithm for switching SSMs. First, we write out the probability density P defined by a switching SSM. For convenience, we express this probability density in the log domain, through its associated energy function or *hamiltonian*, H. The probability density is related to the hamiltonian through the usual Boltzmann distribution (at a temperature of 1),

$$P(\cdot) = \frac{1}{Z} \exp\{-H(\cdot)\},$$

where Z is a normalization constant required such that $P(\cdot)$ integrates to unity. Expressing the probabilities in the log domain does not affect the resulting algorithm. We then similarly express the approximating distribution Q through its hamiltonian H_Q. Finally, we obtain the variational fixed-point equations by setting to zero the derivatives of the KL divergence between Q and P with respect to the variational parameters of Q.

The joint probability of observations and hidden states in a switching SSM is (see equation 3.1)

$$
P(\{S_t, X_t, Y_t\}) = \left[P(S_1) \prod_{t=2}^{T} P(S_t|S_{t-1}) \right] \prod_{m=1}^{M} \left[P\left(X_1^{(m)}\right) \prod_{t=2}^{T} P\left(X_t^{(m)}|X_{t-1}^{(m)}\right) \right]
$$
$$
\cdot \prod_{t=1}^{T} P(Y_t|X_t, S_t). \tag{B.1}
$$

We proceed to dissect this expression into its constituent parts. The initial probability of the switch variable at time $t = 1$ is given by

$$
P(S_1) = \prod_{m=1}^{M} \left(\pi^{(m)}\right)^{S_1^{(m)}}, \tag{B.2}
$$

where S_1 is represented by an $M \times 1$ vector $[S_1^{(1)} \ldots S_1^{(M)}]$ where $S_1^{(m)} = 1$ if the switch state is in state m, and 0 otherwise. The probability of transitioning from a switch state at time $t - 1$ to a switch state at time t is given by

$$
P(S_t|S_{t-1}) = \prod_{m=1}^{M} \prod_{n=1}^{M} \left(\Phi^{(m,n)}\right)^{S_t^{(m)} S_{t-1}^{(n)}}. \tag{B.3}
$$

The initial distribution for the hidden state variable in SSM m is gaussian with mean $\mu_{X_1}^{(m)}$ and covariance matrix $Q_1^{(m)}$:

$$
P\left(X_1^{(m)}\right) = \left|2\pi Q_1^{(m)}\right|^{-\frac{1}{2}}
$$
$$
\exp\left\{-\frac{1}{2}\left(X_1^{(m)} - \mu_{X_1}^{(m)}\right)'\left(Q_1^{(m)}\right)^{-1}\left(X_1^{(m)} - \mu_{X_1}^{(m)}\right)\right\}. \tag{B.4}
$$

The probability distribution of the state in SSM m at time t given the state at time $t - 1$ is gaussian with mean $A^{(m)} X_{t-1}^{(m)}$ and covariance matrix $Q^{(m)}$:

$$
P\left(X_t^{(m)}|X_{t-1}^{(m)}\right) = \left|2\pi Q^{(m)}\right|^{-\frac{1}{2}} \exp\left\{-\frac{1}{2}\left(X_t^{(m)} - A^{(m)} X_{t-1}^{(m)}\right)'(Q^{(m)})^{-1}\right.
$$
$$
\left. \cdot \left(X_t^{(m)} - A^{(m)} X_{t-1}^{(m)}\right)\right\}. \tag{B.5}
$$

Finally, using equation 3.2, we can write:

$$P(Y_t|X_t, S_t) = \prod_{m=1}^{M} \left[|2\pi R|^{-\frac{1}{2}} \right.$$

$$\left. \exp\left\{ -\frac{1}{2} \left(Y_t - C^{(m)} X_t^{(m)} \right)' R^{-1} \left(Y_t - C^{(m)} X_t^{(m)} \right) \right\} \right]^{S_t^{(m)}} \quad (B.6)$$

since the terms with exponent equal to 0 vanish in the product.

Combining equations B.1 through B.6 and taking the negative of the logarithm, we obtain the hamiltonian of a switching SSM (ignoring constants):

$$H = \frac{1}{2} \sum_{m=1}^{M} \log \left| \mathcal{Q}_1^{(m)} \right| + \frac{1}{2} \sum_{m=1}^{M} \left(X_1^{(m)} - \mu_{X_1}^{(m)} \right)' \left(\mathcal{Q}_1^{(m)} \right)^{-1} \left(X_1^{(m)} - \mu_{X_1}^{(m)} \right)$$

$$+ \frac{(T-1)}{2} \sum_{m=1}^{M} \log \left| \mathcal{Q}^{(m)} \right|$$

$$+ \frac{1}{2} \sum_{m=1}^{M} \sum_{t=2}^{T} \left(X_t^{(m)} - A^{(m)} X_{t-1}^{(m)} \right)' (\mathcal{Q}^{(m)})^{-1} \left(X_t^{(m)} - A^{(m)} X_{t-1}^{(m)} \right)$$

$$+ \frac{T}{2} \log |R| + \frac{1}{2} \sum_{m=1}^{M} \sum_{t=1}^{T} S_t^{(m)} \left(Y_t - C^{(m)} X_t^{(m)} \right)' R^{-1} \left(Y_t - C^{(m)} X_t^{(m)} \right)$$

$$- \sum_{m=1}^{M} S_1^{(m)} \log \pi^{(m)} - \sum_{t=2}^{T} \sum_{m=1}^{M} \sum_{n=1}^{M} S_t^{(m)} S_{t-1}^{(n)} \log \Phi^{(m,n)}. \quad (B.7)$$

The hamiltonian for the approximating distribution can be analogously derived from the definition of Q (see equation 4.6):

$$Q(\{S_t, X_t\}) = \frac{1}{Z_Q} \left[\psi(S_1) \prod_{t=2}^{T} \psi(S_{t-1}, S_t) \right] \prod_{m=1}^{M} \psi(X_1^{(m)}) \prod_{t=2}^{T} \psi(X_{t-1}^{(m)}, X_t^{(m)}). \quad (B.8)$$

The potentials for the initial switch state and switch state transitions are

$$\psi(S_1) = \prod_{m=1}^{M} (\pi^{(m)} q_1^{(m)})^{S_1^{(m)}} \quad (B.9)$$

$$\psi(S_{t-1}, S_t) = \prod_{m=1}^{M} \prod_{n=1}^{M} \left(\Phi^{(m,n)} q_t^{(m)} \right)^{S_t^{(m)} S_{t-1}^{(n)}}. \quad (B.10)$$

The potential for the initial state of SSM m is

$$\psi(X_1^{(m)}) = P(X_1^{(m)}) \left[P(Y_1|X_1^{(m)}, S_1 = m) \right]^{h_1^{(m)}}, \quad (B.11)$$

344   Zoubin Ghahramani and Geoffrey E. Hinton

and the potential for the state at time t given the state at time $t - 1$ is

$$\psi(X_{t-1}^{(m)}, X_t^{(m)}) = P(X_t^{(m)}|X_{t-1}^{(m)}) \left[P(Y_t|X_t^{(m)}, S_t = m) \right]^{h_t^{(m)}}. \tag{B.12}$$

The hamiltonian for Q is obtained by combining these terms and taking the negative logarithm:

$$
\begin{aligned}
H_Q = &\frac{1}{2} \sum_{m=1}^{M} \log |Q_1^{(m)}| + \frac{1}{2} \sum_{m=1}^{M} \left(X_1^{(m)} - \mu_{X_1}^{(m)} \right)' (Q_1^{(m)})^{-1} \left(X_1^{(m)} - \mu_{X_1}^{(m)} \right) \\
&+ \frac{(T-1)}{2} \sum_{m=1}^{M} \log |Q^{(m)}| \\
&+ \frac{1}{2} \sum_{m=1}^{M} \sum_{t=2}^{T} \left(X_t^{(m)} - A^{(m)} X_{t-1}^{(m)} \right)' (Q^{(m)})^{-1} \left(X_t^{(m)} - A^{(m)} X_{t-1}^{(m)} \right) \\
&+ \frac{T}{2} \sum_{m=1}^{M} \log |R| + \frac{1}{2} \sum_{m=1}^{M} \sum_{t=1}^{T} h_t^{(m)} \left(Y_t - C^{(m)} X_t^{(m)} \right)' R^{-1} \left(Y_t - C^{(m)} X_t^{(m)} \right) \\
&- \sum_{m=1}^{M} S_1^{(m)} \log \pi^{(m)} - \sum_{t=2}^{T} \sum_{m=1}^{M} \sum_{n=1}^{M} S_t^{(m)} S_{t-1}^{(n)} \log \Phi^{(m,n)} \\
&- \sum_{t=1}^{T} \sum_{m=1}^{M} S_t^{(m)} \log q_t^{(m)}. \tag{B.13}
\end{aligned}
$$

Comparing H_Q with H, we see that the interaction between the $S_t^{(m)}$ and the $X_t^{(m)}$ variables has been eliminated, while introducing two sets of variational parameters: the responsibilities $h_t^{(m)}$ and the bias terms on the discrete Markov chain, $q_t^{(m)}$. In order to obtain the approximation Q that maximizes the lower bound on the log-likelihood, we minimize the KL divergence $KL(Q\|P)$ as a function of these variational parameters:

$$KL(Q\|P) = \sum_{\{S_t\}} \int Q(\{S_t, X_t\}) \log \frac{Q(\{S_t, X_t\})}{P(\{S_t, X_t\}|\{Y_t\})} d\{X_t\} \tag{B.14}$$

$$= \langle H - H_Q \rangle - \log Z_Q + \log Z, \tag{B.15}$$

where $\langle \cdot \rangle$ denotes expectation over the approximating distribution Q and Z_Q is the normalization constant for Q. Both Q and P define distributions in the exponential family. As a consequence, the zeros of the derivatives of KL with respect to the variational parameters can be obtained simply by equating derivatives of $\langle H \rangle$ and $\langle H_Q \rangle$ with respect to corresponding sufficient statistics (Ghahramani, 1997):

$$\frac{\partial \langle H_Q - H \rangle}{\partial \langle S_t^{(m)} \rangle} = 0 \tag{B.16}$$

$$\frac{\partial \langle H_Q - H \rangle}{\partial \langle X_t^{(m)} \rangle} = 0 \qquad\qquad\qquad\qquad\qquad (B.17)$$

$$\frac{\partial \langle H_Q - H \rangle}{\partial \langle P_t^{(m)} \rangle} = 0 \qquad\qquad\qquad\qquad\qquad (B.18)$$

where $P_t^{(m)} = \langle X_t^{(m)} X_t^{(m)'} \rangle - \langle X_t^{(m)} \rangle \langle X_t^{(m)} \rangle'$ is the covariance of $X_t^{(m)}$ under Q. Many terms cancel when we subtract the two hamiltonians,

$$H_Q - H = \sum_{m=1}^{M} \sum_{t=1}^{T} \frac{1}{2} \left(h_t^{(m)} - S_t^{(m)} \right) \left(Y_t - C^{(m)} X_t^{(m)} \right)' R^{-1}$$
$$\cdot \left(Y_t - C^{(m)} X_t^{(m)} \right) - S_t^{(m)} \log q_t^{(m)}. \qquad (B.19)$$

Taking derivatives, we obtain

$$\frac{\partial \langle H_Q - H \rangle}{\partial \langle S_t^{(m)} \rangle} = -\log q_t^{(m)} - \frac{1}{2} \left\langle \left(Y_t - C^{(m)} X_t^{(m)} \right)' R^{-1} \left(Y_t - C^{(m)} X_t^{(m)} \right) \right\rangle$$
$$(B.20)$$

$$\frac{\partial \langle H_Q - H \rangle}{\partial \langle X_t^{(m)} \rangle} = -\left(h_t^{(m)} - \langle S_t^{(m)} \rangle \right) \left((Y_t - C^{(m)} \langle X_t^{(m)} \rangle)' R^{-1} C^{(m)} \right) \quad (B.21)$$

$$\frac{\partial \langle H_Q - H \rangle}{\partial P_t^{(m)}} = \frac{1}{2} \left(h_t^{(m)} - \langle S_t^{(m)} \rangle \right) \left(C^{(m)'} R^{-1} C^{(m)} \right) \qquad (B.22)$$

From equation B.20, we get the fixed-point equation, 4.12, for $q_t^{(m)}$. Both equations B.21 and B.22 are satisfied when $h_t^{(m)} = \langle S_t^{(m)} \rangle$. Using the fact that $\langle S_t^{(m)} \rangle = Q(S_t = m)$ we get equation 4.11.

References

Ackerson, G. A., & Fu, K. S. (1970). On state estimation in switching environments. *IEEE Transactions on Automatic Control*, AC-15(1):10–17.

Anderson, B. D. O., & Moore, J. B. (1979). *Optimal filtering*. Englewood Cliffs, NJ: Prentice-Hall.

Athaide, C. R. (1995). *Likelihood evaluation and state estimation for nonlinear state space models*. Unpublished doctoral dissertation, University of Pennsylvania.

Baldi, P., Chauvin, Y., Hunkapiller, T., & McClure, M. (1994). Hidden Markov models of biological primary sequence information. *Proc. Nat. Acad. Sci. (USA)*, 91(3), 1059–1063.

Bar-Shalom, Y., & Li, X.-R. (1993). *Estimation and tracking*. Boston: Artech House.

Baum, L., Petrie, T., Soules, G., & Weiss, N. (1970). A maximization technique occurring in the statistical analysis of probabilistic functions of Markov chains. *Annals of Mathematical Statistics*, 41, 164–171.

Bengio, Y., & Frasconi, P. (1995). An input-output HMM architecture. In G. Tesauro, D. S. Touretzky, & T. K. Leen (Eds.), *Advances in neural information processing systems, 7* (pp. 427–434). Cambridge, MA: MIT Press.

Cacciatore, T. W., & Nowlan, S. J. (1994). Mixtures of controllers for jump linear and non-linear plants. In J. D. Cowan, G. Tesauro, & J. Alspector (Eds.), *Advances in neural information processing systems, 6* (pp. 719–726). San Mateo: Morgan Kaufmann Publishers.

Carter, C. K., & Kohn, R. (1994). On Gibbs sampling for state space models. *Biometrika, 81,* 541–553.

Chaer, W. S., Bishop, R. H., & Ghosh, J. (1997). A mixture-of-experts framework for adaptive Kalman filtering. *IEEE Trans. on Systems, Man and Cybernetics.*

Chang, C. B., & Athans, M. (1978). State estimation for discrete systems with switching parameters. *IEEE Transactions on Aerospace and Electronic Systems, AES-14*(3), 418–424.

Cover, T., & Thomas, J. (1991). *Elements of information theory.* New York: Wiley.

Dean, T., & Kanazawa, K. (1989). A model for reasoning about persistence and causation. *Computational Intelligence, 5*(3), 142–150.

Dempster, A., Laird, N., & Rubin, D. (1977). Maximum likelihood from incomplete data via the EM algorithm. *J. Royal Statistical Society Series B, 39,* 1–38.

Deng, L. (1993). A stochastic model of speech incorporating hierarchical nonstationarity. *IEEE Trans. on Speech and Audio Processing, 1*(4), 471–474.

Digalakis, V., Rohlicek, J. R., & Ostendorf, M. (1993). ML estimation of a stochastic linear system with the EM algorithm and its application to speech recognition. *IEEE Transactions on Speech and Audio Processing, 1*(4), 431–442.

Elliott, R. J., Aggoun, L., & Moore, J. B. (1995). *Hidden Markov models: Estimation and control.* New York: Springer-Verlag.

Fraser, A. M., & Dimitriadis, A. (1993). Forecasting probability densities by using hidden Markov models with mixed states. In A. S. Wiegand & N. A. Gershenfeld (Eds.), *Time series prediction: Forecasting the future and understanding the past* (pp. 265–282). Reading, MA: Addison-Wesley.

Ghahramani, Z. (1997). *On structured variational approximations* (Tech. Rep. No. CRG-TR-97-1). Toronto: Department of Computer Science, University of Toronto. Available online at: http://www.gatsby.ucl.ac.uk/~zoubin/papers/struct.ps.gz.

Ghahramani, Z., & Hinton, G. E. (1996a). *Parameter estimation for linear dynamical systems* (Tech. Rep. No. CRG-TR-96-2). Toronto: Department of Computer Science, University of Toronto. Available online at: http://www.gatsby.ucl.ac.uk/~zoubin/papers/tr-96-2.ps.gz.

Ghahramani, Z., & Hinton, G. E. (1996b). *The EM algorithm for mixtures of factor analyzers* (Tech. Rep. No. CRG-TR-96-1). Toronto: Department of Computer Science, University of Toronto. Available online at: http://www.gatsby.ucl.ac.uk/~zoubin/papers/tr-96-1.ps.gz.

Ghahramani, Z., & Jordan, M. I. (1997). Factorial hidden Markov models. *Machine Learning, 29,* 245–273.

Goodwin, G., & Sin, K. (1984). *Adaptive filtering prediction and control.* Englewood Cliffs, NJ: Prentice-Hall.

Hamilton, J. D. (1989). A new approach to the economic analysis of nonstationary time series and the business cycle. *Econometrica, 57,* 357–384.

Hamilton, J. D. (1994). *Time series analysis.* Princeton, NJ: Princeton University Press.

Harrison, P. J., & Stevens, C. F. (1976). Bayesian forecasting (with discussion). *J. Royal Statistical Society B, 38,* 205–247.

Hinton, G. E., Dayan, P., & Revow, M. (1997). Modeling the manifolds of images of handwritten digits. *IEEE Transactions on Neural Networks, 8,* 65–74.

Jacobs, R. A., Jordan, M. I., Nowlan, S. J., & Hinton, G. E. (1991). Adaptive mixture of local experts. *Neural Computation, 3,* 79–87.

Jordan, M. I., Ghahramani, Z., Jaakkola, T. S., & Saul, L. K. (1998). An introduction to variational methods in graphical models. In M. I. Jordan (Ed.), *Learning in graphical models.* Norwell, MA: Kluwer.

Jordan, M. I., & Jacobs, R. (1994). Hierarchical mixtures of experts and the EM algorithm. *Neural Computation, 6,* 181–214.

Juang, B. H., & Rabiner, L. R. (1991). Hidden Markov models for speech recognition. *Technometrics, 33,* 251–272.

Kadirkamanathan, V., & Kadirkamanathan, M. (1996). Recursive estimation of dynamic modular RBF networks. In D. Touretzky, M. Mozer, and M. Hasselmo (Eds.), *Advances in neural information processing systems, 8* (pp. 239–245). Cambridge, MA: MIT Press.

Kalman, R. E., & Bucy, R. S. (1961). New results in linear filtering and prediction. *Journal of Basic Engineering (ASME), 83D,* 95–108.

Kanazawa, K., Koller, D., & Russell, S. J. (1995). Stochastic simulation algorithms for dynamic probabilistic networks. In P. Besnard & S. Hanks (Eds.), *Uncertainty in artificial intelligence. Proceedings of the Eleventh Conference* (pp. 346–351). San Mateo, CA: Morgan Kaufmann.

Kehagias, A., & Petrides, V. (1997). Time series segmentation using predictive modular neural networks. *Neural Computation, 9*(8), 1691–1710.

Kim, C.-J. (1994). Dynamic linear models with Markov-switching. *J. Econometrics, 60,* 1–22.

Lauritzen, S. L., & Spiegelhalter, D. J. (1988). Local computations with probabilities on graphical structures and their application to expert systems. *J. Royal Statistical Society B,* 157–224.

Ljung, L., & Söderström, T. (1983). *Theory and practice of recursive identification.* Cambridge, MA: MIT Press.

Meila, M., & Jordan, M. I. (1996). Learning fine motion by Markov mixtures of experts. In D. S. Touretzky, M. C. Mozer, & M. E. Hasselmo (Eds.), *Advances in neural information processing systems, 8.* Cambridge, MA: MIT Press.

Neal, R. M., & Hinton, G. E. (1998). A new view of the EM algorithm that justifies incremental, sparse, and other variants. In M. I. Jordan (Ed.), *Learning in graphical models.* Norwell, MA: Kluwer.

Parisi, G. (1988). *Statistical field theory.* Redwood City, CA: Addison-Wesley.

Pawelzik, K., Kohlmorgen, J., & Müller, K.-R. (1996). Annealed competition of experts for a segmentation and classification of switching dynamics. *Neural Computation, 8*(2), 340–356.

Pearl, J. (1988). *Probabilistic reasoning in intelligent systems: Networks of plausible inference.* San Mateo, CA: Morgan Kaufmann.

Rabiner, L. R., & Juang, B. H. (1986). An introduction to hidden Markov models. *IEEE Acoustics, Speech & Signal Processing Magazine, 3,* 4–16.

Rauch, H. E. (1963). Solutions to the linear smoothing problem. *IEEE Transactions on Automatic Control, 8,* 371–372.

Rigney, D., Goldberger, A., Ocasio, W., Ichimaru, Y., Moody, G., & Mark, R. (1993). Multi-channel physiological data: Description and analysis. In A. Weigend & N. Gershenfeld (Eds.), *Time series prediction: Forecasting the future and understanding the past* (pp. 105–129). Reading, MA: Addison-Wesley.

Roweis, S., & Ghahramani, Z. (1999). A unifying review of linear gaussian models. *Neural Computation, 11*(2), 305–345.

Saul, L. and Jordan, M. I. (1996). Exploiting tractable substructures in intractable networks. In D. Touretzky, M. Mozer, & M. Hasselmo (Eds.), *Advances in neural information processing systems, 8.* Cambridge, MA: MIT Press.

Shumway, R. H., & Stoffer, D. S. (1982). An approach to time series smoothing and forecasting using the EM algorithm. *J. Time Series Analysis, 3*(4), 253–264.

Shumway, R. H., & Stoffer, D. S. (1991). Dynamic linear models with switching. *J. Amer. Stat. Assoc., 86,* 763–769.

Smyth, P. (1994). Hidden Markov models for fault detection in dynamic systems. *Pattern Recognition, 27*(1), 149–164.

Smyth, P., Heckerman, D., & Jordan, M. I. (1997). Probabilistic independence networks for hidden Markov probability models. *Neural Computation, 9,* 227–269.

Ueda, N., & Nakano, R. (1995). Deterministic annealing variant of the EM algorithm. In G. Tesauro, D. Touretzky, & J. Alspector (Eds.), *Advances in neural information processing systems, 7* (pp. 545–552). San Mateo, CA: Morgan Kaufmann.

Weigend, A., & Gershenfeld, N. (1993). *Time series prediction: Forecasting the future and understanding the past.* Reading, MA: Addison-Wesley.

14

Nonlinear Time-Series Prediction with Missing and Noisy Data

Volker Tresp
Reimar Hofmann
Siemens AG, Corporate Technology, Department of Information and Communications, 81730 Munich, Germany

We derive solutions for the problem of missing and noisy data in nonlinear time-series prediction from a probabilistic point of view. We discuss different approximations to the solutions—in particular, approximations that require either stochastic simulation or the substitution of a single estimate for the missing data. We show experimentally that commonly used heuristics can lead to suboptimal solutions. We show how error bars for the predictions can be derived and how our results can be applied to K-step prediction. We verify our solutions using two chaotic time series and the sunspot data set. In particular, we show that for K-step prediction, stochastic simulation is superior to simply iterating the predictor.

1 Introduction

Neural networks have been applied successfully in numerous applications to nonlinear time-series prediction (Weigend & Gershenfeld, 1994). Common problems in time-series prediction are missing and noisy data. The goal is to obtain optimal predictions even if some measurements are unavailable, are not recorded, or are uncertain. For linear systems, efficient algorithms exist for prediction with missing data (Kalman, 1960; Shumway & Stoffer, 1982). In particular, the Kalman filter is based on a state-space formulation and achieves optimal predictions with arbitrary patterns of missing data. For nonlinear systems, the extended Kalman filter, based on a first-order series expansion of the nonlinearities, can be employed. The extended Kalman filter is suboptimal (Bar-Shalom & Li, 1993) and summarizes past data by an estimate of the means and the covariances of the variables involved. The extended Kalman filter fails to give good predictions if the system is not approximated well by a localized linearization, that is, for highly nonlinear systems, in particular if the inaccuracies in the approximations propagate through several iterations, as in K-step prediction. In this article, we propose stochastic sampling, which converges to the optimal solution as the number of samples approaches infinity and can handle arbitrary patterns of noisy and missing data. We demonstrate the benefits of stochastic sampling using three examples.

The related issue of training a time-series model with missing and noisy data will be addressed in a companion article (Tresp & Hofmann, 1997).

In section 2 we derive equations for prediction with missing data. As in the case of regression and classification with missing data (Little & Rubin, 1987; Ahmad & Tresp, 1993; Buntine & Weigend, 1991), the solution consists of integrals over the unknown variables weighted by the conditional probability density of the unknown variables given the known variables. In time-series prediction, we can use the fact that the unknown data themselves are part of the time series. By unfolding the time series in time, we obtain a Bayesian network (Pearl, 1988; Jensen, 1996) (a probabilistic graph with directed arcs) that allows us to clarify dependencies between the variable to be predicted and the measurements that provide information about that variable. In section 3 we generalize the results toward noisy measurements. For nonlinear systems, the integrals cannot be solved in closed form and have to be approximated numerically. In section 4 we propose stochastic sampling, which has the advantage that asymptotically (i.e., with the number of samples approaching infinity) we obtain the optimal prediction. As an alternative approximation, we propose that maximum likelihood estimates can be substituted for the missing data. Furthermore, we discuss solutions based on an iterative approximation of the information provided by past data using probability density estimates. In section 5 we present experimental results demonstrating the superiority of the stochastic sampling approach. In particular, we show that for K-step prediction, stochastic sampling is superior to both simply iterating the system and the extended Kalman filter (the latter two turn out to be identical for K-step prediction). In section 6 we present conclusions.

2 Prediction with Missing Data

2.1 An Illustrative Example. Consider the situation depicted in Figure 1 (top). The time-series model is

$$y_t = f(y_{t-1}, y_{t-2}) + \epsilon_t,$$

where ϵ_t is additive independent, identically distributed (i.i.d.) noise and $f()$ is a nonlinear function. The goal is to predict y_t based on past measurements. Let us assume that y_{t-2} is missing. A common procedure is to obtain an estimate $\hat{y}_{t-2}$ of the missing value and then substitute that estimate in the predictive model,

$$\hat{y}_t = f(y_{t-1}, \hat{y}_{t-2}).$$

In some applications, it might make sense to substitute for the missing value the previous value $\hat{y}_{t-2} = y_{t-3}$ or to substitute the predicted value

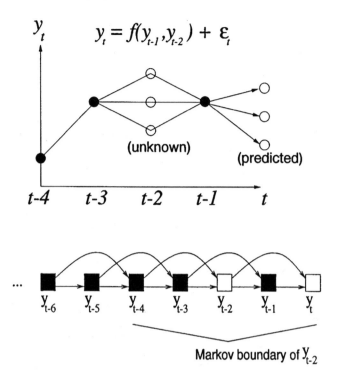

Figure 1: (Top) y_{t-2} is missing, and the goal is to predict y_t. The estimate $\hat{y}_t$ is dependent on the substituted value for y_{t-2}. (Bottom) A time series unfolded in time. Open squares indicate unknown variables, and filled squares indicate measured variables. The arrows indicate that the next realization of the time series can be predicted from only the two most recent values, $y_t = f(y_{t-1}, y_{t-2}) + \epsilon_t$. Here, y_{t-2} is assumed to be missing. The bracket indicates the nodes in the Markov boundary of y_{t-2} (see section 4.1).

$\hat{y}_{t-2} = f(y_{t-3}, y_{t-4})$. Both heuristics might often work in practice, but note the following two points:

1. Since in our example y_{t-1} is known, it should improve our estimate of y_{t-2}.

2. Since y_{t-2} is only estimated, it should be possible to achieve better predictions by substituting not just one estimate but several estimates and then averaging the predictions based on those estimates.

In the following sections, we show that a theoretical analysis confirms these intuitions.

2.2 Theory. Let y_t be the value of the discrete time series at time t. We assume that the underlying probabilistic model of the time series is of order N and can be described by

$$y_t = f(y_{t-1}, y_{t-2}, \ldots, y_{t-N}) + \epsilon_t, \qquad (2.1)$$

where $f()$ is either known or approximated sufficiently well by a function approximator such as a neural network. ϵ_t is assumed to be additive i.i.d. zero-mean noise with probability density $P_\epsilon(\epsilon)$ and typically represents unmodeled dynamics. The conditional probability density of the predicted value of the time series is then

$$P(y_t | y_{t-1}, y_{t-2}, \ldots, y_{t-N}) = P_\epsilon(y_t - f(y_{t-1}, y_{t-2}, \ldots, y_{t-N})). \qquad (2.2)$$

Often gaussian noise is assumed such that

$$P(y_t | y_{t-1}, y_{t-2}, \ldots, y_{t-N}) = G(y_t; f(y_{t-1}, \ldots, y_{t-N}), \sigma^2), \qquad (2.3)$$

where $G(x; c, \sigma^2)$ is our notation for a normal density evaluated at x with center c and variance σ^2.

It is convenient to unfold the system in time which leads to the system shown in Figure 1 (bottom). The realizations of the time series can now be considered random variables or nodes in a Bayesian network, in which directed arcs indicate direct dependencies (Pearl, 1988). The joint probability density in a Bayesian network is the product of all conditional densities and the prior probabilities

$$P(y_1, y_2, \ldots, y_t) = P(y_1, \ldots, y_N) \prod_{l=N+1}^{t} P(y_l | y_{l-1}, \ldots, y_{l-N}), \qquad (2.4)$$

where $P(y_1, \ldots, y_N)$ is the prior probability of the first N values of the time series.

We use the following notation: $Y^u_{t_2,t_1} \subseteq \{y_{t_1}, y_{t_1+1}, \ldots, y_{t_2}\}$ is the set of missing variables from t_1 to t_2, $Y^m_{t_2,t_1} \subseteq \{y_{t_1}, y_{t_1+1}, \ldots, y_{t_2}\}$ is the set of measurements between t_1 and t_2, and $Y_{t_2,t_1} = Y^m_{t_2,t_1} \cup Y^u_{t_2,t_1}$ $(t_1 \le t_2)$.

The theory of Bayesian networks is helpful to decide which past measurements provide information about y_t. Let A and B be nodes in a directed acyclic graph D (in our case, a Bayesian network). A and B are independent given the evidence entered into the network if they are d-separate. The definition of d-separation (Pearl, 1988; Jensen, 1996) follows.

Definition (d-separation).   Two variables A and B in a directed acyclic graph are *d-separated* if for all paths between A and B there is an intermediate variable V such that either (1) the connection is serial or diverging and the state of V is known or (2) the connection is converging and neither V nor any of V's descendants has received evidence.[1]

In other words, A and B are d-separated if every path between both nodes is blocked by condition 1 or 2. An example of a serial connection is $\rightarrow V \rightarrow$, of a diverging connection is $\leftarrow V \rightarrow$, and of a converging connection is $\rightarrow V \leftarrow$. We now apply the concept of d-separation to time-series prediction. Let y_{t-L} be the most recent case, where N consecutive measurements are known; that is, $y_{t-L}, y_{t-L-1}, \ldots, y_{t-L-N+1}$ are all known. In this case, y_t is d-separate from measurements previous to $t - L - N + 1$ given $y_{t-L}, y_{t-L-1}, \ldots, y_{t-L-N+1}$. Consider Figure 1 (bottom). Here, y_{t-5} is d-separated from y_t by y_{t-3} and y_{t-4} since these nodes block all paths from y_{t-5} to y_t. The same d-separation is true for all measurements previous to y_{t-5}. y_{t-4}, on the other hand is not blocked by y_{t-3} and y_{t-1} since the path $y_{t-4} \rightarrow y_{t-2} \rightarrow y_t$ is not blocked.

Following the discussion in the previous paragraph, y_t is independent of measurements earlier than $y_{t-L-N+1}$ given $y_{t-L}, y_{t-L-1}, \ldots, y_{t-L-N+1}$. This means that we have to condition y_t only on measurements $Y^m_{t-1,t-L-N+1}$, and we obtain for the expected value of the next realization of the time series,

$$
\begin{aligned}
E(y_t | Y^m_{t-1,1}) &= \int y_t P(y_t | Y^m_{t-1,t-L-N+1}) dy_t \\
&= \int f(y_{t-1}, \ldots, y_{t-k}, \ldots, y_{t-N}) \\
&\quad \times P(Y^u_{t-1,t-N} | Y^m_{t-1,t-L-N+1}) \, dY^u_{t-1,t-N} \\
&= \int f(y_{t-1}, \ldots, y_{t-k}, \ldots, y_{t-N}) \\
&\quad \times P(Y^u_{t-1,t-L+1} | Y^m_{t-1,t-L-N+1}) \, dY^u_{t-1,t-L+1},
\end{aligned}
\tag{2.5}
$$

where (assuming $t - L \geq N$)

$$
P(Y^u_{t-1,t-L+1} | Y^m_{t-1,t-L-N+1}) = \frac{1}{const} \times \prod_{l=t-L+1}^{t-1} P(y_l | y_{l-1}, \ldots, y_{l-N}),
$$

and $const = P(Y^m_{t-1,t-L+1} | Y^m_{t-L,t-L-N+1})$ is a normalization constant independent of the unknown variables.

3 Prediction with Noisy Measurements

Let again $y_t = f(y_{t-1}, y_{t-2}, \ldots, y_{t-N}) + \epsilon_t$, but now we assume that we have no access to y_t directly. Instead, we measure $z_t = y_t + \delta_t$ where δ_t is independent zero-mean noise (see Figure 2) with probability density $P_\delta(\delta)$.

---

[1] In our case this means that neither V nor any of V's descendants are known.

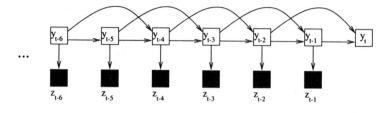

Figure 2: The Bayesian network corresponding to the problem of time-series prediction with noisy measurements ($N = 2$). Open squares indicate unknown variables, and filled squares indicate measured variables.

Let $Z_{t-1,1} = \{z_1 \ldots z_{t-1}\}$ and $Y_{t,1} = \{y_1 \ldots y_t\}$. The joint probability density is

$$P(Y_{t,1}, Z_{t-1,1}) = P(y_1, \ldots, y_N) \prod_{l=N+1}^{t} P(y_l | y_{l-1}, \ldots, y_{l-N})$$

$$\times \prod_{l=1}^{t-1} P(z_l | y_l), \tag{3.1}$$

with $P(z_l | y_l) = P_\delta(z_l - y_l)$. The corresponding Bayesian network is shown in Figure 2. Note that for each known variable z_{t-k}, there is a path to y_t that is not blocked by any of the other known variables and has no converging arrows; that is, the path $z_{t-k} \leftarrow y_{t-k} \rightarrow y_{t-k+1} \rightarrow \cdots \rightarrow y_t$. This means that y_t is dependent on all past measurements.

The expression for the expected value of the next instance of the time series (prediction) is then

$$E(y_t | Z_{t-1,1}) = \int f(y_{t-1}, \ldots, y_{t-N}) \, P(Y_{t-1,t-N} | Z_{t-1,1}) \, dY_{t-1,t-N}$$

$$= \int f(y_{t-1}, \ldots, y_{t-N}) \, P(Y_{t-1,1} | Z_{t-1,1}) \, dY_{t-1,1}, \tag{3.2}$$

where $P(Y_{t-1,1} | Z_{t-1,1}) = 1/const \times P(Y_{t-1,1}, Z_{t-1,1})$ which is obtained from equation 3.1. $const = P(Z_{t-1,1})$ is a normalization constant independent of $Y_{t-1,1}$. Note that the case of noisy measurements includes the case of missing data. In particular, if we allow the measurement noise to be time dependent (which does not introduce any additional complexity), we can use $\sigma_\delta^2(t) = 0$ for certain measurements and $\sigma_\delta^2(t) = \infty$ for unknown data.

4 Approximations to the Theoretical Solutions

In general, if $f()$ is a nonlinear function, the equations we obtained for prediction—equations 2.5 and 3.2—cannot be solved analytically and must be approximated numerically. First, we propose an approximation based on stochastic simulation that provides the optimal prediction when the number of samples approaches infinity. As a second approximation, we discuss an approach where the most likely values are substituted for the missing data. The latter approach tends to be computationally less expensive but provides biased predictions. Finally, we discuss the extended Kalman filter, which can be used on-line and is based on a first-order series expansion of the nonlinearities.

4.1 Stochastic Simulation. We will discuss a solution based on stochastic simulation. Note that all solutions have the general form $\int h(U, M) P(U|M) \, dU$, where U is a set of unknown variables and M is a set of known variables. An integral of this form can be solved by drawing random samples of the unknown variables following $P(U|M)$. Let $U^1, \ldots, U^S$ denote these samples. Then we can approximate

$$\int h(U, M)P(U|M) \, dU \approx \frac{1}{S} \sum_{s=1}^{S} h(U^s, M).$$

The problem now reduces to sampling from $P(U|M)$. Let us first assume that only one variable is missing. Then the problem reduces to sampling from a one-variate distribution, which can be done using sampling-importance-resampling or other sampling techniques (Bernardo & Smith, 1994).

If more than one realization is missing, the situation becomes more complicated. The reason is that the unknown variables are in general dependent, and we have to draw from the joint probability distribution of all unknowns. A general solution to this problem is Markov chain Monte Carlo sampling, with the Metropolis-Hastings algorithm and Gibbs sampling being the two most important representatives. We briefly describe the last.

In Gibbs sampling, we initialize the unknown variables either randomly or better with reasonable initial values. Then we select one of the unknown variables $u_i \in U$ and pick a sample from the one-dimensional conditional density $P(u_i|MB(i))$ and set u_i to that value. $MB(i)$ is the Markov boundary of u_i.[2]

Then we repeat the procedure for another unknown variable, and so on. In this way, repeated samples of all unknowns are drawn. Discard the first samples since they strongly depend on which initial values were chosen. Then, for strictly positive distributions, samples are produced with the correct distribution, that is, for $s \to \infty$, U^s tends in distribution to a joint

---

[2] We have to condition only on the nodes in the Markov boundary since, by definition of the Markov boundary, under the assumption that all nodes in the Markov boundary are unknown, the node u_i is d-separated from the remaining variables in a Bayesian network. The Markov boundary of a node consists of its direct parents, its direct successors, and all direct parents of its direct successors (Pearl, 1988) (as an example, see Figure 1).

random vector whose joint density is $P(U|M)$ (Bernardo & Smith, 1994). Gibbs sampling reduces the problem of drawing a sample from the joint density of all unknowns to sequentially drawing samples from the univariate densities of each unknown conditioned on the variables in its Markov boundary.

In the case of missing data, we have to generate samples from all missing data $Y^u_{t-1,t-L+1}$. In the case of noisy measurements, we even have to sample from all $Y_{t-1,1}$. In practice, one would restrict the sampling to a reasonably chosen time window in the past.

For independent samples, the variance of an estimated mean is equal to σ_s^2/S, where σ_s^2 is the variance of an individual sample. Unfortunately, samples generated by Gibbs sampling and other Markov chain Monte Carlo sampling techniques are typically highly correlated such that, depending on the particular problem, a large number of samples might be required for a good estimate. This is particularly true if regions of high probability are separated by regions of low probability such that the transition between regions has low probability. Another disadvantage is that for each new prediction, we have to perform a separate sampling process. Neal (1993) discusses hybrid Monte Carlo methods and other advanced sampling techniques that try to overcome some of the difficulties associated with dependent samples.

Sampling is simple if only samples of future values are required as in K-step prediction (for details, see section 5.1). The reason is that we can sample forward in time by simply simulating the system. In this procedure, independent samples are generated.

The idea of generating multiple samples from the unknown variables and averaging the responses using those samples confirms the intuition formulated in section 2.1 and is known as multiple imputation in statistical approaches to regression and classification with missing data (Little & Rubin, 1987).

The samples can also be used to estimate variances and covariances from which error bars can easily be derived. As examples, if $\{y_t^s\}_{s=1}^S$ are samples generated from y_t, the standard deviation of y_t can be estimated as

$$stdev(y_t) \approx \sqrt{\frac{1}{S-1}\sum_{s=1}^{S}(y_t^s - \hat{y}_t)^2},$$

and the standard deviation of the estimated $\hat{y}_t = 1/S\sum_{s=1}^S y_t^s$ can be estimated as

$$stdev(\hat{y}_t) \approx \sqrt{\frac{1}{S(S-1)}\sum_{s=1}^{S}(y_t^s - \hat{y}_t)^2}.$$

4.2 Maximum Likelihood Substitution. The approach consists of substituting the most likely values,

$$Y_{t-1,1}^{ml} = \arg \max_{Y_{t-1,1}^u} P(Y_{t-1,1}),$$

for the missing variables. Then we estimate

$$\hat{y}_t = f(Y_{t-1,t-N}^{ml}, Y_{t-1,t-N}^{m}). \tag{4.1}$$

Considering the case with one missing variable y_{t-k} and assuming gaussian noise,

$$y_{t-k}^{ml} = \arg \min_{y_{t-k}} \sum_{l=t-k}^{t-1} (y_l - f(y_{l-1}, y_{l-2}, \ldots, y_{l-N}))^2, \tag{4.2}$$

we simply find the substitution that minimizes the sum of the squared errors. As another interesting case, consider noisy measurements and gaussian noise distributions,

$$Y_{t-1,1}^{ml} = \arg \min_{Y_{t-1,1}^u} \Big[- \log P(Y_{N,1})$$

$$+ \frac{1}{2\sigma_\epsilon^2} \sum_{l=N+1}^{t-1} (y_l - f(y_{l-1}, y_{l-2}, \ldots, y_{l-N}))^2$$

$$+ \frac{1}{2\sigma_\delta^2} \sum_{l=1}^{t-1} (y_l - z_l)^2 \Big],$$

where σ_ϵ^2 and σ_δ^2 are the variances of the two noise sources (see section 3). This is a multidimensional optimization problem. Note that for highly nonlinear systems, equation 4.1 can be a crude estimate of the expected value, and the prediction based on a maximum likelihood estimate of the unknowns can therefore be highly biased.

4.3 Solutions Based on Iterative Density Estimation and the Extended Kalman Filters. We consider the case of prediction with noisy measurements. A solution based on stochastic simulation of equation 3.2 (noisy measurements) means that we have to sample from the space of all unknown variables, $y_1, \ldots, y_t$. This becomes intractable for large t. To summarize the information about past measurements more efficiently, we can use that

$$P(Y_{t-1,t-N}|Z_{t-1,1}) =$$
$$\frac{P(z_{t-1}|y_{t-1}) \int P(Y_{t-2,t-N-1}|Z_{t-2,1}) P(y_{t-1}|Y_{t-2,t-N-1}) dy_{t-N-1}}{\int P(z_{t-1}|y_{t-1}) P(Y_{t-2,t-N-1}|Z_{t-2,1}) P(y_{t-1}|Y_{t-2,t-N-1}) dY_{t-1,t-N-1}}. \tag{4.3}$$

This equation can be derived from the Chapman-Kolmogorov equation and by applying Bayes' rule (Lewis, 1986). The update equation implies that we can summarize all information provided by the past measurements by approximating $P(Y_{t-1,t-N}|Z_{t-1,1})$ and use equation 4.3 to update the estimates on-line as time progresses and more measurements become available.

If the system is linear and the noise is normally distributed, equation 4.3 can be solved analytically, and the probability densities can be represented by a multidimensional normal distribution. This is the well-known Kalman filter.

In general, the integral in equation 4.3 must be solved numerically, and an appropriate representation for the conditional density has to be found. Neural network techniques for approximating joint and conditional densities exist (Neuneier, Hergert, Finnoff, & Ormoneit, 1994; Bishop, 1994).

In Lewis (1986) it is shown that for continuous time systems, the time update leads to the Fokker-Planck equation, which can be solved in only a few simple cases. The problem can be simplified by requiring only that the iterative estimates of the mean and the covariance be found. Unfortunately, this approach leads to computationally intractable solutions (Lewis, 1986). The update equations become tractable by using a first-order series expansion of the nonlinearities (Lewis, 1986; Bar-Shalom & Li, 1993), which leads to the extended Kalman filter. The extended Kalman filter can be used for both discrete and continuous time systems and summarizes past data by an estimate of the mean and the covariance of the variables involved; it is suboptimal in the sense that even with a perfect model, due to the linearization of the system, it does not provide optimal predictions (Lewis, 1986; Bar-Shalom & Li, 1993). The Kalman filter is an iterative algorithm and has the great advantage that it can be used on-line. The Kalman filter has been used for training neural networks and for neural control (Singhal & Wu, 1989; Kadirkamanathan & Niranjan, 1991; Puskorius & Feldkamp, 1994).

5 Experiments

5.1 K-Step Prediction. K-step prediction can be considered a special case of prediction with missing data: y_t must be predicted with $y_{t-1}, \ldots, y_{t-K+1}$ missing. In this case, stochastic simulation is very simple: generate a sample y_{t-K+1}^s of the first missing value using the distribution $P(y_{t-K+1}|y_{t-K}, \ldots, y_{t-K-N+1})$. Using that sample and the previous measurements, generate a sample of y_{t-K+2} following $P(y_{t-K+2}|y_{t-K+1}^s, \ldots, y_{t-K-N+2})$, and so on until a sample of each unknown is produced. Repeat this procedure S times and approximate

$$E(y_t|Y_{t-K,1}) \approx \frac{1}{S} \sum_{s=1}^{S} f(y_{t-1}^s, y_{t-2}^s, \ldots, y_{t-N}^s),$$

where we have assumed that $K > N$. If $K \leq N$, substitute measured values

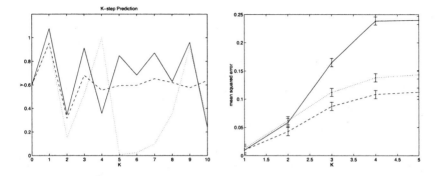

Figure 3: (Left) The noisy logistic map (solid line), the K-step prediction using stochastic simulation (dashed line) and the K-step prediction by simply iterating the logistic map (dotted line). The prediction based on stochastic simulation converges for large K toward the mean of the time series (which is the optimal solution, since chaotic time series quickly become unpredictable for large K). (Right) The mean squared error as a function of K in K-step prediction. The iterated solution (solid line) and the approximation based on stochastic simulation with 3 (dotted line) and 20 samples (dashed line) are shown. For K = 1 (one-step prediction), the iterated system gives the optimal prediction. For K > 1, the accuracy of the prediction of the iterated solution quickly deteriorates. The error bars (± one standard deviation) are derived from 2000 independent runs.

for y_{t-k} for $k \geq K$. In this procedure, samples are simply generated by simulating the system, including the noise model.

5.1.1 *Logistic Map.* In the first experiment, we used the noisy logistic map $y_t = 4q_{t-1}(1 - q_{t-1}) + \epsilon_t$ with $0 \leq q_{t-1} < 1$ and where

$$
q_t = \begin{cases} y_t & \text{if } 0 \leq y_t < 1 \\ y_t - 1 & \text{if } y_t \geq 1 \\ y_t + 1 & \text{if } y_t < 0 \end{cases}
$$

where ϵ_t is uncorrelated gaussian noise with a variance of $\sigma^2 = 0.01$.[3]
     The left panel of Figure 3 shows a realization of the time series and the predictions based on stochastic simulation and a simple iteration of the map. The right panel shows the mean squared error as a function of K averaged over 2000 realizations. Shown are the iterated system (continuous line) and

---

[3] Here and in the following experiments, q_t is introduced only for notational convenience to differentiate the cases when additive noise results in a value of the time series for which the iteration is not defined. q_t is therefore not a "real" hidden variable.

solutions following the stochastic sampling approach (dotted and dashed). As expected, for $K = 1$ the iterated solution is optimal, but for $K > 1$, stochastic simulation with even only a few samples is far superior. This indicates that for highly nonlinear stochastic time series, simply iterating the model K-times as it is usually done in K-step prediction is suboptimal if $K > 1$. Note that the K-step prediction of the extended Kalman filter, which is based on a local linearization of the nonlinearities, is identical to the iterated system (and therefore is suboptimal as well).

5.1.2 Sunspot Data. The second experiment uses records of yearly sunspot activities from the year 1700 to 1979. First, a multilayer perceptron was trained to predict the sunspot activity based on the 12 previous years of sunspot activity. The neural network had 12 inputs and one hidden layer with 8 hidden units. Following other authors, we trained on data from 1700 to 1920. We used a weight decay parameter of 0.2.[4]

After training, the mean squared error on the training set is 51.6, on test set 1 (data from 1921 to 1955) the mean squared error is 161.5, and on test set 2 (data from 1956 to 1979) the mean squared error is 682.0. We assumed normally distributed additive noise with a variance equal to the average error on the whole data set $\sigma^2 = 124$. Figure 4 shows the sunspot data (dots) from $T = 1738$ to $T = 1987$. In the experiment, we perform K-step prediction starting from $T = 1738$ (i.e., $T = 1738$ corresponds to one-step prediction and $T = 1987$ corresponds to 250-step prediction). The top panel of the figure displays the prediction of the iterated system, and the second panel shows the prediction by stochastic simulation using 1000 samples. The bottom panel shows one simulated run (including the noise model). Since the last includes the simulated noise, it is noisier than the iterated system, but the noisier time series is more similar to the true time series (dots). Unlike the prediction based on the iterated system, the prediction based on stochastic simulation converges toward a constant for large K and gives the correct estimate in predicting the mean if K is large.

Figure 5 shows the mean squared prediction error as a function of K. We see that for $K \gg 1$, stochastic simulation is clearly superior. Recall that for $K = 1$, the iterated prediction is optimal.

5.2 Prediction with Missing Data. In this experiment we used the Henon map[5] $y_t = 1 - aq_{t-1}^2 + bq_{t-2} + \epsilon_t$ with $a = 1.4$, $b = 0.3$ and where

$$q_t = \begin{cases} y_t & \text{if } -1.26 \leq y_t < 1.26 \\ y_t - 1.26 & \text{if } y_t \geq 1.26 \\ y_t + 1.26 & \text{if } y_t < 1.26 \end{cases}$$

---

[4] Readers who are unfamiliar with weight decay or the multilayer perceptron should consult Bishop (1994).

[5] A variation of this experiment has been presented by Tresp and Hofmann (1995).

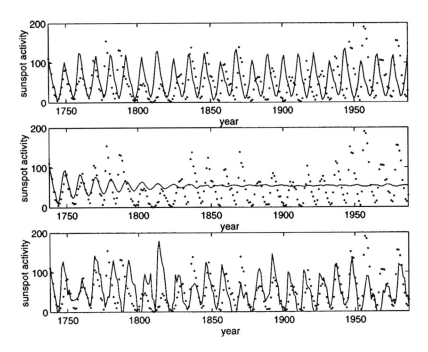

Figure 4: Sunspot data from $T = 1738$ to $T = 1987$ (dots). The continuous lines show the K-step predicted value (K increasing with T) based on three different methods. The top plot shows the iterated system, the middle plot shows the prediction based on stochastic simulation using $S = 1000$ samples, and the bottom plot shows one run of the stochastic simulation.

and where ϵ_t is uncorrelated gaussian noise with a variance of $\sigma^2 = 0.1$. The goal is to predict y_t with different patterns of $y_{t-1}, y_{t-2}, y_{t-3}, y_{t-4}$ missing, and y_{t-5}, y_{t-6} known. We used stochastic simulation (here, Gibbs sampling) of equation 2.5 for prediction. Figure 6 shows the results.

The considerable reduction in error for the solution based on stochastic simulation compared to the heuristic solution is apparent.

6 Conclusions

We have shown how the problem of missing and noisy data can be approached in a principled way in time series prediction. By unfolding the time series in time, we could apply ideas and methods from the theory of Bayesian networks. We proposed approximations based on stochastic simulations. Experimental results using the logistic map, the Henon map, and the sunspot data confirmed that stochastic sampling leads to excellent

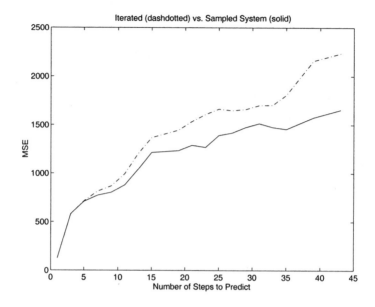

Figure 5: Mean squared error for K-step prediction for the iterated system (dash-dotted line) and the prediction based on stochastic simulation (solid line) for the sunspot data. It is apparent that for $K \gg 1$, the prediction based on stochastic simulation is superior. Shown are averages over all possible experiments, where in each experiment the prediction was started from a different point in time. For 1-step prediction, we used 250 different starting times, which means we averaged over 250 experiments; for 50-step prediction, we used 200 possible starting times and consequently could average over 200 experiments.

predicitions which are clearly superior to simple heuristic approaches. The main drawback of stochastic sampling is that generated samples are often highly correlated and a large number of samples might be required to obtain good approximations. For the problem of noisy measurements, the solution would require generating samples from the joint probability space of all past realizations of the time series, which is clearly unfeasible. In practice, one would sample only from realizations of the time series up to a reasonably chosen time window into the past, which, as a drawback, would lead to suboptimal solutions even with a large number of samples. In this article, we focused on univariate time-series prediction. The results can easily be extended to multivariate times series (see the appendix).

Appendix: Multivariate Nonlinear Time Series

The results can easily be generalized to general nonlinear multivariate models. It is convenient to switch to a state-space representation where $y_t \in \Re^{D_y}$

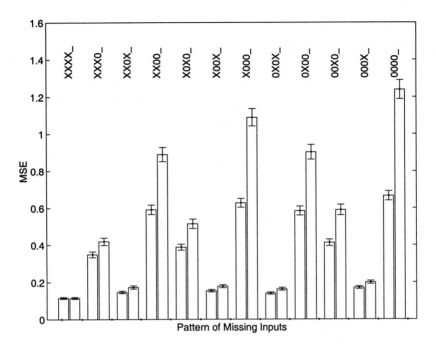

Figure 6: Time-series prediction with missing data. The patterns of the missing data are indicated using X for known, 0 for unknown values, and "_" for the value to be predicted. For example, $XXOO\_$ indicates that y_{t-4} and y_{t-3} are known and that y_{t-1} and y_{t-2} are missing. y_{t-5} and y_{t-6} are always known. The goal is to predict y_t using either stochastic sampling (left bars) or a heuristic where predicted values are substituted for the missing data (right bars). The height of the bars indicates the squared prediction error averaged over 1000 experiments. The error bars show $\pm$ their standard deviation. For stochastic sampling, we used 200 samples for each prediction. Except for one-step prediction ($XXXX\_$) the stochastic sampling solution is significantly better than the heuristic.

is a D_y-dimensional state-space vector containing all relevant states of all time series involved. Typically, y_t will be the present and past realizations of all time series involved, up to a time window in the past. The nonlinear state-space model is

$$y_t = f(y_{t-1}) + \epsilon_t,$$

where ϵ_t is a D_y-dimensional vector of possibly correlated noise and with probability density P_ϵ. We assume that we have access to a D_z-dimensional measurement vector $z_t \in \Re^{D_z}$ with

$$z_t = g(y_t) + \delta_t,$$

where δ_t is a D_z-dimensional vector of possibly correlated noise and with probability density P_δ. Recall from the discussion in section 3 that the problem of missing data can be considered a special case of noisy data. The joint density of the time series up to time t (not including z_t, since we consider predictions) is

$$P(Y_{t,1}, Z_{t-1,1}) = P(y_1) \prod_{l=2}^{t} P_\epsilon(y_l - f(y_{l-1})) \prod_{l=1}^{t-1} P_\delta(z_l - g(y_l)), \qquad \text{(A.1)}$$

with $Z_{t-1,1} = \{z_1 \ldots z_{t-1}\}$ and $Y_{t,1} = \{y_1 \ldots y_t\}$. Now

$$E(y_t|Z_{t-1,1}) = \int f(y_{t-1}) \, P(Y_{t-1,1}|Z_{t-1,1}) \, dY_{t-1,1},$$

where $P(Y_{t-1,1}|Z_{t-1,1}) = P(Y_{t-1,1}, Z_{t-1,1})/P(Z_{t-1,1})$ is obtained from equation A.1.

Acknowledgments

This work was supported by grant 01 IN 505 A9 from the Bundesministerium für Bildung, Wissenschaft, Forschung und Technologie.

References

Ahmad, S., & Tresp, V. (1993). Some solutions to the missing feature problem in vision. In S. J. Hanson, J. D. Cowan, & C. L. Giles (Eds.), *Neural information processing systems, 5* (pp. 393–440). San Mateo, CA: Morgan Kaufmann.

Bar-Shalom, Y., & Li, X.-R. (1993). *Estimation and tracking*. Boston: Artech House.

Bernardo, J. M., & Smith, A. F. M. (1994) *Bayesian theory*. New York: Wiley.

Bishop, C. M. (1994). *Neural networks for pattern recognition*. New York: Oxford University Press.

Buntine, W. L., & Weigend, A. S. (1991). Bayesian back-propagation. *Complex Systems, 5*, 605–643.

Jensen, F. V. (1996). *An introduction to Bayesian networks*. New York: Springer-Verlag.

Kalman, R. E. (1960). A new approach to linear filtering and prediction problems. *Trans. ASME J. Basic Eng., 8*, 35–45.

Kadirkamanathan, V., & Niranjan, M. (1991). Nonlinear adaptive filtering in nonstationary environments. *ICASSP 91*.

Lewis, F. L. (1986). *Optimal estimation with an introduction to stochastic control theory*. New York: Wiley.

Little, R. J. A., & Rubin, D. B. (1987). *Statistical analysis with missing data*. New York: Wiley.

Neal, R. M. (1993). *Probabilistic inference using Markov chain Monte Carlo methods* (Tech. Rep. No. CRG-TR-93-1). Department of Computer Science, University of Toronto.

Neuneier, R., Hergert, F., Finnoff, W., & Ormoneit, D. (1994). Estimation of conditional densities: A comparison of neural network approaches (pp. 689–692). *Proc. of ICANN 94*, Sorrento.

Pearl, J. (1988). *Probabilistic reasoning in intelligent systems*. San Mateo, CA: Morgan Kaufmann.

Puskorius, G. V., & Feldkamp, L. A. (1994). Neurocontrol of nonlinear dynamical systems with Kalman filter trained recurrent networks. *IEEE Transactions on Neural Networks, 5*(2), 279–297.

Shumway, R. H., & Stoffer, D. S. (1982). An approach to time series smoothing and forecasting using the EM algorithm. *Journal of Time Series Analysis, 3,* 253–264.

Singhal, S., & Wu, L. (1989). Training multi-layer perceptrons with the extended Kalman algorithm. In D. S. Touretzky (Ed.), *Advances in neural information processing systems, 1* (pp. 133–140). San Mateo, CA: Morgan Kaufman.

Tresp, V., & Hofmann, R. (1995). Missing and noisy data in nonlinear time-series prediction. In F. Girosi, J. Makhoul, E. Manolakos, & E. Wilson (Eds.), *Neural networks for signal processing 5* (pp. 1–10). New York: IEEE.

Tresp, V., & Hofmann, R. (1997). *Missing and noisy data in nonlinear time-series modeling*. Unpublished manuscript.

Weigend, A. S., & Gershenfeld, N. (Eds.). (1994). *Time-series prediction*. Reading, MA: Addison-Wesley.

15

Correctness of Local Probability Propagation in Graphical Models with Loops

Yair Weiss
Department of Brain and Cognitive Sciences, MIT, Cambridge, MA 02139, U.S.A.

Graphical models, such as Bayesian networks and Markov networks, represent joint distributions over a set of variables by means of a graph. When the graph is singly connected, local propagation rules of the sort proposed by Pearl (1988) are guaranteed to converge to the correct posterior probabilities. Recently a number of researchers have empirically demonstrated good performance of these same local propagation schemes on graphs with loops, but a theoretical understanding of this performance has yet to be achieved.

For graphical models with a single loop, we derive an analytical relationship between the probabilities computed using local propagation and the correct marginals. Using this relationship we show a category of graphical models with loops for which local propagation gives rise to provably optimal maximum a posteriori assignments (although the computed marginals will be incorrect). We also show how nodes can use local information in the messages they receive in order to correct their computed marginals.

We discuss how these results can be extended to graphical models with multiple loops and show simulation results suggesting that some properties of propagation on single-loop graphs may hold for a larger class of graphs. Specifically we discuss the implication of our results for understanding a class of recently proposed error-correcting codes known as turbo codes.

1 Introduction

Problems involving probabilistic belief propagation arise in a wide variety of applications, including error-correcting codes, speech recognition, and medical diagnosis. Typically, a probability distribution is assumed over a set of variables, and the task is to infer the values of the unobserved variables given the observed ones. The assumed probability distribution is described using a graphical model (Lauritzen, 1996); the qualitative aspects of the distribution are specified by a graph structure. Figure 1 shows two examples of such graphical models: a Bayesian network (Pearl, 1988; Jensen, 1996) (see Figure 1a) and Markov networks (Pearl, 1988; Geman & Geman, 1984) (see Figures 1b–c).

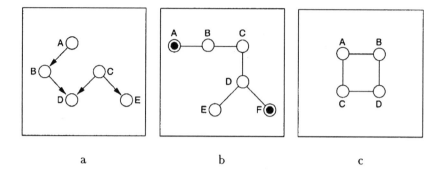

a   b   c

Figure 1: Examples of graphical models. Nodes represent variables, and the qualitative aspects of the joint probability function are represented by properties of the graph. Shaded nodes represent observed variables. (a) Singly connected Bayesian network. (b) Singly connected Markov network (A and F are observed). (c) Markov network with a loop. This article analyzes the behavior of local propagation rules in graphical models with a loop.

If the graph is singly connected—there is only one path between any two given nodes—then there exist efficient local message-passing schemes to calculate the posterior probability of an unobserved variable given the observed variables. Pearl (1988) derived such a scheme for singly connected Bayesian networks and showed that this "belief propagation" algorithm is guaranteed to converge to the correct posterior probabilities (or "beliefs"). However, as Pearl noted, the same algorithm will not give the correct beliefs for multiply connected networks:

> When loops are present, the network is no longer singly connected and local propagation schemes will invariably run into trouble. . . . If we ignore the existence of loops and permit the nodes to continue communicating with each other as if the network were singly connected, messages may circulate indefinitely around the loops and the process may not converge to a stable equilibrium. . . . Such oscillations do not normally occur in probabilistic networks. . . . which tend to bring all messages to some stable equilibrium as time goes on. However, this asymptotic equilibrium is not coherent, in the sense that it does not represent the posterior probabilities of all nodes of the network. (p. 195)

Despite these reservations, Pearl advocated the use of belief propagation in loopy networks as an approximation scheme (J. Pearl, personal communication), and one of the exercises in Pearl (1988) investigates the quality of the approximation when it is applied to a particular loopy belief network.

Several groups (Frey, 1998; MacKay & Neal, 1995; Weiss, 1996) have recently reported excellent experimental results by running algorithms equivalent to Pearl's algorithm on networks with loops. Perhaps the most dramatic instance of this performance is in an error-correcting code scheme known as turbo codes (Berrou, Glavieux, Thitimajshima, 1993), described as "the most exciting and potentially important development in coding theory in many years" (McEliece, Rodemich, & Cheng, 1995) and have recently been shown to use an algorithm equivalent to belief propagation in a network with loops (Wiberg, 1996; Kschischang & Frey, 1998; McEliece, MacKay, & Cheng, 1998). Although there is widespread agreement in the coding community that these codes "represent a genuine, and perhaps historic, breakthrough" (McEliece et al., 1995), a theoretical understanding of their performance has yet to be achieved.

Here we lay a foundation for an understanding of belief propagation in networks with loops. For networks with a single loop, we derive an analytic expression relating the steady-state beliefs to the correct posterior probabilities. We discuss how these results can be extended to networks with multiple loops and show simulation results for networks with multiple loops. Specifically we discuss the implication of our results for understanding the performance of turbo codes.

2 Formulation: Bayes Nets, Markov Nets, and Belief Propagation _____

Bayesian networks and Markov networks are graphs that represent the qualitative nature of a distribution over a set of variables; the structure of the graph implies a product form for the distribution. See Pearl (1988, chap. 3) for a more exhaustive treatment.

A Bayesian network is a directed acyclic graph in which the nodes represent variables, the arcs signify the existence of direct influences among the linked variables, and the strength of these influences is expressed by forward conditional probabilities. Using the chain rule, the full probability distribution over the variables can be expressed as a product of conditional and prior probabilities. Thus, for example, for the network in Figure 1a, we can write:

$$P(ABCDEF) = P(A)P(B \mid A)P(C)P(D \mid B, C)P(E \mid C). \tag{2.1}$$

A Markov network is an undirected graph in which the nodes represent variables, and arcs represent compatability constraints between them. Assuming that all probabilities are nonzero, the Hammersley-Clifford theorem (Pearl, 1988) guarantees that the probability distribution will factorize into a product of functions of the maximal cliques of the graph. Thus, for example, in the network in Figure 1c we have:

$$P(ABCD) = \frac{1}{Z}\Psi(AB)\Psi(AC)\Psi(CD)\Psi(DB). \tag{2.2}$$

Different communities tend to prefer different graphical models (see Smyth, 1997, for a recent review). Directed graphs are more common in artificial intelligence, medical diagnosis, and statistics, and undirected graphs are more common in image processing, statistical physics, and error-correcting codes. In both cases, however, a full specification of the probability distribution involves specifying the graph and numerical values for the conditional probabilities (in Bayes nets) or the clique potentials (in Markov nets).

Given a full specification of the probability, the inference task in graphical models is simply to infer the values of the unobserved variables given the observed ones. Figure 1b shows an example. The observed nodes A, F are represented by shaded circles in the graph. We use $\mathcal{O}$ to denote the set of observed variables. There are actually three distinct subtasks for the inference problem:

- *Marginalization*: Calculating the marginal probability of a variable given the observed variables—for example $P(C = c \mid \mathcal{O})$.

- *Maximum a posteriori (MAP) assignment*: Finding assignments to the unobserved variables that are most probable given the observed variables—for example, finding (b, c, d, e) such that $P(B = b, C = c, D = d, E = e \mid \mathcal{O})$ is maximized.

- *Maximum marginal (MM) assignment*: Finding assignments to the unobserved variables that maximize the marginal probability of the assignment—for example, finding (b, c, d, e) such that $P(B = b \mid \mathcal{O}), P(C = c \mid \mathcal{O}), P(D = d \mid \mathcal{O}), P(E = e \mid \mathcal{O})$ are all maximized.

2.1 Message-Passing Algorithms for Graphical Models. For singly connected graphical models, there exist various message-passing schemes for performing inference (see Smyth, Heckerman, & Jordan, 1997 for a review). Here we present such a scheme for pairwise Markov nets—ones in which the maximal cliques are pairs of units. This choice is not as restrictive as it may seem. First, any singly connected Markov net is a pairwise Markov network, and a Markov network with larger cliques can be converted into a pairwise Markov network by merging larger cliques into cluster nodes. Furthermore, as we show in the appendix, any Bayesian network can be converted into a pairwise Markov net. When this conversion is performed, the update rules given here reduce to Pearl's original algorithm for inference in Bayesian networks. The main advantage of the pairwise Markov net formulation is that it enables us to write the message-passing scheme in terms of matrix and vector operations, and this makes the subsequent analysis simpler.

To derive the message-passing algorithm, consider first the naive way of performing inference: by exhaustive enumeration. Referring again to

Figure 1b, calculating the marginal of C merely involves computing:

$$P(C = c \mid A = a, F = f) = \alpha \sum_{b,d,e} P(a, b, c, d, e, f), \qquad (2.3)$$

where α is a normalizing factor.

This exhaustive enumeration is, of course, exponential in the number of unobserved nodes, but for the particular factorized distributions of Markov nets, we can write:

$$
\begin{aligned}
P(C = c \mid A &= a, F = f) \\
&= \alpha \sum_{b} \sum_{d} \sum_{e} \Psi(ab)\Psi(bc)\Psi(cd)\Psi(df)\Psi(de) \qquad (2.4) \\
&= \alpha \left(\sum_{b} \Psi(ab)\Psi(bc) \right) \left(\sum_{d} \Psi(cd)\Psi(df) \sum_{e} \Psi(de) \right). \qquad (2.5)
\end{aligned}
$$

Note that the exponential enumeration is now converted into a series of enumerations over each variable separately and that many of the terms (e.g., $\sum_b \Psi(ab)\Psi(bc)$) are equivalent to matrix multiplication. This forms the basis for the message-passing algorithm.

The messages that nodes transmit to each other are vectors, and we denote by $\vec{v}_{XY}$ the message that node X sends to node Y. We define the transition matrix of an edge in the graph by

$$M_{XY}(i, j) \overset{\text{def}}{=} \Psi(X = i, Y = j). \qquad (2.6)$$

Note that the matrix going in one direction on an edge is equal by definition to the transpose of the matrix going in the other direction: $M_{XY} = M_{YX}^T$. We denote by $\vec{b}_X$ the belief vector at node X.

Following the terminology of Pearl (1988) we call the message-passing scheme for calculating marginals *belief update*. In belief update, the message that node X sends to node Y is updated as follows:

- Combine all messages coming into X except for that coming from Y into a vector $\vec{v}$. The combination is done by multiplying all the message vectors element by element.

- Multiply $\vec{v}$ by the matrix M_{XY} corresponding to the link from X to Y.

- Normalize the product $M_{XY}\vec{v}$ so it sums to 1. The normalized vector is sent to Y.

The belief vector for a node X is obtained by combining all incoming messages to X (again by multiplying the message vectors element by element) and normalizing.

By introducing a symbol $\odot$ for the componentwise multiplication operator, the updates can be rewritten:

$$\vec{v}_{XY} \leftarrow \alpha M_{XY} \underset{Z \in N(X) \backslash Y}{\bigodot} \vec{v}_{ZX} \tag{2.7}$$

$$\vec{b}_X \leftarrow \alpha \underset{Z \in N(X)}{\bigodot} \vec{v}_{ZX}, \tag{2.8}$$

where $\vec{z} = \vec{x} \odot \vec{y} \leftrightarrow \vec{z}(i) = \vec{x}(i)\vec{y}(i)$. Throughout this article $\alpha\vec{v}$ denotes normalizing the components of $\vec{v}$ so they sum to 1.

The procedure is initialized with all message vectors set to $(1, 1, \ldots, 1)$. Observed nodes do not receive messages, and they always transmit the same vector. If X is observed to be in state x, then $\vec{v}_{XY}(i) = \Psi(X = x, Y = i)$. The normalization of $\vec{v}_{XY}$ in equation 2.7 is not theoretically necessary; whether the message are normalized or not, the belief vector $\vec{b}_X$ will be identical. Thus one could use an equivalent algorithm where the messages are not normalized. However, as Pearl (1988) has pointed out, normalizing the messages avoids numerical underflow and adds to the stability of the algorithm. Equation 2.7 does not specify the order in which the messages are updated. For simplicity, we assume throughout this article that all nodes simultaneously update their messages in parallel.

For a singly connected network, the belief update equations (equations 2.7–2.8) solve two of the three inference tasks mentioned earlier. It can be shown that the the belief vectors reach a steady state after a number of iterations equal to the length of the longest path in the graph. Furthermore, at convergence, the belief vectors are equal to the posterior marginal probabilities. Thus for singly connected networks, $\vec{b}_X(j) = P(X = j \mid \mathcal{O})$.

We define the belief update (BU) assignment by assigning each variable X to the state j that maximizes $\vec{b}_X(j)$. Since $\vec{b}_X$ converges to the correct posteriors for a singly connected network, the BU assignment is guaranteed to give the MM assignment. Thus two of the three inference tasks mentioned earlier can be solved using the belief update procedure.

To calculate the MAP assignment, however, calculating the posterior marginals is insufficient. In order to calculate the MAP assignment, the nodes need to calculate the posterior when the other unobserved nodes are maximized rather than summed. In Figure 1 this corresponds to calculating

$$P^*(C = c \mid A = a, F = f) = \alpha \max_{b,d,e} P(a, b, c, d, e, f) \tag{2.9}$$

(we use the notation P^* to denote the fact that P^* does not correspond to a marginal probability).

In complete analogy to equation 2.4 the maximization over the unobserved variables can be replaced by a series of maximizations over individual variables. This leads to an alternative message-passing scheme that we call, following Pearl (1988), *belief revision*.

The procedure is almost identical to that described earlier for belief update. The only difference is that the matrix multiplication in equation 2.7 needs to be replaced with a nonlinear matrix operator. For a matrix M and a vector $\vec{x}$, we define the operator $\overset{\infty}{M}$ such that $\vec{y} = \overset{\infty}{M} \vec{x}$ if

$$\vec{y}(i) = \max_j M(i, j)\vec{x}(j). \qquad (2.10)$$

Note that the $\overset{\infty}{M}$ operator is similar to regular matrix multiplication, with the sum replaced with the maximum operator.

The belief revision update rules are

$$\vec{v}_{XY} \leftarrow \alpha \overset{\infty}{M}_{XY} \underset{Z \in N(X) \setminus Y}{\bigodot} \vec{v}_{ZX} \qquad (2.11)$$

$$\vec{b}_X \leftarrow \alpha \underset{Z \in N(X)}{\bigodot} \vec{v}_{ZX}, \qquad (2.12)$$

with initialization identical to belief update.

Again, it can be shown that for singly connected networks, the belief vector $\vec{b}_X(i)$ at a node will converge to the modified belief $P^*(X = i)$. We define the belief revision (BR) assignment as assigning each node X the value j that maximizes $\vec{b}_X(j)$ after belief revision has converged. From the definition of P^*, it follows that the BR assignment is equal to the MAP assignment for singly connected networks. Thus, all three inference tasks can be accomplished by local message passing.

Update rules such as equations 2.7–2.8 and Equations 2.11–2.12 have appeared in many areas of applied mathematics and optimization. In the hidden Markov model literature, the belief update equations (2.7–2.8) are equivalent to the forward-backward algorithm, and the BR equations (2.11–2.12) are equivalent to the Viterbi algorithm (Rabiner, 1989). In a general optimization context, equations 2.11–2.12 are a distributed implementation of standard dynamic programming (Bertsekas, 1987). If the nodes represent continuous gaussian random variables, equations 2.7–2.8 are equivalent to the Kalman filter and optimal smoothing (Gelb, 1974). In error-correcting codes, both belief revision and belief update can be thought of as special cases of a general class of decoding algorithms for codes defined on graphs (Kschischang & Frey, 1998; Forney, 1997; Aji & McEliece, in press).

In nearly all the contexts surveyed above, belief propagation has been analyzed only for singly connected graphs. Note, however, that these procedures are perfectly well defined for any pairwise Markov network. This raises questions, including:

- How far is the steady-state belief from the correct posterior when the update rules (equations 2.7–2.8) are applied in a loopy network?

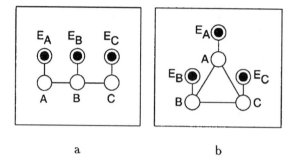

a   b

Figure 2: Intuition behind loopy belief propagation. In singly connected networks (a), the local update rules avoid double counting of evidence. In multiply
connected networks (b), double counting is unavoidable. However, as we show
in the text, certain structures lead to equal double counting.

- What are the conditions under which the BU assignment equals the
  MM assignment when the update rules are applied in a loopy network?

- What are the conditions under which the BR assignment equals the
  MAP assignment when the update rules are applied in a loopy network?

Answering these questions is the goal of this article.

3 Intuition: Why Does Loopy Propagation Work? _____

Before launching into the details of the analysis, let us consider the examples
in Figure 2. In both graphs, there is an observed node connected to every
unobserved nodes; we will refer to the observed node connected to X as
the local evidence at X. Intuitively, the message-passing algorithm can be
thought of as a way of communicating local evidence between nodes such
that all nodes calculate their beliefs given all the evidence.

As Pearl (1988) has pointed out, in order for a message-passing scheme
to be successful, it needs to avoid double counting—a situation in which
the same evidence is passed around the network multiple times and mis-
taken for new evidence. In a singly connected network (such as Figure 2a)
this is accomplished by update rules such as those in equation 2.7. Thus
in Figure 2a, node B will receive from A a message that involves the local evidence at A and send that information to C. The message it sends
to A will involve the local evidence at C but *not* the local evidence at A.
Thus, A never receives its own evidence back again, and double counting
is avoided.

In a loopy graph (such as Figure 2b), double counting cannot be avoided. Thus, B will send A's evidence to C, but in the next iteration, C will send that same information back to A. Thus, it seems that belief propagation in such a net will invariably give the wrong answer. How, then, can we explain the good performance reported experimentally?

Intuitively, the explanation is that double counting may still lead to correct inference if all evidence is double counted in equal amounts. Because nodes mistake existing evidence for new evidence, they are overly confident in their beliefs regarding which values should be assigned to the unobserved variables. However, if all evidence is equally double counted, the assignment, although based on overly confident beliefs, may still be correct. Indeed, as we show in this article, this intuition can be formalized for belief revision. For all networks with a single loop, the BR assignment gives the maximum a posteriori (MAP) assignment even though the numerical values of the beliefs are wrong.

The notion of equal double counting can be formalized by means of what we call the unwrapped network corresponding to a loopy network. The unwrapped network is a singly connected network constructed such that performing belief propagation in the unwrapped network is equivalent to performing belief propagation in the loopy network. The exact construction method of the unwrapped network is discussed in section 5, but the basic idea is to replicate the nodes and the transition matrices as shown in the examples in Figure 3. As we show, (see also Weiss, 1996; MacKay & Neal, 1995; Wiberg, 1996; Frey, Koetter, & Vardy, 1998), for any number of iterations of belief propagation in the loopy network, there exists an unwrapped network such that the final messages received by a node in the unwrapped network are equivalent to those that would be received by a corresponding node in the loopy network. This concept is illustrated in Figure 3. The messages received by node B after one, two, and three iterations of propagation in the loopy network are identical to the final messages received by node B in the unwrapped networks shown in Figure 3.

It seems that all we have done is to convert a finite, loopy problem into an infinite network without loops. What have we gained? The importance of the unwrapped network is that since it is singly connected, belief propagation on it is guaranteed to give the correct beliefs. Thus, belief propagation on the loopy network gives the correct answer for the unwrapped network. The usefulness of this estimate now depends on the similarity between the probability distribution induced by the unwrapped problem and the original loopy problem.

In subsequent sections we formally compare the probability distribution induced by the loopy network to that induced by the original problem. Roughly speaking, if we denote the original probability induced on the hidden nodes in Figure 1b by

$$P(a, b, c) = \alpha e^{-J(a,b,c)}, \tag{3.1}$$

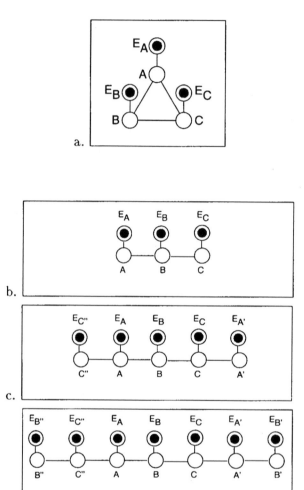

Figure 3: (a) Simple loopy network. (b–d) Unwrapped networks corresponding to the loopy network. The unwrapped networks are constructed by replicating the evidence and the transition matrices while preserving the local connectivity of the loopy network. They are constructed so that the messages received by node B after t iterations in the loopy network are equivalent to those that would be received by B in the unwrapped network. The unwrapped networks for the first three iterations are shown.

then MAP assignment for the unwrapped problem maximizes

$$\tilde{P}(a, b, c) = \alpha e^{-kJ(a,b,c)} \tag{3.2}$$

for some positive constant k. That is, if we are considering the probability of assignment, the unwrapped problem induces a probability that is a monotonic transformation of the true probability. In statistical physics terms, the unwrapped network has the same energy function but at different temperature. This is the intuitive reason that belief revision, which finds the MAP assignment in the unwrapped network, also finds the MAP assignment in the loopy network. However, belief update, which finds marginal distributions of particular nodes, may not find the MM assignment; the marginals of $\tilde{P}$ are not necessarily a monotonic transformation of the marginals of P.

Since every iteration of loopy propagation gives the correct beliefs for a different problem, it is not immediately clear why this scheme should ever converge. Note, however, that the unwrapped network of iteration $t + 1$ is simply the unwrapped network of size t with an additional finite number of nodes added at the boundary. Thus, loopy belief propagation will converge when the addition of these nodes at the boundary will not alter the posterior probability of the node in the center. In other words, convergence is equivalent to the independence of center nodes and boundary nodes in the unwrapped network. In the subsequent sections, we formalize this intuition.

4 Belief Update in Networks with a Single Loop

Consider a network composed of N unobserved nodes arranged in a loop and N observed nodes, one attached to each unobserved node (see Figure 4). We denote by $U_1, U_2, \ldots, U_N$ the unobserved variables, and $O_1, O_2, \ldots, O_N$ the corresponding observed variables. In this section we derive a relationship between the belief at a given node $\vec{b}_{U_1}$ and the correct posterior probability, which we denote by $\vec{p}_{U_1}$.

First, let us find what the messages received by node U_1 converge to. By the belief update equations (see equation 2.7), the message that U_N sends to U_1 depends on the message U_N receives from U_{N-1}

$$\vec{v}_{U_N U_1} \leftarrow \alpha M_{U_N U_1} \left(\vec{v}_{O_N U_N} \odot \vec{v}_{U_{N-1} U_N} \right), \tag{4.1}$$

and similarly the message U_{N-1} sends to U_N depends on the message U_{N-1} receives from U_{N-2}:

$$\vec{v}_{U_{N-1} U_N} \leftarrow \alpha M_{U_{N-1} U_N} \left(\vec{v}_{O_{N-1} U_{N-1}} \odot \vec{v}_{U_{N-2} U_{N-1}} \right) \tag{4.2}$$

We can continue expressing each message in terms of the one received from the neighbor until we go back in the loop to U_1:

$$\vec{v}_{U_1 U_2} \leftarrow \alpha M_{U_1 U_2} \left(\vec{v}_{O_1 U_1} \odot \vec{v}_{U_N U_1} \right). \tag{4.3}$$

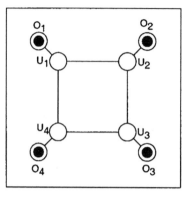

Figure 4: Simple network with a single loop. We label the unobserved nodes $U_1, \ldots, U_N$ and the observed nodes $O_1, \ldots, O_N$. We derive an analytical relationship between the belief vector at each node in the loop (e.g., $\vec{b}_{U_1}$) and its correct marginal probability (e.g., $\vec{p}_{U_1}$).

Thus, the message U_N sends to U_1 at a given time step depends on the message U_N sent to U_1 at a previous time step (N time steps ago),

$$\vec{v}_{U_N U_1}^{(t+N)} = \alpha C_{N1} \vec{v}_{U_N U_1}^{(t)}, \tag{4.4}$$

where the matrix C_{N1} summarizes all the operations performed on the message as it is passed around the loop,

$$C_{N1} = M_{U_N U_{N-1}} D_N M_{U_{N-1} U_{N-2}} D_{N-1}, \ldots, M_{U_1 U_2} D_1, \tag{4.5}$$

and we define the matrix D_i to be a diagonal matrix whose elements are the constant messages sent from observed node O_i to unobserved U_i. A diagonal matrix is used because it enables us to rewrite the componentwise multiplication of two vectors as a multiplication of a matrix and a vector. For any vector $\vec{x}$, $D_i \vec{x} = \vec{v}_{O_i U_i} \odot \vec{x}$.

Using the matrix C_{N1} we can formally state the claims of this section.

Claims. Consider a pairwise Markov network consisting of a single loop of unobserved variables $\{U_i\}_{i=1}^N$, each of which is connected to an observed variable O_i. Define C_{N1} as in equation 4.5 where D_i a diagonal matrix whose entries are the messages $\vec{v}_{O_i U_i}$. If all elements of C_{N1} are nonzero, then:

1. $\vec{v}_{U_N U_1}$ converges to the principal eigenvector of C_{N1}.

2. $\vec{v}_{U_2 U_1}$ converges to the principal eigenvector of $D_1^{-1} C_{N1}^T D_1$.

3. The convergence rate of the messages is governed by the ratio of the largest eigenvalue of C_{N1} to the second-largest eigenvalue.

4. The diagonal elements of C_{N1} give the correct posteriors: $\vec{p}_{U_1}(i) = \alpha C_{N1}(i, i)$.

5. The steady-state belief $\vec{b}_{U_1}$ is related to the correct posterior marginal $\vec{p}_{U_1}$ by: $\vec{b}_{U_1} = \beta \vec{p}_{U_1} + (1 - \beta)\vec{q}_{U_1}$, where β is the ratio of the largest eigenvalue of C_{N1} to the sum of all eigenvalues and $\vec{q}_{U_1}$ depends on the eigenvectors of C_{N1}.

The first claim follows from the recursion (see equation 4.4). Recursions of this type form the basis of the power method for finding eigenvalues of matrices (Strang, 1986). The method is based on the following lemma (Strang, 1986).

Power method lemma. *Let C be a matrix with eigenvalues $\lambda_1, \ldots, \lambda_n$ sorted by decreasing magnitude and eigenvectors $\vec{u}_1, \ldots, \vec{u}_n$. If $|\lambda_1| > |\lambda_2|$, then the recursion $\vec{x}^{(t+1)} = \alpha C \vec{x}^{(t)}$ converges to a multiple of $\vec{u}_1$ from any initial vector $\vec{x}^{(0)} = \sum_i \beta_i \vec{u}_i$ s.t. $\beta_1 \neq 0$. The convergence factor r is given by $r = |\lambda_2/\lambda_1|$ (the distance to the steady-state vector decreases by $r\%$ at every iteration).*

Proof. If $\vec{v}$ is a fixed point for the recursion (see equation 4.4), then $\vec{v} = \alpha C_{N1}\vec{v}$ or $C_{N1}\vec{v} = 1/\alpha\vec{v}$ so that $\vec{v}$ is an eigenvector of C_{N1}. The power method lemma guarantees that in general, the method will converge to the principal eigenvector—the one with the largest eigenvalue.

It is not trivial to check for a given matrix and initial condition whether the assumptions of the power method lemma are satisfied. A sufficient (but not necessary) condition is that all elements of the matrix C and the initial vector $\vec{x}^{(0)}$ be positive. The Perron-Frobenius theorem (Minc, 1988) guarantees that for such matrices $\lambda_1 > \lambda_2$ and that C will have only one eigenvector whose elements are nonnegative: $\vec{u}_1$. Thus for C with positive elements, the iterations will converge to $\alpha\vec{u}_1$ for any initial vector $\vec{x}^{(0)}$ with positive elements. If the matrix contains nonnegative values, conditions for guaranteed convergence from arbitrary initial condition are more complicated (Minc, 1988).

In the context of graphical models, the matrix C_{N1} is a product of matrices with nonnegative elements (the elements are either conditional probabilities or potential functions), but it may contain zeros. Indeed, it is possible to construct examples of graphical models for which the messages do not converge. These examples, however, are extremely rare (e.g., when all the transition matrices are deterministic).

To summarize, if the matrix C_{N1} has only positive elements, then $\vec{v}_{U_N U_1}$ converges to the principal eigenvector of C_{N1}.

Proof. To prove the second claim, we define

$$C_{21} = M_{U_2 U_1} D_2 M_{U_3 U_2} D_3, \ldots, M_{U_1 U_N} D_1, \tag{4.6}$$

and in complete analogy to the previous proof, this defines a recursion for
$\vec{v}_{U_2 U_1}$ and therefore the steady-state message is the principal eigenvector of
C_{21}. Furthermore, C_{21} can be expressed as

$$C_{21} = D_1^{-1} C_{N1}^T D_1, \tag{4.7}$$

where we have used the fact that for any two nodes X, Y $M_{XY} = M_{YX}^T$.

Proof. The third claim, regarding the convergence rate of the messages,
also follows from the power method lemma. Thus the convergence rate
of $\vec{v}_{U_N U_1}$ is governed by the ratio of the largest eigenvalue to the second
largest eigenvalue of C_{N1} and that of $\vec{v}_{U_2 U_1}$ by the ratio of eigenvalues of
C_{21}. Furthermore, by equation 4.7, C_{21} and C_{N1} have the same eigenvalues.

Proof. To prove the fourth claim, we denote by $\vec{e}_i$ the vector that is zero
everywhere except for a 1 at the ith component; then:

$$\vec{p}_{U_1}(i) = \alpha \sum_{U_2,\ldots,U_N} P(U_1 = i, U_2, \ldots, U_N) \tag{4.8}$$

$$= \alpha \sum_{U_2,\ldots,U_N} \Psi(i, U_2)\Psi(i, O_1)\Psi(U_2, U_3) \tag{4.9}$$

$$\Psi(U_2, O_2), \ldots, \Psi(U_N, i)\Psi(U_N, O_N)$$
$$= \alpha \sum_{U_2} \Psi(i, U_2)\Psi(U_2, O_2) \sum_{U_3} \Psi(U_2, U_3) \tag{4.10}$$

$$\cdots \sum_{U_N} \Psi(U_N, O_N)\Psi(U_N, i)\Psi(i, O_1)$$

$$= \alpha \vec{e}_i^T M_{U_2 U_1} D_2 M_{U_3 U_2} D_3, \ldots, M_{U_1 U_N} D_1 \vec{e}_i \tag{4.11}$$

$$= \alpha \vec{e}_i^T C_{21} \vec{e}_i \tag{4.12}$$

$$= \alpha C_{21}(i, i). \tag{4.13}$$

Note that we can also calculate the normalizing factor α in terms of the
matrix C_{21}; thus:

$$\vec{p}_{U_1}(i) = \frac{C_{21}(i, i)}{trace(C_{21})}. \tag{4.14}$$

Again, by equation 4.7, C_{21} and C_{N1} have the same diagonal elements so
$\vec{p}_{U_1}(i) = \alpha C_{N1}(i, i)$.

Proof. To prove the fifth claim, we denote by $\{\vec{w}_i, \lambda_i\}$ the eigenvectors and
eigenvalues of the matrix C_{N1} and by $\{\vec{s}_i, \lambda_i\}$ the eigenvectors and eigenvalues of matrix C_{21}. Now, recall from the belief update rules equation 2.7,
that:

$$\vec{b}_{U_1} = \alpha \vec{v}_{U_2 U_1} \odot \vec{v}_{U_N U_1} \odot \vec{v}_{O_1 U_1}, \tag{4.15}$$

Using the first two claims, we can rewrite this in terms of the diagonal matrix D_1 and the principal eigenvectors of C_{21} and C_{N1},

$$\vec{b}_{U_1} = \alpha D_1 \vec{s}_1 \odot \vec{w}_1, \tag{4.16}$$

or, in component notation,

$$\vec{b}_{U_1}(i) = \alpha D_1(i, i)\vec{s}_1(i)\vec{w}_1(i). \tag{4.17}$$

However, to obtain an expression analogous to equation 4.14 we want to rewrite $\vec{b}_{U_1}$ solely in terms of C_{21}.

First we write $C_{21} = S\Lambda S^{-1}$ where the columns of S contain the eigenvectors of C_{21} and the diagonal elements of Λ contain the corresponding eigenvalues. We order S such that the principal eigenvector is in the first column; thus $S(i, 1) = \beta \vec{s}_1(i)$. Surprisingly, the first *row* of S^{-1} is related to the product $D_1\vec{w}_1$, where $\vec{w}_1$ is the principal eigenvector of C_{N1}:

$$C_{21} = S\Lambda S^{-1} \tag{4.18}$$

$$C_{N1} = D_1^{-1}C_{21}^T D_1 = D_1^{-1}(S^{-1})^T \Lambda S^T D_1. \tag{4.19}$$

Thus the first row of $S^{-1}D_1^{-1}$ gives the principal eigenvector of C_{N1}, or

$$D_1(i, i)\vec{w}_1(i) = \gamma S^{-1}(1, i), \tag{4.20}$$

where the constant γ is independent of i. Substituting into equation 4.17 gives:

$$\vec{b}_{U_1}(i) = \alpha S(i, 1)S^{-1}(1, i), \tag{4.21}$$

where α is again a normalizing constant. In fact, this constant is equal to unity since for any invertible matrix S:

$$\sum_i S(i, 1)S^{-1}(1, i) = 1. \tag{4.22}$$

Finally, we can express the relationship between $\vec{p}_{U_1}$ and $\vec{b}_{U_1}$:

$$\vec{p}_{U_1}(i) = \frac{\vec{e}_i^T C_{21} \vec{e}_i}{trace(C_{21})} \tag{4.23}$$

$$= \frac{\vec{e}_i^T S\Lambda S^{-1}\vec{e}_i}{\sum_j \lambda_j} \tag{4.24}$$

$$= \frac{\sum_j S(i, j)\lambda_j P^{-1}(j, i)}{\sum_j \lambda_j} \tag{4.25}$$

$$= \frac{\lambda_1 \vec{b}_{U_1}(i) + \sum_{j=2} S(i, j)\lambda_j S^{-1}(j, i)}{\sum_j \lambda_j}. \tag{4.26}$$

Thus $\vec{p}_{U_1}$ can be written as a weighted average of $\vec{b}_{U_1}$ and a second term, which we will denote by $\vec{q}_{U_1}$,

$$\vec{p}_{U_1} = \frac{\lambda_1}{\sum_j \lambda_j}\vec{b}_{U_1} + \left(1 - \frac{\lambda_1}{\sum_j \lambda_j}\right)\vec{q}_{U_1} \qquad (4.27)$$

with:

$$\vec{q}_{U_1} = \frac{\sum_{j=2} S(i, j)\lambda_j S^{-1}(j, i)}{\sum_{j=2} \lambda_j}. \qquad (4.28)$$

The weight given to $\vec{b}_{U_1}$ is proportional to the maximum eigenvalue λ_1. Thus the error in loopy belief propagation is small when the maximum eigenvalue dominates the eigenvalue spectrum:

$$\vec{p}_{U_1} - \vec{b}_{U_1} = \left(1 - \frac{\lambda_1}{\sum_j \lambda_j}\right)(\vec{q}_{U_1} + \vec{p}_{U_1}). \qquad (4.29)$$

Note again the importance of the ratio between the subdominant eigenvalue and the dominant one. When this ratio is small, loopy belief propagation converges rapidly, and furthermore the approximation error is small.

The preceding discussion has made no assumption about the range of possible values that variables in the networks can take. If we now assume that the variables are binary, we can show that the belief update assignment is guaranteed to give the maximum marginal assignment.

Claim. Consider a pairwise Markov network consisting of a single loop of unobserved variables U_i, each connected to an observed variable O_i. Assume the unobserved variables are binary; then the belief update assignment gives the maximum marginal assignment.

Proof. Note that in this case,

$$\vec{p}_{U_1}(i) = \frac{\lambda_1 S(i, 1)S^{-1}(1, i) + \lambda_2 S(i, 2)S^{-1}(2, i)}{\lambda_1 + \lambda_2} \qquad (4.30)$$

$$= \frac{\lambda_1 \vec{b}_{U_1}(i) + \lambda_2(1 - \vec{b}_{U_1}(i))}{\lambda_1 + \lambda_2}. \qquad (4.31)$$

Thus:

$$\vec{p}_{U_1}(i) - \vec{p}_{U_1}(j) = \frac{\lambda_1 - \lambda_2}{\lambda_1 + \lambda_2}(\vec{b}_{U_1}(i) - \vec{b}_{U_1}(j)). \qquad (4.32)$$

Thus $\vec{p}_{U_1}(i) - \vec{p}_{U_1}(j)$ will be positive if and only if $\vec{b}_{U_1}(i) - \vec{b}_{U_1}(j)$ is positive ($\lambda_1 > \lambda_2$, $\lambda_1 > 0$ and $trace(C_{12}) > 0$). In other words the calculated beliefs may be wrong but are guaranteed to be on the correct side of 0.5.

4.1 Correcting the Beliefs Using Locally Available Information. Equation 4.26 suggests that if node U_1 was able to estimate the higher-order eigenvalues and eigenvectors of the matrix C_{21} from the messages it receives, it would be able to correct the belief vector. Indeed, there exist several numerical algorithms to estimate all eigenvectors of a matrix using recursions similar to equation 4.4 (Strang, 1986).

Claim. Consider a pairwise Markov network consisting of a single loop of unobserved binary variables $\{U_i\}_{i=1}^N$, each of which is connected to an observed variable O_i. For node U_i define the temporal difference $\vec{d}_i^{(t)} = \vec{v}_{U_2 U_1}^{(t)} - \vec{v}_{U_2 U_1}^{(t-N)}$, and the ratio r as the solution to $\vec{d}_i^{(t)} = r\vec{d}_i^{(t-N)}$. Then $\vec{p}_{U_i} = \frac{1}{1+r}\vec{b}_{U_i} + \frac{r}{1+r}(1 - \vec{b}_{U_i})$.

The proof is based on the following lemma:

Temporal difference lemma. *Let C be a matrix with eigenvalues $\lambda_1, \ldots, \lambda_n$ sorted by decreasing magnitude and eigenvectors $\vec{u}_1, \ldots, \vec{u}_n$. Assume that the eigenvectors are normalized so they sum to 1. Define the recursion $\vec{x}^{(t+1)} = \alpha C \vec{x}^{(t)}$ and the temporal difference $\vec{d}^{(t)} = \vec{x}^{(t)} - \vec{x}^{(t-1)}$. Assume that the conditions of the power method lemma hold, and in addition, $|\lambda_2| > |\lambda_3|$, then $\vec{d}^{(t)}$ approaches a multiple of $\vec{u}_2 - \vec{u}_1$, and furthermore $\vec{d}^{(t)}$ approaches $\frac{\lambda_2}{\lambda_1}\vec{d}^{(t-1)}$.*

Proof. This lemma can be proved by linearizing the relationship between $\vec{x}^{(t+1)}$ and $\vec{x}^{(t)}$ around the steady-state value $\vec{x}^\infty$ and then applying the power-method lemma.

The temporal difference lemma guarantees that each component of $\vec{d}$ in the claim will decrease geometrically in magnitude, and the rate of decrease gives the ratio $r = \lambda_2/\lambda_1$. Substituting $r = \lambda_2/\lambda_1$ into equation 4.31 gives:

$$\vec{p}_{U_1} = \frac{1}{1+r}\vec{b}_{U_1} + \frac{r}{1+r}(1 - \vec{b}_{U_1}). \tag{4.33}$$

More complicated correction schemes are possible. In the case of ternary nodes, the nodes can use the direction of the vector $\vec{d}$ to calculate the second eigenvector and obtain a better estimate of the correct probability. In general, all eigenvectors and eigenvalues can be calculated by performing operations on the stream of messages a node receives.

4.2 Illustrative Examples. Figure 5a shows a network of four nodes, connected in a single loop. Figure 5b shows the local probabilities—the probability of a node's being in state 1 or 2 given only its local evidence. The transition matrices were set to:

$$M = \begin{pmatrix} 0.9 & 0.1 \\ 0.1 & 0.9 \end{pmatrix}. \tag{4.34}$$

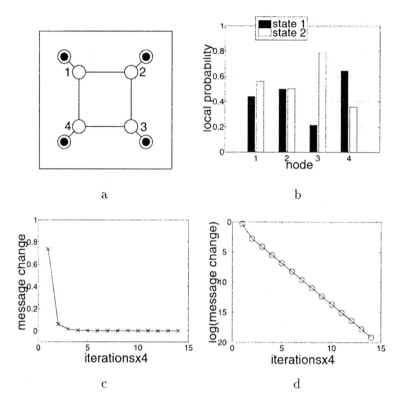

a   b

c   d

Figure 5: (a) Simple loop structure. (b) Local evidence probabilities ($\vec{v}_{O_i U_i}$) used in the simulations. (c) Differences between messages at four iterations ($|\vec{v}^{(t)}_{U_2 U_1} - \vec{v}^{(t-4)}_{U_2 U_1}|$). Note the geometric convergence. (d) Log of the magnitude of the differences plotted in c. The slope of this line determines the ratio of the second and first eigenvalues.

Figure 5c shows the convergence rate of one of the messages as a function of iteration. We plot $\|\vec{d}^{(t)}\|$ as a function of iteration, and the magnitude can be seen to decrease geometrically (or linearly in the log plot in Figure 5d). The rate at which the components of $\vec{d}^{(t)}$ decrease gives the value of r that the nodes can use to correct the beliefs.

   Figure 6a shows the correct posteriors (calculated by exhaustive enumeration) and the steady-state beliefs estimated by loopy propagation. Note that the estimated beliefs are on the correct side of 0.5 as guaranteed by the theory but are numerically wrong. In particular, the estimated beliefs are overly confident (closer to 1 and 0, and further from 0.5). Intuitively, this is due to the fact that the loopy network involves counting each evidence multiple

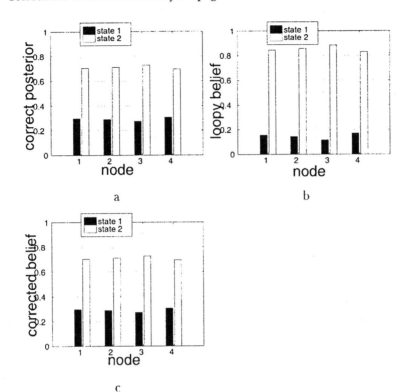

Figure 6: (a) Correct marginals (calculated by exhaustive enumeration) for the data in Figure 5. (b) Beliefs estimated at convergence by the loopy belief propagation algorithm. Note that the estimated beliefs are on the correct side of 0.5 as guaranteed by the theory but are numerically wrong. In particular, the estimated beliefs are overly confident (closer to 1 and 0, and further from 0.5). (c) Estimated beliefs after correction based on the convergence rates of the messages (see equation 4.33). The beliefs are identical to the correct beliefs up to machine precision.

times rather than a single time, thus leading to an overly confident estimate. More formally, this is a result of λ_2 being positive (see equation 4.31). Figure 6c shows the estimated beliefs after the correction of equation 4.33 has been added. The beliefs are identical to the correct beliefs up to machine precision.

Figure 7 illustrates the relationship between the asymptotic convergence ratio $|r| = \|\vec{d}^{(t+4)}\| / \|\vec{d}^{(t)}\|$ and the approximation error $\|\vec{b}_X - \vec{p}_X\|$ at a given node. Each data point represents the results on a simple loop network (see

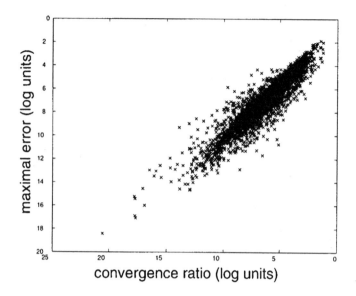

Figure 7: Maximal error between the beliefs estimated using loopy belief update and the true beliefs, plotted as a function of the convergence ratio. As predicted by the theory, the error is small when convergence is rapid.

Figure 5a) with randomly selected transition matrices. Consistent with equation 4.26 the error is small when convergence is rapid and large when convergence is slow.

4.3 Networks Containing a Single Loop and Additional Trees. The results of the previous section can be extended to networks that contain a single loop and additional trees. An example is shown in Figure 8a. These networks include arbitrary combinations of chains and trees, except for a single loop. The nodes in these networks can be divided into two categories: those in the loop and those not in the loop. For example in Figure 8, nodes 1–4 are part of the loop, while nodes 5–7 are not.

Let us focus first on nodes inside the loop. If all we are interested in is obtaining the correct beliefs for these nodes, then the situation is equivalent to a graph that has only the loop and evidence nodes. That is, after a finite number of iterations, the messages coming into the loop nodes from the nonloop nodes will converge to a steady-state value. These messages can be thought of as messages from observed nodes, and the analysis of the previous section holds.

For nodes outside the loop, however, the relationship derived in the previous section between $\vec{p}_X$ and $\vec{b}_X$ does not hold. In particular, there is no

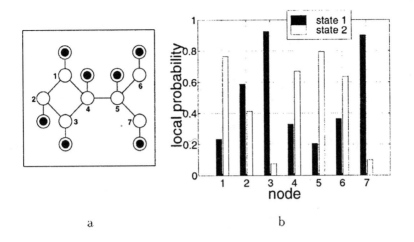

Figure 8: (a) A network including a tree and a loop. (b) The probability of each node given its local evidence used in the simulations.

guarantee that the BU assignment will give the MM assignment, even in the case of binary nodes. Consider node 5 in the figure. Its posterior probability can be factored into three independent sources: the probability given the evidence at node 6, at node 7, and the evidence in the loop. The messages that node 5 receives from nodes 6 and 7 in the belief update algorithm will correctly give the probability given the evidence at these nodes. However, the message it receives from node 4 will be based on the messages passed around the loop multiple times; that is, evidence in the loop will be counted more times than evidence outside the loop.

Nevertheless, if nodes in the loop use the convergence rate to correct their beliefs, they can also correct the messages they send to nodes outside the loop in a similar way. One way to do this is to calculate outgoing messages $\vec{v}_{XY}$ by dividing the belief vector $\vec{b}_X$ componentwise by the vector $\vec{v}_{YX}$ and multiplying the result by M_{XY}. If $\vec{b}_X$ is as defined by equation 2.8 then this procedure gives the exact same messages as equation 2.7. However, if $\vec{b}_X$ represents the corrected beliefs, then the outgoing messages will also be corrected, and the beliefs in all nodes will be correct.

To illustrate these ideas, consider Figures 8 and 9. Figure 8b shows the local probabilities for each of the seven nodes. The transition matrix was identical to that used in the previous example (see equation 4.33). Figure 9a shows the correct posterior probabilities calculated using exhaustive enumeration and Figure 9b the beliefs estimated using regular belief update on the loopy network. Note that the beliefs for the nodes inside the loop are on the correct side of 0.5 but overly confident. But the belief of node 6 is *not* on

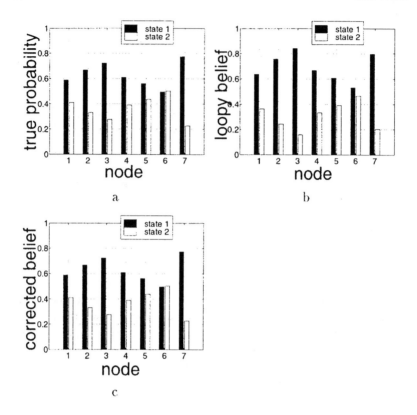

Figure 9: (a) Correct posterior probabilities calculated using exhaustive enumeration. (b) Beliefs estimated using regular belief update on the loopy network. Note that the beliefs for the nodes inside the loop are on the correct side of 0.5 but overly confident. The belief of node 6 is *not* on the correct side of 0.5. (c) Results of the corrected belief propagation algorithm, modified by using equation 4.33 for nodes in the loop. The results are identical to the correct posteriors up to machine precision.

the correct side of 0.5. Finally, Figure 9c shows the results of the corrected belief propagation algorithm, by using equation 4.33 for nodes in the loop. The results are identical to the correct posteriors up to machine precision.

5 Belief Revision in Networks with a Single Loop

For belief revision the situation is simpler than belief update. In belief update we had to distinguish between binary nodes versus nonbinary nodes, and between networks consisting of a single loop versus networks with a loop and additional trees. For belief revision we can prove the optimality of the BR assignment for any net with a single loop.

Claim. Consider a pairwise Markov net with a single loop. If all potentials Ψ are positive and belief revision converges, then the BR assignment gives the MAP assignment.

The proof uses the notion of the "unwrapped" network introduced in section 3. Recall that for every loopy net, node X, and iteration t, there exists an unwrapped network such that the messages received by node X in the loopy net after t iterations are identical to the final messages received by the corresponding node in the unwrapped network after convergence. This means that the BR assignment at node X after t iterations corresponds to the MAP assignment for the corresponding X in the unwrapped network. It does not, however, tell us anything directly about the MAP assignment for other replicas of X in the unwrapped network. When belief revision converges, however, the BR assignment at X gives us the MAP assignment at nearly all replicas of X in the unwrapped network. This is shown in the following two lemmas.

Unwrapped network lemma. *For every node X in a loopy network and iteration time t, we can construct an unwrapped network such that all messages $\vec{v}_{YX}^{(t)}$ that X receives from a neighboring node Y at time t in the loopy network are equal to the final messages $\vec{v}_{YX}$ that X receives from the corresponding node in the unwrapped network.*

Proof. The proof is by construction. We construct an unwrapped tree by setting X to be the root node and then iterating the following procedure t times:

- Find all leafs of the tree (nodes that have no children).

- For each leaf, find all k nodes in the loopy graph that neighbor the node corresponding to this leaf.

- Add $k-1$ nodes as children to each leaf, corresponding to all neighbors except the parent node.

The transition matrices are set to be identical to those in the loopy network. Likewise, if a node X in the loopy network is observed to be in state i, then all replicas of X are also set to be observed in state i. Thus, any node in the interior of the unwrapped tree has the same neighbors as the corresponding node in the loopy network and the same transition matrices. It is easy to verify that the messages that the root node receives in the unwrapped tree are identical to those received by the corresponding node in the loopy network after t iterations.

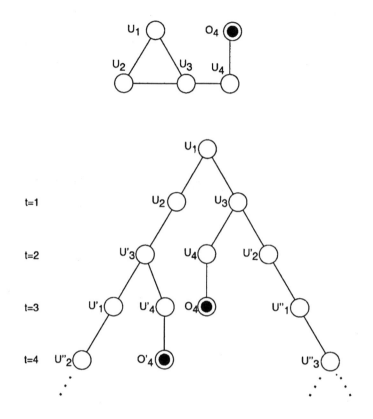

Figure 10: Illustration of the procedure for generating an unwrapped network. At every iteration, we examine all leaf nodes in the tree and find the neighbors of the corresponding node in the loopy network. We add nodes as children to each leaf corresponding to all neighbors except the parent node.

Figure 10 illustrates the construction of the unwrapped network for a network with a single loop. Although we have used a tree structure to generate the unwrapped network, for the case of a single-loop network, the unwrapped network is equivalent to an increasingly long chain (corresponding to the loop nodes) and additional tree nodes connected to the chain at the corresponding nodes. Figure 11a shows the same unwrapped network as in Figure 10 but drawn as a long chain. We define the end point nodes of the unwrapped network as the two loop nodes that are most distant from the root. Thus, in Figure 11a, U_2'' and U_3'' are end point nodes.

Any unwrapped network defines a joint probability distribution, and we can therefore define the MAP assignment of the unwrapped network. Although the unwrapped network is constructed so that all replicas of X have identical neighbors, there is no constraint that their MAP assignment is identical. Thus in Figure 11a, the MAP assignment in the unwrapped network requires assigning values to 11 variables. There is no guarantee that replicas of the same node (e.g., U_1, U_1') will have the same assignment. However, as we show in the following lemma, if belief revision converges the MAP assignment for the unwrapped network is guaranteed to be semiperiodic. All replicas of a given node in the unwrapped network will have the same MAP assignment as long as they are far away from the end point nodes.

Periodic assignment lemma. *Assume all messages in a network with a single loop converge to their steady-state values after t_c iterations: $\vec{v}_{XY}^{(t)} = \vec{v}_{XY}^{\infty}$ for $t > t_c$. If Y is a node in the unwrapped network such that the distance of Y to both end points is greater than t_c, then the MAP assignment at Y is equal to the BR assignment of the corresponding node in the loopy network.*

Proof.   We first show that all messages transmitted in the unwrapped network are equal to the steady-state messages in the loopy network. To show this, we divide the nodes in the unwrapped network into two categories: chain nodes, which form part of the infinite chain (corresponding to nodes in the loop in the loopy network), and nonchain nodes (corresponding to nodes outside the loop in the loopy network). This gives four types of messages in the unwrapped network. Leftward and rightward messages are the two directions of propagation inside the chain, outward are propagated in the nonchain nodes away from the chain nodes, and inward messages go toward the chain nodes. Thus in Figure 11a, $\vec{v}_{U_2 U_1}$ is a rightward message, $\vec{v}_{U_3 U_1}$ is a leftward message, $\vec{v}_{U_3 U_4}$ is an outward message, and $\vec{v}_{U_4 U_3}$ is an inward message.

The inward messages depend on only other inward messages and the evidence at the nonchain nodes. Thus, they are identical at all replicas of the nonchain nodes. Since the transition matrices and evidences are replicated from the loopy network, the inward messages are identical to the corresponding messages in the loopy network.

The leftward messages depend on only other leftward messages to the right of them and the inward message. By construction of the unwrapped network, if X is a node in the unwrapped network whose distance from the right-most end point is d and Y is its neighbor on the left, then $\vec{v}_{XY} = \vec{v}_{XY}^{(d)}$; that is, the message is identical to the message that X sends to Y in the loopy network at time d. Since $d > t_c$ $\vec{v}_{XY} = \vec{v}_{XY}^{\infty}$.

The proof for the rightward messages is analogous to that of the leftward messages. Finally, the outward messages that a chain node sends to a nonchain node depend on only the leftward and rightward messages. Thus if both leftward and rightward messages that it receives are equal to the steady-state messages in the loopy network, so will the outward message it sends out.

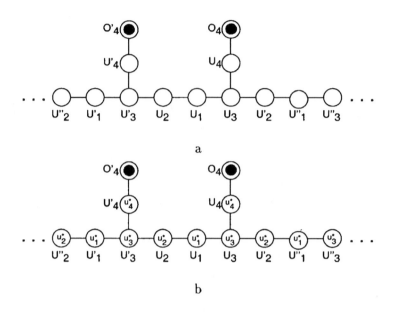

Figure 11: (a) For networks with a single loop, the unwrapped network is equivalent to an increasingly long chain (corresponding to the loop nodes) and additional trees connected at the corresponding nodes. (b) When belief revision converges, the MAP assignment of the unwrapped network contains periodic replicas of the MAP assignment in the loopy network.

If X is a node in the unwrapped tree whose distance from the end point is more than t_c, all incoming messages to X are identical to the steady-state messages in the loopy network in the corresponding node. Therefore, the belief vector at X is identical to the corresponding steady-state belief in the loopy network, and the MAP assignment at X is equal to the BR assignment in the corresponding node.

The periodic assignment lemma guarantees that if belief revision converges, then the MAP assignment in the unwrapped tree will have replicas of the BR assignment for all nodes whose distance from the end points is greater than t_c. The importance of this result is that we can now relate optimality in the unwrapped tree to optimality in the loopy network.

It is easier here to work with log probabilities than with probabilities. We define $J(X, Y) = -\log \Psi(X, Y)$. For any Markov network with observed variables, we refer to the network cost function J as the negative log posterior of the unobserved variables. Thus in Figure 10a,

$$J(\{u_i\}) = J(u_1, u_2) + J(u_2, u_3) + J(u_3, u_1) + J(u_3, u_4) + J(u_4, o_4), \quad (5.1)$$

where o_4 is the observed value of O_4.

Optimality relationship lemma. *Assume that belief revision converges in a network with a single loop and u_i^* is the BR assignment in the loopy network. Assume furthermore that all potentials $\Psi(X, Y)$ are nonzero, and define J as the negative log posterior of the loopy network. For any n, u_i^* must minimize*

$$J_n(\{u_i\}) = nJ(\{u_i\}) + \tilde{J},   \tag{5.2}$$

where $\tilde{J}$ is finite and independent of n.

Proof. To prove this, note that for any n there exists a t such that the unwrapped network at iteration t contains a subnetwork with n copies of all links in the loopy network. Furthermore, by choosing a sufficiently large t, the distance of all nodes in the subnetwork from the end points can be made sufficiently large. By the periodic assignment lemma, the MAP assignment will have replicas of the BR assignment for all nodes within the subnetwork. Furthermore, by the definition of the MAP assignment, the assignment within the subnetwork maximizes the posterior probability when nodes outside the subnetwork are clamped to their MAP assignment values. We denote by J_n the cost function that the assignment of the subnetwork minimizes. The cost function decomposes into a sum of pairwise costs, one for each link in the subnetwork. For a periodic assignment, the cost function can be rewritten as

$$J_n(\{u_i\}) = nJ(\{u_i\}) + \tilde{J},   \tag{5.3}$$

where the $\tilde{J}$ term captures the existence of links between the boundaries of the chain and its observed neighbors. This term is independent of n (the distance of the neighboring nodes to the end points is also greater than t_c). Since periodic copies of $\{u_i^*\}$ form the MAP assignment for the subnetwork, $\{u_i^*\}$ must minimize J_n.

Figure 12 illustrates the optimality relationship lemma for $n = 2$. The subnetwork encircled by the dotted line includes two copies of all links in the original loopy network. Therefore the subnetwork cost J_n is given by

$$J_n(\{u_i\}) = 2J(\{u_i\}) + \tilde{J}(\{u_i\}),   \tag{5.4}$$

with $\tilde{J}(\{u_i\})$ a sum of the two links that connect the subnetwork to the larger unwrapped network: $J(u_2^*, u_1) + J(u_1, u_3^*)$.

Proof. The optimality relationship lemma essentially proves the main claim of this section. Since the BR assignment minimizes J_n for arbitrarily large n and $\tilde{J}$ is independent of n, the BR assignment must minimize J and hence is the MAP assignment for the loopy network.

To illustrate this analysis, Figure 13 shows two network structures for which there is no guarantee that the BU assignment will coincide with the

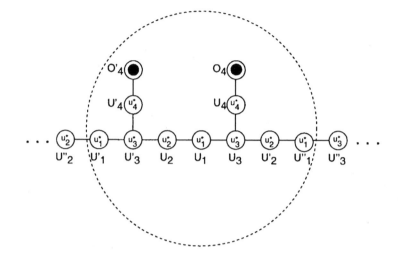

Figure 12: Proof of the optimality relationship lemma for networks with a single loop. For any n there exists a t such that the unwrapped network of size t includes a subnetwork that contains exactly n copies of all links in the original loopy network.

MM assignment. The loop structure has ternary nodes, while the added tree on the right means that the BU assignment even for binary variables will not necessarily give the MM assignment.

However, due to the claim proved above, the BR assignment should always coincide with the MAP assignment. We selected 5000 random transition matrices for the two structures and calculated the correct beliefs using exhaustive enumeration. We then counted the number of correct assignments using belief update and belief revision by comparing the BU assignment to the MM assignment and the BR assignment to the MAP assignment. We considered assignment only when belief revision converged (about 95% of the simulations).

The results are shown in Figure 13. In both of these structures, the BU assignment is not guaranteed to give the MM assignment, and indeed the wrong assignment is sometimes observed. However, an incorrect BR assignment is never observed.

6 Discussion: Single Loop

The analysis enables us to categorize a given network with a loop into one of two categories: (1) structures for which both belief update and belief revision are guaranteed to give the correct assignment or (2) those for which only belief revision is guaranteed to give the correct assignment.

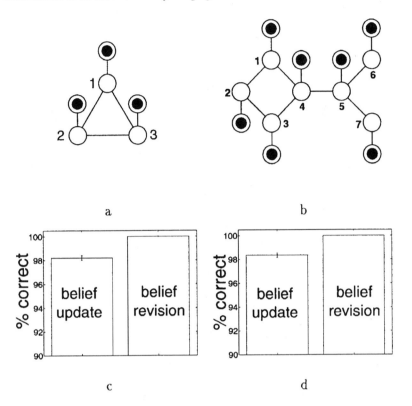

a

b

c

d

Figure 13: (a–b) Two structures for which the BU assignment need not coincide with the MM assignment, but the BR assignment is guaranteed to give the MAP assignment. (a) Simple loop structure with ternary nodes. (b) Loop adjoined to a tree. (c–d) Number of correct assignments using belief update and belief revision in 5000 networks of these structure with randomly generated transition matrices. Consistent with the analysis, the BU assignment may be incorrect, but an incorrect BR assignment is never observed.

The crucial element determining the performance of belief update is the eigenspectrum of the matrix C_{N1}. Note that this matrix depends on both the transition matrices and the observed data. Thus belief update may give very exact estimates for certain observed data even in structures for which it is not guaranteed to give the correct assignment.

We have primarily dealt here with discrete state spaces, but the analysis can also be carried out for continuous spaces. For the case of gaussian posterior probabilities, it is easy to show that belief update assignment will give the correct MAP assignment for all gaussian Markov networks with single loop (this is due to the fact that belief update and revision are identical for a gaussian).

We emphasize again that our choice of Markov nets with pairwise potentials as the primary object of analysis was based mainly on notational convenience. Due to the equivalence between Pearl's algorithm on Bayesian nets and our update rules on Markov nets, our results also hold for applications of Pearl's original update rules on Bayesian nets with a single loop. In particular, this means that one can perform exact inference on a Bayesian net with a single loop by running Pearl's propagation algorithm and then using a correction analogous to equation 4.33. More generally, if the Bayesian network can be converted into a Markov network with a single loop, our results show how to perform exact inference. Exact inference in networks containing a single loop, however, can also be performed using cut-set conditioning (Pearl, 1988). Our goal in analyzing belief propagation in networks with a single loop is primarily to understand loopy belief propagation in general, with single-loop networks being the simplest special case.

Independent of our work, several groups working in the context of error-correcting codes have recently obtained results on probability propagation in networks with a single loop. Aji, Horn, and McEliece (1998) have shown that iterative decoding (equivalent to belief update) of a single-loop code will converge to a correct decoding for binary nodes. They also showed that the messages will converge to the principal eigenvectors of a matrix analogous to our matrix C_{21}. Forney, Kschischang, and Marcus (1998) have also shown the convergence of the messages to the principal eigenvectors and have additionally analyzed the "max-sum" decoding algorithm (analogous to belief revision) on a network consisting of a single loop, showing that it will converge to the dominant pseudocodeword—a periodic assignment on the unwrapped network such that the average cost per period is minimal. To the best of our knowledge, the analytical relationship between the correct beliefs and the steady-state ones, the analysis of networks including a single loop and arbitrary trees, and the correction of beliefs using locally available information have not been discussed elsewhere.

One of the important distinctions that arise from analyzing networks containing a single loop and arbitrary trees is the difference in performance between belief update and belief revision when both converge. The BR assignment is always guaranteed to give the MAP assignment, while the BU assignment is guaranteed to give the MM assignment only when there are no additional trees attached to the loop and the nodes are binary. As we show in subsequent sections, this difference in performance is also apparent in networks with multiple loops.

7 Networks with Multiple Loops

The basic intuition that explains why belief propagation works in networks with a single loop is the notion of equal double counting. Essentially, while evidence is double counted, all evidence is double counted equally, as can be seen in the unwrapped network, and hence belief revision is guaranteed to give the correct assignment. Furthermore, by using recursion expressions for the messages, we could quantify the "amount" of double counting, and derive a relationship between the estimated beliefs and the true ones.

For networks with multiple loops, the situation is more complex. In particular, the relationship between the messages sent at time t and at time $t + n$ is not as simple as in the single loop case, and tools such as the power method lemma or the temporal difference lemma are of no immediate use. However, the notion of the unwrapped tree is equally well applied to networks with multiple loops. Figure 14 shows an example. The unwrapped network lemma of the previous section holds; that is, the messages received by node A in the loopy network after four iterations are identical to the final messages received by node A in the unwrapped network. Furthermore, a version of the periodic assignment lemma of the previous section holds for any network; if belief revision converges, then the MAP assignment for arbitrarily large unwrapped networks contains periodic replicas of the BR assignment.

Thus for a network with multiple loops, if BR converges, then one can construct arbitrarily large problems such that periodic copies of the BR assignment give the optimal assignment for that problem. For example, for the network in Figure 14, the periodic assignment lemma guarantees that if $\{u_i^*\}$ is the BR assignment, then it minimizes

$$J_n(\{u_i\}) = nJ(\{u_i\}) + \tilde{J}_n \qquad (7.1)$$

for arbitrarily large n. As in the single-loop case, $\tilde{J}_n$ is a boundary cost reflecting the constraints imposed on the end points of the unwrapped network. Note that unlike the single-loop case, the boundary cost here may increase with increasing n.

Because the boundary cost may grow with n, we cannot automatically assume that if an assignment minimizes J_n, it also minimizes J; that is, the assignment may be optimal only because of the boundary cost. We have not been able to determine analytically the conditions under which the steady-state assignment is due to $\tilde{J}$ as opposed to J. However, the fact that equation 7.1 holds for arbitrarily large subnetworks (such that the boundary can be made arbitrarily far from the center node) leads us to hypothesize that for positive potentials Ψ loopy belief revision will give the correct assignment for the network in Figure 14.

Although we have not been able to prove this hypothesis, extensive simulation results are consistent with it. We performed loopy belief revision on the structure shown in Figure 14 using randomly selected transition matrices and local evidence probabilities. We repeated the experiment 10,000 times and counted the number of correct assignments. As in the previous section, a correct assignment for belief revision is one that is identical to the MAP

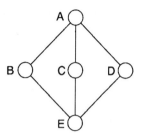

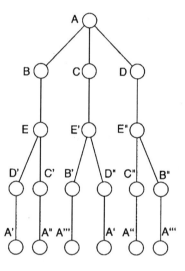

Figure 14: (Top) A Markov network with multiple loops. (Bottom) Unwrapped network corresponding to this structure. Note that all nodes and connections in the loopy structure appear equal numbers of time in the unwrapped network, except the boundary nodes A.

assignment, and a correct assignment for belief update is one that is identical to the MM assignment. Again, we considered only runs in which belief revision converged. We never observed a convergence of belief revision to an incorrect assignment for this structure, while belief update gave 247 incorrect assignments (error rate 2.47%). Since these rates are based on 10,000 trials, the difference is highly significant. While by no means a proof, these simulation results suggest that some of our analytic results for single-loop networks may also hold for a subclass of multiple loop networks. Trying to extend the proofs for a broader class of networks is a topic of current research.

7.1 Turbo Codes. Turbo codes are a class of error-correcting codes whose decoding algorithm has recently been shown to be equivalent to belief propagation on a network with loops. To make the connection to the update rules (equations 2.7–2.8) explicit, we briefly review this equivalence.

We use the formulation of turbo decoding presented in (McEliece et al., 1995). An unknown binary vector $\vec{U}$ is encoded using two codes, each of which is easy to decode by itself, and the results are transmitted over a noisy channel. The task of turbo decoding is to infer the values of every bit of $\vec{U}$ from two noisy versions $\vec{Y}_1, \vec{Y}_2$ that are received after transmission. The decoder knows the prior distribution over $\vec{U}$ (which we assume here is uniform) and the two conditional probabilities $p_i(\vec{y} \mid \vec{u}) = P(\vec{Y}_i = \vec{y} \mid \vec{U} = \vec{u})$.

Since both noisy versions are assumed to be conditionally independent, the marginal probability ratio is simply

$$\frac{P(U(i) = 1)}{P(U(i) = 0)} = \frac{\sum_{\vec{u}:\, U(i)=1} P(\vec{Y}_1 \mid \vec{U})P(\vec{Y}_2 \mid \vec{U})}{\sum_{\vec{u}:\, U(i)=0} P(\vec{Y}_1 \mid \vec{U})P(\vec{Y}_2 \mid \vec{U})}. \tag{7.2}$$

In the typical error-correcting code application, the sum in equation 7.2 is intractable. Rather, the Turbo decoder approximates the ratio by the iterative algorithm outlined in Figure 15.

The algorithm consists of two turbo decision modules, each of which considers only one "noisy version" $\vec{Y}_i$. Each module receives a likelihood ratio vector as input and outputs a modified likelihood ratio vector that takes into account the observed $\vec{Y}_i$. If $\vec{T} = TDM_1(\vec{S})$, then:

$$\vec{T}(i) = \frac{\sum_{\vec{u}:\, \vec{u}(i)=1} p(\vec{y}_1 \mid \vec{u}) \prod_{j \neq i} \vec{S}(j)^{\vec{u}(j)}}{\sum_{\vec{u}:\, \vec{u}(i)=0} p(\vec{y}_1 \mid \vec{u}) \prod_{j \neq i} \vec{S}(j)^{\vec{u}(j)}}. \tag{7.3}$$

The output of module 2 is identical with $\vec{y}_1$ replaced by $\vec{y}_2$. Note that each module still requires summing over all $\vec{u}$, but the codes are constructed so that $p_i(\vec{y} \mid \vec{u})$ have a factorized structure that enables calculation of $TDM_i(\vec{S})$ efficiently.

The turbo decoding iterations can be written as

$$\vec{T} \leftarrow TDM_1(\vec{S}) \tag{7.4}$$
$$\vec{S} \leftarrow TDM_2(\vec{T}), \tag{7.5}$$

and the likelihood ratio is approximated as

$$\vec{R} = \vec{T} \odot \vec{S}. \tag{7.6}$$

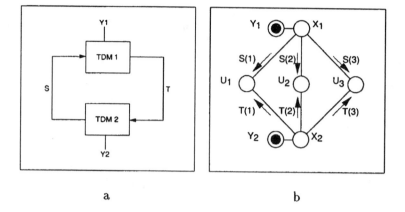

a   b

Figure 15: (a) The Turbo decoding algorithm consists of two Turbo decision modules such that the output of each module serves as the input to the other one. The posterior likelihood ratio is approximated by multiplying the outputs S, T at convergence. (b) The Turbo decoding algorithm as belief update in a loopy Markov network. Each unknown bit is represented by a node U_i. The belief of a node is approximated by multiplying the two incoming messages (corresponding to S and T). When the link matrices are set as explained in the text, the update rules for the messages (equation 2.7–2.8) reduce to the turbo decoding algorithm.

To see the equivalence of this scheme to belief update in Markov nets, consider Figure 15b. We assume that the unknown vector $\vec{U}$ is of length 3 and represent the value of the ith bit with a node U_i in the graph. Each U_i is connected to exactly two nodes, X_1, X_2, that are in turn connected to the received "noisy versions" Y_1, Y_2. By the belief update equations (see equation 2.8), the belief of node U_i is equal to the pointwise multiplication of the messages it receives from X_1 and X_2. Note the similarity to equation 7.6, where the likelihood ratio for $U(i)$ is obtained by multiplying $S(i)$ and $T(i)$. Indeed, we now show that when the potentials in the graph in Figure 15b are set in a particular form, $S(i)$ is equivalent to the message that X_1 sends to U_i and $T(i)$ is equivalent to the message that X_2 sends to U_i.

X_i are meant to represent copies of the unknown binary message $\vec{U}$ and hence in the example (of message length 3), X_i can take on eight possible values. We set $\Psi(\vec{x}_i, u_j) = 1$ if $\vec{x}_i(j) = u_j$ and zero otherwise. Furthermore, we set $\Psi(\vec{x}_i, \vec{y}_i) = p_i(\vec{y}|\vec{x})$.

When the potentials are set in this form, the belief update equations (see equation 2.7) give the turbo decoding algorithm. Denote the message $\vec{v}_{X_2 U_i}$ sent by node X_2 to U_i by the vector $\alpha(T_i, 1)$. The message $\vec{v}_{U_i X_1}$ that U_i sends to X_1 is a vector of length 8. It is obtained by taking the message U_i receives from X_2 and multiplying it by the transition matrix $M_{U_iX_1}$:

$$\vec{v}_{U_1X_1}(x_1) = \alpha \sum_{u_1} \Psi(x_1, u_i)\vec{v}_{X_2U_i}(u_i) \tag{7.7}$$

$$= \alpha T_i^{X_1(i)}. \tag{7.8}$$

Now, the message $\vec{v}_{X_1U_i}$ sent from X_1 to U_1 is a vector of length 2 that is obtained by multiplying all incoming messages except the one coming from U_i and then passing the result through the transition matrix $M_{X_1U_i}$:

$$\vec{v}_{X_1U_i}(u_i) = \sum_{x_1} \Psi(x_1, u_i)p_1(y_1 \mid x_1) \prod_{j \neq i} T_j^{x_1(j)}. \tag{7.9}$$

If we denote by $\vec{S}(i)$ the ratio of components of $\vec{v}_{X_1U_i}$, then equation 7.9 is equivalent to equation 7.3. Thus the belief update rules in equations 2.7–2.8 give the turbo decoding algorithm.

McEliece et al. (1995) showed several examples where the turbo decoding algorithm converges to an incorrect decoding. Since the turbo decoding algorithm is equivalent to belief update, we wanted to see how well a decoding algorithm equivalent to belief revision will perform.

We randomly selected the probability distributions $p_1(u)$ and $p_2(u)$ and calculated the MAP assignment (often referred to as the ML decoding in coding applications) and the MM assignment (referred to as the optimal bitwise decoding, or OBD, in coding applications). We compared these assignments to the BU and BR assignments. As in previous sections, the BU assignment was judged correct if it agreed with the MM assignment, and the BR assignment was judged correct if it agreed with the MAP assignment. We repeated the experiment for 10,000 randomly selected probability distributions. Only trials in which belief revision converged were considered.

Results are shown in Figure 16. As observed by McEliece et al. (1995) turbo decoding is quite likely to converge to an incorrect decoding (16% of the time). In contrast, belief revision converges to an incorrect answer less than 0.1% of the runs. Note that this difference is based on 10,000 trials and is highly significant. However, the results considered only cases where belief revision converged, and in general belief revision converged less frequently than did belief update.

A turbo decoding algorithm that used maximization rather than summation in equation 7.3 was presented in Benedetto, Montorsi, Divsalar, and Pollara (1996), where the maximization was presented as an approximation to the full sum in equation 7.3. The decoding performance of the approximate algorithm was shown to be slightly worse than standard turbo decoding. In our simulations, however, we considered only decodings where belief revision converged, whereas in Benedetto et al. (1996), the decoding

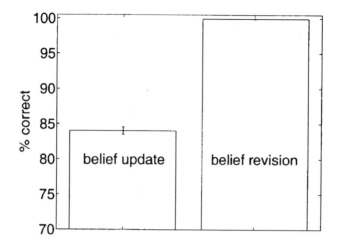

Figure 16: Results of belief revision and update on the turbo code problem.

obtained after a fixed number of iterations was used, regardless of whether the algorithm converged. Our motivation in considering only decodings at convergence was based on our analysis of single-loop networks. The simulation results suggest that turbo codes exhibit a similar difference in performance between belief update and belief revision.

From a practical point of view, of course, errors due to failures in convergence are as troubling as errors due to a convergence to a wrong answer. Thus understanding the behavior of the decoding algorithms when they do not converge is an important question for further research. Forney et al. (1998) have obtained some encouraging results in this regard.

Unlike the networks considered in the previous sections, the turbo code Markov net has deterministic links (between the X_i and U_j), and hence the log of the potential functions Ψ may be infinite. We believe this may be the reason for the existence of a few incorrect decodings with the belief revision. The deterministic links make it difficult to relate optimality in the unwrapped tree to optimality in the original loopy network.

7.2 Discussion. Turbo codes are not the only error-correcting code whose decoding is equivalent to belief propagation. Indeed one of the first derivations of an algorithm equivalent to belief propagation appears in Gallager (1963) as a means of decoding codes known as low-density parity check codes. Gallager's decoding algorithm is equivalent to probability propagation on a network with loops, and Gallager discussed the fact that his decoding algorithm is not guaranteed to give the optimal decoding because it considers replicas of the same evidence as if they were independent. Gallager also showed that his algorithm will give the MAP decoding for a computation tree, equivalent to our unwrapped network. He noted that if the number of iterations is small compared to the size of the loops in the graph, the computation tree will not contain replicas of the same evidence. He presented a method of constructing codes such that the size of the loops in the network will be large.

Indeed, if double counting is to be avoided, we would expect performance of belief propagation in loopy nets to be best when the size of the loops is large or (equivalently) the number of iterations is small. Turbo codes, however, contradict both of these expectations. The Markov network corresponding to turbo decoding (see Figure 15b) contains many loops of size 4. Furthermore, it has been well established (McEliece et al., 1996; Benedetto et al., 1996) that turbo decoding performance improves as the number of iterations is increased.

The performance of turbo codes is consistent, however, with the expectation based on the notion of equal double counting emphasized throughout this article. As we saw in the analysis of networks with a single loop, the BR assignment at convergence is guaranteed to give the MAP assignment regardless of the size of the loop. Furthermore, as we discussed in section 3, for any finite number of iterations, the unwrapped network will not contain an equal number of replicas of all nodes and connections. It is only as the size of the unwrapped network approaches infinity that the influence of the boundary nodes can be neglected. Thus, additional iterations are expected, based on our analysis, to increase the decoding performance.

Despite the importance of turbo codes, one should use caution in generalizing from their performance to general loopy belief propagation. In the typical turbo decoding setting, the probabilities $P(\vec{y}_i \mid \vec{u})$ in equation 7.3 are highly peaked around the correct $\vec{u}$. Thus the sum in equation 7.3 is typically dominated by a single term, and therefore belief revision (in which the sum is approximated by its largest value) and belief update behave quite similarly. As we have shown throughout this article, this is not the case for general loopy belief propagation, nor is it the case for Turbo decoding when the probabilities $P(\vec{y}_i \mid \vec{u})$ are chosen randomly in simulations. We believe that additional insights into Turbo decoding will be obtained by comparing the performance of the algorithm at different probability regimes.

8 Conclusion

As many authors have observed, in order for belief propagation to be exact, we must find a way to avoid double counting. Since double counting is unavoidable in networks with loops, belief propagation in such networks may seem to be a bad idea. The excellent performance of turbo codes motivates a closer look at belief propagation in loopy networks. Here we have shown a class of networks for which, even though the evidence is double counted, all evidence is equally double counted. For networks with a single loop, we have obtained an analytical expression relating the beliefs estimated by loopy belief propagation and the correct beliefs. This allows us to find structures in which belief update may give the wrong beliefs, but the BU assignment is guaranteed to give the correct MM assignment. We have also shown that for networks with a single loop, the BR assignment is guaranteed to give the MAP assignment. For networks with multiple loops we have presented simulation results suggesting that some of the results we have obtained analytically for single-loop networks may hold for a large class of networks. These results are an encouraging first step toward understanding belief propagation in networks with loops.

Appendix: Converting a Bayesian Net to a Pairwise Markov Net _____

There are various ways to convert a Bayesian network into a Markov network that represents the same probability distribution. Indeed one of the most popular inference algorithms for Bayesian networks is to convert them into a Markov network known as the join tree or the junction tree (Pearl, 1988; Jensen, 1996) and perform inference on the junction tree. Here we present a method to convert a Bayesian network into a Markov net with pairwise potentials, such that the update rules described in the article reduce to Pearl's algorithm on the original Bayesian network. In particular, if the Bayesian network has loops in it, so will the corresponding Markov network constructed using this method. This should be contrasted with the junction tree construction in Jensen (1996) which constructs a singly connected Markov network for any Bayesian network.

For concreteness, consider the Bayesian network in Figure 8a. The joint probability is given by:

$$P(ABCDEF) = P(A)P(B \mid A)P(C \mid A)P(D \mid BC)P(F \mid C)P(E \mid D) \quad (A.1)$$

The procedure is simple. For any node that has multiple parents, we create a compound node into which the common parents are clustered. This compound node is then connected to the individual parent nodes as well as the child. For all nodes that have single parents, we drop the arrows and leave the topology unchanged. Figure 17 shows an example. Since D has two parents B and C, we create a compound node $Z = (B', C')$ and connect it to D, B, and C.

Having created a new graph, we need to set the pairwise potentials so that the probability distributions are identical. The potentials are the conditional probabilities of children given parents, with the exception of the potentials between the parent nodes and a compound node. These are set to one if the nodes have a consistent estimate of the parent node and zero otherwise. Thus in the example, if $Z = (B', C')$ then $\Psi(BZ) = 1$ if $B' = B$ and zero otherwise.

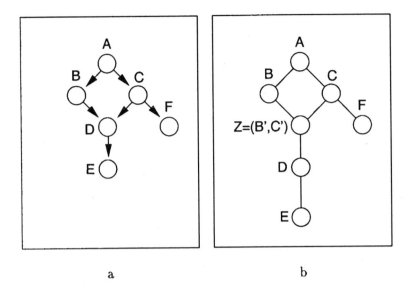

a   b

Figure 17: Any Bayesian netowrk can be converted into a pairwise Markov network by adding cluster nodes for all parents that share a common child. (a) Bayesian network. (b) Corresponding pairwise Markov network. A cluster node for (B, C) has been added. When the potentials are set in the way detailed in the text, the update rules presented in this article reduce to Pearl's propagation rules in the original Bayesian network.

To complete the example, we set $\Psi(AB) = P(A)P(B \mid A)$, $\Psi(AC) = P(C \mid A)$, $\Psi(FC) = P(F \mid C)$, $\Psi(ZD) = P(D \mid B'C')$ and then the joint probability of the Markov net,

$$P(ABCDEFZ) = \Psi(AB)\Psi(AC)\Psi(FC)\Psi(BZ)\Psi(DE)\Psi(ZB)\Psi(ZC), \text{(A.2)}$$

which contains only pairwise potentials but is identical to the probability distribution of the original Bayes net (see equation A.1).

We now describe the equivalence between the messages passed in the Markov net and those that are passed in the Bayes net using Pearl's algorithm. If X is a single parent of Y, then the message X sends to Y in the Bayes net is given by $\pi_x(y)$. The message that X sends to Y in the Markov net is given by $\vec{v}_{XY}$. The messages are related by multiplication by the link matrix: $\vec{v}_{XY} = \alpha M_{XY}\pi_x(y)$. Thus, in Pearl's formulation, the matrix multiplication is performed at the child node, while in the algorithm described here, it is performed in the parent node. The message that Y sends to X in Pearl's algorithm is denoted by $\lambda_Y(x)$ and is equal to $\vec{v}_{YX}$ in the Markov net algorithm up to normalization. In Pearl's algorithm the π messages are normalized, but the λ ones are not, and in the algorithm presented here, all messages are normalized. If X is one of many parents of Y, then in the Markov net, X is connected to Y by means of a cluster node Z. As before, $\vec{v}_{XZ} = M_{XZ}\pi_X(y)$ but since the M_{XZ} matrix contains only ones or zeros, the message in the Markov net is simply a replication of elements in the Bayesian net message. As before $\lambda_Y(x)$ is given by $\alpha\vec{v}_{ZX}$.

Every message in Pearl's algorithm in the Bayes net can be identified with an equivalent message in the Markov net using the algorithm presented here. Furthermore, by substituting the equivalent messages into the update rules presented here, one can derive Pearl's update rules.

Acknowledgments

This work was supported by NEI R01 EY11005 to E. H. Adelson. I thank the anonymous reviewers, E. Adelson, M. Jordan, P. Dayan, M. Meila, Q. Morris, and J. Tenenbaum for helpful discussions and comments. After a preliminary version of this work appeared (Weiss, 1997), I had the pleasure of several discussions with D. Forney and F. Kschischang regarding related work they have been pursuing independently. I thank them for their comments and suggestions.

References

Aji, S., Horn, G., & McEliece, R. (1998). On the convergence of iterative decoding on graphs with a single cycle. In *Proc. 1998 ISIT.*

Aji, S. M., & McEliece, R. (in press). The generalized distributive law. *IEEE Trans. Inform. Theory.* Available at: http://www.systems.caltech.edu/EE/Faculty/rjm.

Benedetto, S., Montorsi, G., Divsalar, D., & Pollara, F. (1996). *Soft-output decoding algorithms in iterative decoding of turbo codes* (Jet Propulsion Laboratory, Telecommunications and Data Acquisition Progress Rep. 42-124). Pasadena, CA: California Institute of Technology.

Berrou, C., Glavieux, A., & Thitimajshima, P. (1993). Near Shannon limit error-correcting coding and decoding: Turbo codes. In *Proc. IEEE International Communications Conference '93.*

Bertsekas, D. P. (1987). *Dynamic programming: Deterministic and stochastic models.* Englewood Cliffs, NJ: Prentice Hall.

Forney, G. (1997). On iterative decoding and the two-way algorithm. In *Intl. Symp. Turbo Codes and Related Topics* (Brest, France).

Forney, G., Kschischang, F., & Marcus, B. (1998). *Iterative decoding of tail-biting trellisses.* Presented at 1998 Information Theory Workshop in San Diego.

Frey, B. J. (1998). *Graphical models for pattern classification, data compression and channel coding.* Cambridge, MA: MIT Press.

Frey, B. J., Koetter, R., & Vardy, A. (1998). Skewness and pseudocodewords in iterative decoding. In *Proc. 1998 ISIT.*

Gallager, R. (1963). *Low density parity check codes.* Cambridge, MA: MIT Press.

Gelb, A.(Ed.). (1974). *Applied optimal estimation*. Cambridge, MA: MIT Press.

Geman, S., & Geman, D. (1984). Stochastic relaxation, Gibbs distributions, and the Bayesian restoration of images. *IEEE Trans. PAMI, 6*(6), 721–741.

Jensen, F. (1996). *An introduction to Bayesian networks*. Berlin: Springer-Verlag.

Kschischang, F. R., & Frey, B. J. (1998). Iterative decoding of compound codes by probability propagation in graphical models. *IEEE Journal on Selected Areas in Communication, 16*(2), 219–230.

Lauritzen, S. (1996). *Graphical models*. New York: Oxford University Press.

MacKay, D., & Neal, R. M. (1995). Good error-correcting codes based on very sparse matrices. In *Cryptography and Coding: 5th IAM Conference. Lecture Notes in Computer Science No. 1025* (pp. 100–111). Berlin: Springer-Verlag.

McEliece, R., MacKay, D., and Cheng, J. (1998). Turbo decoding as an instance of Pearl's "belief propagation" algorithm. *IEEE Journal on Selected Areas in Communication, 16*(2), 140–152.

McEliece, R., Rodemich, E., & Cheng, J. (1995). The Turbo decision algorithm. In *Proc. 33rd Allerton Conference on Communications, Control and Computing* (pp. 366–379). Monticello, IL.

Minc, H. (1988). *Nonnegative matrices*. New York: Wiley.

Pearl, J. (1988). *Probabilistic reasoning in intelligent systems: Networks of plausible inference*. San Mateo, CA: Morgan Kaufmann.

Rabiner, L. (1989). A tutorial on hidden Markov models and selected applications in speech recognition. *Proc. IEEE, 77*(2), 257–286.

Smyth, P. (1997). Belief networks, hidden Markov models, and Markov random fields: A unifying view. *Pattern Recognition, 18*(11), 1261–1268.

Smyth, P., Heckerman, D., & Jordan, M. I. (1997). Probabilistic independence networks for hidden Markov probability models. *Neural Computation, 9*(2), 227–269.

Strang, G. (1986). *Introduction to applied mathematics*. Wellesley, MA: Wellesley-Cambridge.

Weiss, Y. (1996). Interpreting images by propagating Bayesian beliefs. In M. Mozer, M. Jordan, & T. Petsche (Eds.), *Advances in neural information processing systems, 9*. Cambridge, MA: MIT Press.

Weiss, Y. (1997). *Belief propagation and revision in networks with loops* (Tech. Rep. No. 1616). Cambridge, MA: MIT Artificial Intelligence Laboratory.

Wiberg, N. (1996). *Codes and decoding on general graphs*. Unpublished doctoral dissertation, University of Linkoping, Sweden.

Received November 11, 1997; accepted November 25, 1998.

Index